SUN, MOON, and EARTH
The Sacred Relationship of
Yoga and Ayurveda

Mas Vidal

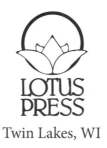

LOTUS
PRESS
Twin Lakes, WI

Disclaimer

This book is an educational manual and information contained herein is in no way to be considered as a substitute for your inner guidance or consultation with a professional physician or any duly licensed health care professional. The publisher and author are not liable for any injury sustained by the use of the information contained herein.

First Edition, 2017.
Printed in the United States of America
Mas Vidal
SUN, MOON, and EARTH –*The Sacred Relationship of Yoga and Ayurveda*
ISBN: 978-0-9406-7640-4
Library of Congress Control Number: 2016959715

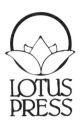

LOTUS
PRESS

Published by:
Lotus Press, P.O. Box 325, Twin Lakes, Wisconsin 53181 USA
Web: www.lotuspress.com
e-mail: lotuspress@lotuspress.com
800-824-6396

TABLE OF CONTENTS

Background

Part One: A Global Perspective

Part Two: The Body as the Vehicle of Consciousness

Part Three: Lifestyle as the New Religion

ILLUSTRATIONS

ABOUT THE COVER

For most of us living on planet earth, the sun and moon are the celestial bodies we look up to, literally and metaphorically. The sun draws our attention in many ways. We bathe in its rays of optimism. The soft luminosity of the moon likewise spawns a mystical quality in our hearts.

In the cover image, the moon appears on Shiva's left side, symbolic of the ida nadi (subtle lunar channel) governing these energies in the mind-body complex. The sun appears on the right side, symbolic of the pingala nadi (subtle solar channel). The essence of yoga lies in the balance or union of these as inner forces.

One of the simplest forms of managing these energies is the practice of pranayama or energy control through Nadi Shodhana (alternate nostril purification). The two nostrils can be seen as channels or rivers where the energies of the sun and moon flow through the nose, our connection to breath of life. The two physical eyes represent fire, and the two physical ears can connect us to the eternal sound or ocean of consciousness through the element of ether.

Shiva is most generally associated with the sun, but is also connected with the darkness of the moon, which appears waning over his head. This shows Shiva's connection to the mind or the unseen and mysterious aspects of our lives. Shiva draws us inward to connect first with subtle cosmic planetary forces, and then beyond these to discover the bliss of the pure awareness.

The Background

The backdrop for the sun and moon is the star symbolic of the spiritual eye or Kutashta, as it is referred to in the Bhagavad Gita. The star's five points can be correlated to the five elements of creation: earth, water, fire, air, and ether. These elements are also influenced by the sun, moon, and earth, as explained in Jyotish, the science of light. The three lotuses sprouting from the earth represent the gunas or qualities of our efforts, which determine the lifestyle we create. When we make choices in our life that originate from the highest capacity of the mind, or sattva guna, the splendor and grace of Shiva is granted to us.

Shiva and the Serpents

Lord Shiva as Mahadeva is the highest attribute of yoga, and is represented in the ultimate union, communion, and state of transcendental consciousness that we as human beings have the power to experience. Shiva as Nageshvara, the lord of the serpents, reflects mastery over the energy of pure consciousness. The halo of the seven Nagas or serpents creates a crown of light, symbolic of the awakened kundalini that arises as the Shakti or power of the individual soul (Jivatman).

The seven serpents can also be correlated to the realms of consciousness (lokas). The pranic energies of the serpent can also carry the dangerous poison of misconduct if they are mismanaged by a reckless lifestyle and not for their real purpose of destroying the conditions of the mind. Krishna in the Bhagavad Gita[1] expresses his connection to the Naga serpents as Ananta (that which is eternal) or Shesha (that which is preserved), symbolic of the eternal forces behind the realms of existence or Mother Nature (prakriti).

The Deeper Meaning of Shiva

In another aspect, Shiva as the cosmic dancer demonstrates mastery over the awakened kundalini. As the lover, Shiva entices us to surrender into the stillness of the soul that is peace, love, and joy arising from the union with the Divine vibration or Pranava, which literally means the everrenewing, eternal ocean of bliss.

Shiva personifies the grace and poise cultivated when we cling to the "spiritual path" or sadhana that cultivates the synergy between mind and body required to unite with spirit. Shiva epitomizes the discipline of a balanced life, the management of our senses and social interactions (kama).

When we can direct the pranic energy to its culmination or bindu at the point of Shiva's Oneness, the aspirant (sadhaka) experiences liberation or moksha. The bindi is the red dot typically worn between the eyebrows by women of the Hindu-Vedic culture. It is also worn by both men and women during various yogic rituals such as pujas. The term originates from the word bindu found in the Nasadiya Sukta of the Rig Veda. It symbolizes the culmination of the three worlds: the body-earth-physical or waking state; the mind-moon-astral or dream state; and the soul-suncausal or deep sleep state. Shiva is the triadic union that reveals the prana or vayu that exists beyond the realm of time and space, the external universe, and is the underling force that sustains life. Humanity's dilemmas and woes lie in the inability to understand the intrinsic relationship the mind and body share with the One creator (Brahma).

---

1 Chapter 10, verses 28-29.

Visualization of Shiva For Meditation

The image of Shiva and the serpents arising out of the lotus flower can be used as a powerful yantra, a vehicle for expanding the prana at each chakra. One can begin at the root chakra (muladhara) and, while silently chanting Om, visualize Shiva as primal sound expanding the lotus petals of awareness in each center, gradually rousing the soul's inherent qualities of peace, contentment, and compassion. Such a purifying practice can bring connection to the five elements.

This can be further expanded through the silent chanting of the auspicious mantra Aum Namah Shivaya to release the amrita (nectar) of devotion in a form of yoga known as Bhakti. This gives rise to the essence of Shiva as the compassionate one. We ultimately understand that Lord Shiva's destruction of attachments, identities, and delusions are essentially his blessings. Shiva is itself the practice of meditation as the highest or Raja yoga, which is often depicted with Shiva seated in the asana or seat of meditation with serene eyes, as seen in this illustration. Shiva as Yogeshvara teaches us how to connect to various asanas or postures as aspects of the Divine Self in creation. While embracing Shiva, the power of surrender is born, allowing us to transcend the poses, the body, and the senses.

Living Shiva

Many consider Mahavatar Babaji of Yogananda's Kriya yoga lineage as a manifestation of Lord Shiva. Babaji is the Maha Guru of Yoga and the guiding force behind many lineages of the modern era that aim to usher us back to the golden era of higher consciousness. During an unassuming pilgrimage to the Dunagiri region of the Almora district of the Himalayas, an area where the Pandavas of the Mahabharata took refuge during the Kurukshetra war, I visited Babaji's cave and experienced a subtle yet profound shift in my consciousness. Although difficult to express in words, I had begun to carry a more consistent feeling of contentment, meaning, and purpose in life. This awoke me from a dark night of the soul or period of transition into my dharma. Unbeknownst to me at the time, these sacred Himalayan hills are the land where the story of the Bhagavad Gita was told, and are permeated with Shiva's heavenly presence, along with that of Babaji and other great yogis preparing to share their sacred relationship with the Divine to all of us in the world.

FOREWORD *by Phil Goldberg*

A survey in early 2016 reported that 36 million Americans claim to be yoga practitioners. It also found that 28% all Americans have taken a yoga class at some point in their lives and 34%--80 million people!--say they are likely to practice yoga in the next twelve months. Even if the numbers are slightly skewed, that is a lot of bending and stretching. And make no mistake, bending and stretching is exactly what "yoga" is coming to mean based on general usage and the images projected by the media.

Those astonishing data are, on the one hand, good news to anyone who appreciates the remarkable benefits that accrue from regular yoga practice *of any authentic kind* and wants them to be shared by as many people as possible. At the same time, the fact that yoga is now defined mainly as a physical fitness regimen, virtually synonymous with the postures known as *asanas,* is deeply troubling to anyone who understands the full depth and breadth of the yogic repertoire of practices, the profundity of yoga philosophy and the spiritually transformative potential of deep, classical yoga.

In this ambiguous atmosphere it is imperative that knowledgeable yoga experts lead a public education campaign to restore the complete meaning of the word yoga and make sure everyone who bends and stretches and purchases chic yoga merchandise knows that there is a lot more to the tradition than meets the eye, if that eye is fixed on the images of hot practitioners looking like Cirque du Soleil performers. Fundamentally speaking, yoga means union, and not just the union of the head to the knee, or even the union of mind and body. The sacred treasury of wisdom and practices that constitute the yoga tradition is designed to produce the unification of our individual selves to the universal Self that is the very origin and essence of all that is. Its aim is liberation, enlightenment, awakening, or whichever of the many terms one prefers for the reaching the highest rungs on the ladder of human development.

With this book, and in his ongoing work as a teacher and practitioner, Mas Vidal is making a significant contribution to the important effort of preserving and disseminating the fullness of yoga. In this clear, intriguing and comprehensive book, he reminds us that for all its important benefits to health, vitality and wellbeing, yoga is about Self-Realization. He knows that we do yoga to achieve Yoga. That is, we engage in the practices that constitute the yogic repertoire to achieve the unified state of consciousness that is the very definition of Yoga, as articulated by the sages who gave us the Bhagavad Gita, the Upanishads, the Yoga Sutras and other illuminating texts.

The sublimely elevating insights and immensely practical methods that have come down to us from the Himalayan rishis have been filtering into American soil ever since Ralph Waldo Emerson and Henry David Thoreau walked the woods of New England in glorious solitude and pondered great ideas with their brother and sister Transcendentalists. What came to be called Emersonian philosophy was marinated in a Vedic sauce, and that influence still resonates with modern students, readers and scholars. Thoreau read the Bhagavad Gita every morning on Walden Pond and pronounced its philosophy "stupendous and cosmogonal" by comparison to the "puny and trivial" literature of his time. He calls himself a yogi in *Walden*, and it should be obvious that he did not mean he performed downward dog each day. Yoga studios wouldn't appear in Concord, or even Cambridge, for at least another century.

The great transmission from India to America was conducted through the medium of books and journals in the 19th century. Then it accelerated with the arrival of bona fide gurus, swamis and yoga masters, beginning in 1893 with Swami Vivekananda's triumphant appearance at the Parliament of the World's Religions in Chicago. Vivekananda set the tone, and it was picked up and amplified by others in the early 20th century. The most notable advocate in that period was Paramahansa Yogananda, who settled in America and broadcast his Kriya Yoga throughout the world with the help of what was then modern technology: trains, planes and mail order.

In the Sixties, the counterculture explosion mixed with mass communication and changes in immigration law to bring us a parade of gurus and yogacharyas with a variety of yogic methods and Vedic wisdom. They included Maharishi Mahesh Yogi, Swami Muktananda, Srila Prabhupada, Swami Vishnudevananda, Swami Satchidananda, and many others, including the pair of teachers who escorted Postural Yoga onto center stage: B.K.S. Iyengar and K. Patthabhi Jois. Throughout the century, the transmission gathered steam and prominent Westerners assimilated yogic teachings and Vedantic philosophy, integrating them into their own areas of expertise and propagated them in modified form to the masses: public intellectuals (Aldous Huxley, Joseph Campbell); psychologists (William James, Abraham Maslow); poets (Yeats, Ginsberg); novelists (Hesse, Salinger); and musicians, most spectacularly the Beatles.

Most of this transpired with philosophy and meditation leading the way and spiritual illumination as the prime motivation. Always, of course, there were instrumental aims as well; people always want to improve their lives in specific ways (the usual suspects: money, work, love, marriage) and Americans found the insights and methods imported from India to be of great pragmatic value.

But spirituality and the elevation of consciousness were seldom neglected or hidden. They were, in fact, understood to be the very instruments through which the practical benefits the teachings accrued. That began to change when scientists conducted experiments on meditation. The early research on Transcendental Meditation, circa 1970, triggered a scientific juggernaut that continues to this day. Science, however, is secular almost by definition, and its nature is to dissect, isolate and reduce complex phenomena to the equivalent of a drug's "active ingredients." Meditation quickly became secularized as a therapeutic practice for stress reduction and other measurable benefits, almost a natural substitute for pharmaceuticals.

It was virtually inevitable that the focus on the quantifiable benefits of meditation (primarily physical almost by definition) would in turn ignite similar interest in the tangible benefits of asana-focused Hatha Yoga, with its emphasis on anatomical rigor. As noted earlier, this reductionist tendency of the West now threatens to make yoga synonymous with physical exercise, if not defined by it entirely.

Like other aspects of culture (art forms, foods, fashions, etc.), spiritual teachings and healthcare technologies have always been refined, reformed and recalibrated over the course of time, as social customs and mores change. Sometimes, in that inevitable adaptive process, things of value get lost or corrupted. In the interest of making products and services accessible to as many people as possible, and to satisfy the needs of a diverse range of individuals, alterations are made that can distort or dilute the very ideas and methods that are being eagerly promoted. This can occur even when the promoters have the best of intentions. When commercial interests, the imperatives of mass media and the cacophony of Internet-sharing enter the picture, the potential for distortion increases. Hence, vigilance has become more and more necessary.

What makes those of us who care about the future of yoga optimistic is the presence of authors and educators like Mas Vidal. Teachers who are rooted in the deepest, most complete yoga, and are linked to a reputable and enduring lineage, offer hope that these precious teachings will be adapted to a new era and a new culture with integrity, skill and discernment.

The book in your hands is comprehensive and far-ranging. Part philosophy, part history and part practical self-improvement, it represents an honest attempt to integrate ancient India and the modern West without compromising either one. A few of its features stand out for me.

One is Vidal's contention that the growing understanding of, and interest in, the mind-body-spirit relationship can be traced to the state of Bengal in eastern India about a century ago, and to the capital city of Calcutta (now Kolkata) in particular. It was, indeed, a remarkable period, especially in the area around Calcutta University, which, like Greenwich Village, was a cauldron for unconventional ideas, innovative art, revolutionary politics and reformist spirituality. I am not expert enough to evaluate the historical veracity of Vidal's narrative, but I found his argument stimulating and convincing.

Swami Vivekananda grew up in that area in the 19th century, and a generation later Mukunda Ghosh, who would become Paramahansa Yogananda, spent the better part of his youth there. As I am currently working on a biography of Yogananda, I was pleased that this book devotes considerable space to him and his guru lineage. Yogananda's immense contribution to the transmission of yoga to the West is often underestimated, and it is illuminating to read how the cultural atmosphere in the Calcutta of his formative years helped prepare him for his mission.

Another aspect of this book I found particularly commendable was its integral approach. Vidal recognizes that yoga is both therapeutically useful and spiritually illuminating. Healing and liberation are linked, as they are in real life. So are mind, body and spirit, as was understood by the yoga masters who taught asana and pranayama mainly as preparation for deep meditation. Also linked integrally are yoga and Ayurveda. The two classical systems are often segregated in the West and treated as if they were unrelated disciplines. Vidal emphasizes their shared pedigree and interrelated applications, as symbolized by the sun (yoga) and moon (Ayurveda).

The challenge faced by those who believe yoga has much to offer the modern world is: to adapt yoga to modern Western culture; avoid diluting, distorting or corrupting the tradition; make the inventory of yogic methods accessible to those whose needs and desires are physical, therapeutic and even narcissistic, and all while promoting awareness of the oceanic depths and astronomical breadth of true yoga. That is a big and important task, and Mas Vidal's book is a worthy addition to the bag of tricks that will, I have no doubt, meet the challenge.

Philip Goldberg, cohost of Spirit Matters podcast and author of *American Veda: From Emerson and the Beatles to Yoga and Meditation, How Indian Spirituality Changed the West.*

INTRODUCTION *By David Frawley*

The Vedic teachings of India are probably the oldest, most extensive and continually used spiritual and healing tradition in the world. From the ancient Himalayan rishis many thousands of years ago to the great gurus of modern India today forms an unbroken lineage of enlightened yogis and sages that is unparalleled anywhere else in the world.

Yoga in all of its many facets originates from the Vedic teachings as a way of spiritual practice aimed at Self-realization in the deepest sense of the term - returning to our true nature as pure consciousness beyond body and mind, time and space. The cosmic sound vibration OM from which the Vedic mantras arise is the indicator of *Ishvara*, the Cosmic Lord, described in the *Yoga Sutras* as the original guru of Yoga. Both Vedic and yogic teachings are said to derive from Cosmic Intelligence, not simply from human invention or the powers of the human mind.

The practice Yoga is closely allied at a theoretical level with Vedanta, the Vedic philosophy of Self-realization and Oneness with all. Vedanta comprises Jnana Yoga or the Yoga of knowledge among the primary Yoga paths, and looks at Yoga practices, including Hatha Yoga, as providing a helpful foundation for its subtle meditation approaches.

At a personal level, this profound Vedic teaching is most easily accessed through Ayurveda, the Vedic system of natural and yogic healing for body and mind. Ayurveda teaches us how cosmic forces like Agni (cosmic light principle) and Vayu (cosmic prana principle) relate to our biological and physiological energies and have medical implications.

Classical Yoga, as taught in the Yoga Sutras, is the Vedic system of spiritual practice aimed at accessing higher consciousness through deep meditation. Ayurveda is the branch of Vedic knowledge for health and well-being at all levels of life and for all types of people and their differing goals and aspirations.

Today, the healing aspect of Yoga is emphasized in Yoga circles, including a new emphasis on Yoga therapy or Yoga Chikitsa. Yet this is often occurring, without understanding the profound Ayurvedic connections behind yogic healing. Ayurveda takes the spiritual and psychological principles of Yoga and extends them to a physical level for understanding the energetics behind body and mind. For this Ayurveda brings to Yoga the important theory of the three *doshas* or biological humors of Vata (air), Pitta (fire) and Kapha (water) for understanding individual constitutional types and the disease process.

Ayurveda comprises a complete yogic system of healing, both for right living practices and for the treatment of serious diseases, both chronic and acute. Notably Ayurveda helps us understand our unique mind-body (doshic) types and how to balance them at all levels including diet, exercise, life-style, creativity and spiritual practice. Ayurveda enables us to integrate all Yoga therapies into a holistic and organic approach that helps us develop greater vitality, longevity, creativity and higher awareness.

Mas Vidal

Mas Vidal is a rare western Yoga teacher, who has studied Yoga in depth and is also trained in Ayurvedic medicine and related Vedic sciences including Vedic astrology. He approaches Yoga and Ayurveda in an integral manner, understanding their deep relationship and mutual efficacy for both health and spirituality. His book explains the extensive Ayurvedic implications of Yoga practices that many Yoga teachers fail to see or do not comprehend.

Yet Mas also understands the deeper spiritual and psychological side of Yoga that goes beyond Yoga postures or techniques to the intricacies of meditation and the unfoldment of a higher consciousness. Yoga asanas calm the body to help us move us within to the core of our being. The body is not the goal or the focus of Yoga practice but its foundation. Yoga aims to take us beyond the limitations of body consciousness to a recognition of our unity with the whole of life.

I have known and worked with Mas for twenty years and noted his dedication to the teaching and practice of Yoga and Ayurveda, and his study with a variety of important teachers and guides. He is not content merely to repeat what the books say but has learned to adapt the teachings in one-to-one consultations and group classes that he offers throughout North America and the world as a whole. His Yoga-Ayurveda programs are unique and transformative.

The Greater Yoga Tradition

Mas Vidal's view of Yoga challenges current theories about the history of Yoga in the West. In this regard one should not forget the foundation that Swami Vivekananda and the disciples of Ramakrishna brought to the West with their projection of Yoga as a universal spiritual path, or the vast integral Yoga that Sri Aurobindo envisioned. For them, Yoga was a system of complete development of mind, heart and character, to bring out the highest Divine potential within each one of us.

Yoga is rooted in the *Yoga Sutras*, Rishi Patanjali's compilation of the principles of Yoga practice, which in turn look back to the *Vedas*, India's older mantric tradition of cosmic and Self-knowledge. Patanjali's Yoga is often called or related to traditions of Raja Yoga and Ashtanga Yoga.

The many branches of Yoga include Shaivite Yoga, like Hatha Yoga, Siddha Yoga and the older Pashupata Yoga. Vaishnava Yoga has many forms, particularly as taught by Krishna in the *Bhagavad Gita*, and the great text of the *Srimad Bhagavatam*. Yoga contains many branches as knowledge (Jnana), devotion (Bhakti), service and ritual (Karma), internal practices (Kriya), Prana, Mantra, Laya and more. Yogic teachings occur in Vedic texts, Yoga Shastras, Mahabharata, Agamas, Puranas, Tantras, extending to Buddhist, Jain and Sikh teachings – a vast and formidable literature, of which only a small portion is accessible in English.

Mas has a special connection with Paramahansa Yogananda and the Kriya Yoga tradition of Yogavatar Babaji. I have called Yogananda "the father of Yoga in the West" as he was the first great Yoga teacher in modern times from India to reside in the West and direct his teachings primarily to a western audience. Yogananda provided the West a firm foundation in classical Yoga, including not simply asana, but pranayama, mantra and meditation, Karma Yoga, Bhakti Yoga, Jnana Yoga and Raja Yoga, following the broader view that Vivekananda had set in motion.

Yogananda's legacy has shaped western Yoga and preserved it from simply falling into an exercise tradition that many have tried to turn it to. Mas helps us understand the integral view and deeper wisdom that Yogananda held, and shares special implications about Yogananda's teachings, particularly relative to asana. Yogananda's understanding of pranayama, not just as an outer energy practice, but an awakening of the subtle powers of consciousness, is an important consideration for all yogis today, along with how Yogananda emphasized the control and inward turning of the senses.

Cosmic Time Cycles or Yugas

Paramahansa Yogananda, through his guru Swami Sri Yukteswar, taught that humanity is entering into a new cycle of civilization, which is called the Dwapara Yuga, an age of electricity, technology and subtle energy, including atomic power. This new era, though not an age of complete enlightenment, indicates major new progress for humanity. It is not without its dangers, as the new technology can also create new and more dangerous weapons of mass destruction, as we have already witnessed, but overall it will impel humanity forward to a more intelligent way of life. It is projected to last until around 4100 AD.

There is some controversy in regard to Sri Yukteswar's cycles as other Yoga groups place us in a spiritual dark age or Kali Yuga, said to have begun around 3100 BCE at the time of Sri Krishna, to continue for 432,000 years. In defense of Sri Yukteswar –whose theory is also examined in my book the *Astrology of the Seers* – the ancient king lists of India, as explained in the *Puranas*, suggest a shorter time cycle such as he indicates. The number of kings listed for the different yugas are too few in number to cover the hundreds of thousand of years needed for the longer yuga cycles.

Role of Asana

Mas, an athlete himself, shows us how to integrate physical Yoga and asana routines into deeper Yoga practices and meditation. Yoga asana traditions are seldom given the same detailed explanations as meditation and pranayama practices in classical texts, making it harder to determine their original background and scope of application. For this we have to look more into the background of the tradition. Asana practices are connected to Vedic martial arts, including those within monastic orders, with classical Indian dance, and the gestures of ritualistic approaches. They are not outside of but an interrelate part of the greater Yoga tradition.

Hindu deities like Lord Shiva, Krishna and Hanuman have long served as icons of yoga practice in India on various levels, with Lord Shiva as regarded as the originator of the asanas and mantras of classical Yoga, a topic covered in my recent book, **Shiva, the Lord of Yoga**.

The great teachers of Ayurveda and the great teachers of Yoga cross over, starting with Patanjali himself who was a famous adept in both disciplines, going back to the Rishis Vasishta and Agastya, among the most famous Vedic seers, renowned as great yogis and healers.

Yoga Beyond Asana

Current views of Yoga in the West put too much emphasis on precision asana practice, as if Yoga were a mere outer physical discipline of structural alignment. Real Yoga leaves body consciousness aside at the early stages of practice and sets the senses and mind aside not long after that. Sri Aurobindo noted that true Yoga begins with a complete silence, calm and surrender of the being, a complete inner orientation to the Divine.

In the Vedic view, the human being is not merely a physical entity limited to the material world. The human being is a spiritual being linked to subtle levels of existence and higher states of consciousness, the ability to access which we have all but forgotten in our current materialistic mindset. The human being is a manifestation of the Purusha, the Cosmic Person, whose body is the physical universe, whose mind is the cosmic mind, and whose nature is Being-Consciousness-Bliss Absolute. Yoga restores our cosmic connection and the greater wholeness of our nature that embraces all of existence in a single vision.

New View of Yoga in the West

It is time for Yoga in the West to embrace the greater Yoga tradition, the deeper concerns of healing the mind and awakening our higher Self-awareness. Yoga is about Self-realization, not about the physical or mental self but our cosmic Self that is one with all.

It is also time for Yoga in the West to embrace Ayurveda, which is the original yogic system of medicine that takes the principles of Yoga and extends them to diagnosis and all factors of natural healing. Yoga without Ayurveda lacks a practical foundation in daily life or a comprehensive means to allow us to access the profound healing energies of prana and consciousness.

Mas Vidal provides an excellent primer in Yoga and Ayurveda with a comprehensive overview of the spiritual life and its important concerns. His book *Sun, Moon and Earth*, shows us how to access the healing and consciousness-promoting energies of the universe in a way that is both simple and profound, explained with clarity and intricacy. His is an in-depth manual of Yoga and Ayurveda that provides a firm foundation for students to apply these Vedic sciences in an authentic and comprehensive manner from physical health to cosmic consciousness.

The book is broad in scope and detailed in application. It has a practical value for anyone interested in health and well-being and a spiritual dimension for those motivated to delve into the deeper yogic quest for unity consciousness. We recommend the book to all students and teachers of Yoga and Ayurveda to deepen their knowledge and expand their scope of practice and healing therapies.

Dr. David Frawley (Pandit Vamadeva Shastri) is a world-renowned teacher of Yoga and Ayurveda and author of fifty books on Vedic topics, including the classic text *Yoga and Ayurveda: Self Healing and Self-realization*. He is a rare recipient of the Padma Bhushan award from the President of India, one of India's highest national honors, for his work as a Vedic educator.

ACKNOWLEDGMENTS

I would like to express my gratitude to a number of people who supported my life in various ways and influenced this book. To both of my parents (Ada Larrea and Raul P. Masvidal) for teaching me to never give up and that hard work is a vital part of life. To Deborah Shelton for her motherly spiritual support in my formative years. To the Dancing Shiva Yoga and Ayurveda center, which I opened in 2001 as a place of pilgrimage for truth seekers, including myself, and to all those who visited there. You all were my teachers and so many have also become my spiritual friends. A special thank you to Vamadeva (David Frawley) for teaching me to see the grandeur of the Vedic tradition through his inspiring books, teachings, mentorship, and friendship, and for writing the Introduction to this, my first book. I am truly blessed. I want to also honor and thank the many Ayurvedic doctors from India whom I have known and with whom I studied over many years, such as Mr. & Mrs Dr. Ranade, Mr. & Mrs. Dr. Lele, Dr. Srikrishna Phadke, and many others whom I have met in my visits to Pune, India. A special thanks to Chakrapani Ullal, my first Vedic Astrology teacher, who humbly demonstrates the importance of lineage, as well as my first Sanskrit mantra teacher, the late Thomas Ashley Farrand (Namadeva).

I am also extremely grateful for the many enlightened Swamis whom I have been fortunate to have counseled with, in both the United States and India, especially Swami Jyotirmayanandaji of Yoga Research Foundation in Miami. Your feeling and attitude are always sacred, and the wisdom of the scriptures you have shared is always consistently Divine. Very distinct gratitude and pronams to the monks of my own lineage at Self-Realization Fellowship (Yogoda Satsanga Society), such as the late Brother Bhaktananda for teaching me the importance of "practicing the presence of God," Brother Anandamoy for his insight, Brother Paramananda for always being a smile millionaire, Brother Tyagananda, Brahmachari Andy, and Brahmachari Shekhar for their brotherly friendship and support, and both Swami Ishwaranandaji and Swami Vishwanandaji for their humble guidance and wisdom.

As will be obvious to any reader of this book, I have been profoundly influenced by the teachings and practice of Paramahansa Yogananda. I am extremely grateful to the Self-Realization Fellowship (SRF) and Yogoda Satsanga Society (YSS), the organizations he founded to disseminate those teachings, both for the sincerity with which they fulfill their mission and the assistance they have given me in so many ways. I would like to thank the Fellowship's Permissions Office for its review of and helpful comments on my manuscript, and also make it clear that I do not serve the Fellowship in any official capacity, nor is this book a sanctioned SRF publication. I sincerely thank SRF for its input. Any remaining differences are, of course, my own.

I also want to give a special thanks to Tom Lane for his patient editing of the manuscript, Bryan Boettcher for his cover art and other drawings in the book, and Shawn Freeman for cover design and layout. Thanks to all of you through out the world who have given support to my classes and workshops, giving my yoga and Ayurveda message a chance to be heard, and helping bring yoga and Ayurveda back together again.

MY STORY

My fascination with nature began at a very young age. I remember that, with the dawn of every rising sun, I felt such a magnetic pull to the outdoors that it ran through my body like electricity. As I could see the sunrise approaching, I felt like a restless monkey in a cage, removed from his playground environment.

In many ways, the vast majority of our culture today has been removed far from its home, its womb of gathering knowledge, its place for healing and uniting with the common thread that connects us all. We live in pressure-sealed, temperature-controlled boxes, out of touch with the elements, the change of seasons, and the songs of wisdom that nature sings and shares with us.

In an age of communication-enhancing technology, the gaps in actually communicating through real contact are growing wider and wider. People are speaking to gadgets and not to each other. Societies are buying their food in boxes, freezers, and sealed wrappers. They are prepared in factories rather than gardens. We are evidently living in a time of global disconnect and disharmony, not just amongst ourselves, but also from our ecology and the knowledge of the Ancients. The Western lifestyle feeds us junk food, pills, bills, television, and recreational drugs, all of which leave us with a residue of toxicity and dependency.

I remember one Christmas morning, a day I have always cherished as sacred, I was feeling empty inside and shedding tears of disillusionment, I tried to comprehend where this feeling was coming from. I realized my dissatisfaction with materialism was something I could no longer ignore. The indirect means of expressing love, through material gifts and holiday rituals that were far from holy, were becoming meaningless. I felt that I had lost the romance I had cherished with the Divine for so many years. My soul was crying for answers to life's biggest questions: Why am I here? What is my purpose? What is love and peace, and where do I find them?

Suddenly, I found myself at a crossroads. Do I indulge more in this life, burying my emotions inside and just letting this feeling pass? Or do I keep inquiring as to the source of my questions? Several years of a toxic lifestyle (wine, intoxicants, sex, and sitcoms) went by, leaving me nowhere but depressed, toxic, and still denying my inner conscience. I realized that all along I had denied identity with who I really was as a person, and ignored the things I enjoyed and the talents I had.

I realized that I needed to reconnect with my body, and began a strict muscle-building regimen by locking myself in a room after school to lift weights and do pull-ups and push-ups. Gradually, my outlook on life started to change. I was so fascinated by how a body can change that, after only about two and a half years of body-building, someone suggested I enter the Mr. Florida contest. I made the decision to enter 21 days before the competition and won first place. I then entered another contest a few weeks later and won it as well.

I had cultivated tremendous strength and size naturally, by training the body and eating the right diet. But those aching, unanswered questions still existed. This led me eventually to reconnect with nature as a guide to help me solve the mystery. I learned to enjoy simplicity and find great pleasure in humble living. I spent a lot of time outdoors, motivating and coaching others, privately and in small groups, on a path of wellness through cross-training and integrative sports classes. While I thoroughly enjoyed bringing greater health to others, I still needed something that satisfied my inner being.

Like many in the West, my health and happiness had been based on the body, people, and external sources of stimulation. Now, I wanted an answer to come from within. I started searching by going to church, synagogues, courses in Buddhism and spirituality—anything that crossed my path. I was terribly hungry for knowledge of a practice that would satisfy my body, mind, and spirit.

Finding Yoga

Now that the seed of yearning for a higher purpose in my life had been planted, I was in search of the water that would allow that seed to sprout and expand into my true nature. My story of finding yoga is a sweet one, and, by no coincidence, the discovery occurred while in pursuit of the "One" love, along with a desire for nature's bounty.

While in a college English literature class at the University of Florida, I was exposed to the philosophical, learned writings of Ralph Waldo Emerson and Henry David Thoreau. These were ideal books for me to read while at university in Gainesville, a small city surrounded by the countryside of north-central Florida. I was so intrigued by the way both Emerson and Thoreau spoke of the relationship that humanity has with nature and of the values of morality, friendship, and love, among many other topics to ponder.

This was also the first time I heard of the Bhagavad Gita and how society conspires against those who begin to ask life's deeper questions. As Emerson said, "Society everywhere is in conspiracy against the manhood of every one of its members. The virtue in most request is conformity. Self-reliance is its aversion. It loves not realities and creators, but names and customs. Whoso would be a man must be a nonconformist." When I read these words, I felt like I was bathing myself in something so grand and vast, yet so present and alive. I felt myself becoming more intrigued by the topics of solitude, the divinity in nature, and the discovery of the soul. These are some of the first insights in a spiritual quest that was burgeoning naturally inside of me.

A couple of years later, after graduating from college, while holding on to the small-town values I had cherished, I found myself living in the mammoth city of Los Angeles, California, a place I had been drawn to since elementary school. I remembered writing book reports about California and having strong visions of beach scenes and palm tree-lined streets. Now, a couple of years later, I was able to fulfill one of my strongest desires.

One of the first things I started doing was meditation. I would sit for five minutes in stillness while listening to new age-type spa music, something I had mocked and ridiculed only years prior. This was a huge change, having grown up an athlete and body-builder who listened to American rock-and-roll music.

One crispy and sunny California day, I decided to go shopping at a natural food grocery store in the very affluent neighborhood of Beverly Hills. I began to push my shopping cart to the usual sections in the store. As I turned the corner to approach the deli counter to place an order, I became mesmerized by the eyes of an attractive young woman with brown hair, who was also pushing her cart past the deli section. This young woman's eyes appeared to me like crystalline pools of infinite love and peace. I was dazzled and oblivious at the same time, but felt such a magnetic pull that I decided to follow her to the produce section, hoping I would meet her.

To me she was certainly the belle of the store, and as she moved over to the next aisle, I continued to follow her, but had no luck connecting. She walked to a register to pay, and off she went. Sad and confused, I stopped for a moment to ponder what I was feeling and why I was so drawn to following someone around a grocery store. Was it because of something that I felt through her eyes? For a moment, I thought to myself how odd it would sound if I shared this story with a friend. But I felt that something profound had attracted me. It was beyond words and much more than a mere physical sensation.

After leaving the store, I still felt mystically attracted to something within this person. Returning to my apartment, which was in another area of the city, I went on with my daily schedule, taking my mind away from the mystical eyes that dazzled my spirit at the grocery store. The next day I went about my activities. As I ended my errands, I headed home. As I was about to pull into the driveway, I had to yield to someone walking down the sidewalk. The young female pedestrian looked familiar. Suddenly, I realized who it was. "Oh, my lord!" I silently screamed in my car. The woman with the mystical eyes was walking right in front of my driveway, the next day, in a completely different part of Los Angeles.

How could this be? I questioned it, and considered for a moment that it was my imagination. I was bewildered as to what she was doing there. Instantly, I was again intrigued to know more about what I was feeling. I rushed into the garage and parked my car. I followed her, again, into an artsy store at the end of my block.

At this point, I was definitely feeling weird about my actions and began to question my motives. But at the same time, I felt that sense of mysticism I had experienced in the grocery store the day before. I wanted to know what was inside of this women that felt so compelling and inspiring at the same time. Unlike the grocery store experience, the moment I walked into the artsy store, we made eye contact, and we immediately engaged in conversation. I was overjoyed. Our conversation was warm and cordial, but I also felt anxious and wanted to know more about the energy I was so drawn to.

In the meanwhile, I learned she was a vegetarian chef and worked at a local eatery in the neighborhood I lived in. She had also been looking for a new place to live. Well, within a week's time, she had become my new roommate. We began to develop a nice friendship as we shared some social time together. I felt that I was beginning to discover more about what I was drawn to.

Interestingly enough, one afternoon we decided to get some lunch at a local health-food eatery. When we sat down to eat, she closed her eyes in front of me, and I was instantly transported into a realm of fascination and excitement. I sat there and peered at her with her closed eyes, wondering where she was going. Was she speaking to God or someone else? I felt a wonderful wave of peace flow over me as she opened her twinkling eyes, and knew that I also wanted to go to that place.

She shared that she had an interest in meditation and had recently begun to practice. She also offered a prayer of gratitude before her meals, so that the food would be blessed. Later that day, in our apartment, I discovered a small magazine and leaflet about yoga meditation that had been left on the kitchen counter. I was intrigued and began to flip through the pages with deep interest and fascination. I did not really understand what this yoga thing was, and approached it with some apprehension.

The next day I met a friend of hers who also meditated. They shared a meditation practice based on the teachings of an Indian mystic. While over at her friend's house, I noticed a picture of this yogi, who had long wavy hair and a very serene and piercing look on his face. As I stared at the picture, he seemed to stare back at me. I did not know what to say to her, except "I kind of look like him," because I also had long hair and dark skin like him. In hindsight, as we were walking out, I realized that this was a very superficial statement.

After about three and half weeks as my roommate, the young woman expressed concern about being able to pay the rent, because her work situation had changed. She was now being forced to move back to her parents' home in the north-eastern United States. Before I knew it, she was gone, and I never heard from her again.

I was concerned now about unexpectedly having to pay the whole rent myself. I even felt some anger towards her. But when I sat to reflect, I found myself closing my eyes and going into meditation. For the first time, I discovered the anger had shifted into gratitude, as I focused on the positive qualities she had left behind.

I continued to meditate for about five minutes each day, feeling like it was an eternity to sit there, although I did begin to feel more peaceful afterwards. But as I read more about the yoga meditation teachings of Paramahansa Yogananda, I discovered how profound they were, answering many of life's questions that I had begun to ponder while I was in college a couple of years before. I knew that what I had discovered was something that could help me find greater contentment within myself, and I became inspired to study the teachings of the East further.

Through this particular exchange with my roommate, as well as others that followed, I learned of the capacity of finding new and old lessons hidden within every experience. The design of this world is such that it mirrors what we are projecting inside of ourselves, and each experience, whether it be physical, mental, or emotional, offers us an opportunity to gain greater insight into the nature of our being. In due course, a series of events and encounters with people kept drawing me to study yoga and explore other mystical teachings. I began to see a link between my consciousness and the outer world I was attracting. I developed a great appreciation for spirituality, and realized that life is a blessing that can teach us that all things do not just happen by chance or coincidence, but are a reminder that we have a relationship with the Divine.

I went on to share many of the interesting experiences from my expanding world of metaphysics with my new friend Deborah, whom I considered to be my "west coast mom." I met her when I was very young at some family gatherings. She had been living in California for many years, was always hospitable, and introduced me to many people. Deborah was a beautiful former Miss USA, and then became an established Hollywood actress. I spent much time with her discussing spirituality, health, and relationships on our morning walks in the Hollywood Hills.

A few weeks after my introduction to meditation through my mystical-eyed roommate, Deborah invited me to my first Hatha Yoga class, and afterwards gave me a brief introduction to the profound wisdom of Ayurveda. As I listened to her speak with such grace and eloquence, I was intrigued by this system, founded on the five elements, which incorporates a vast understanding of nature's laws. For years, I continued my practice of Hatha Yoga both with Deborah and on my own, exploring different classes and teachers.

It was not until many years later that I learned about the close relationship between yoga and Ayurveda. As I researched this further, I was attracted to the wisdom behind these traditions, and how they comprise a profound and detailed teaching on all aspects of life, health, natural living, relationships, and even astrology.

During a period of deep searching for more direction into my life purpose or dharma, I became enraptured with a book entitled *Yoga and Ayurveda* by David Frawley, which demonstrated the connection between these two systems in a simple yet enticing manner. Almost instantaneously, I felt a surge of ideas that began to stretch my consciousness in many directions. I was overwhelmed and found myself asking so many questions. Where has Ayurveda been? Why has yoga been without Ayurveda for so long? These and many more questions were eventually answered during my first trip to India, where I could experience first-hand the energy that has sustained these systems for thousands of years.

Over a period of many years, I immersed myself in deep research and the study of yoga and Ayurveda, expanding my interest into many related topics like Sanskrit chanting (*mantra*), energy work (*Tantra*), herbology, diet, astrology and the ancient teachings (*Vedas*), in all of which I received much guidance and support from David Frawley. The more I studied, the more I discovered the need for healing from the inside out, a need to unite with something beyond the material world, and a way to develop an eternal and Divine relationship between my spirit and nature.

I was not looking for something quick and simple. What I yearned for was profound. The wisdom of this sacred relationship, although rooted in sciences from an ancient civilization such as India, offers a very practical means for healing the body and mind, and provides all the necessary guidance for anyone to evolve in a harmonious way. In practicing yoga with its equally important counterpart Ayurveda, the two sciences unite as a divine couple. But for many of us, one very important factor remains: the willingness to change.

In the Bhagavad Gita, Krishna states, "That which is born of the clear perceptive discrimination of self-realization—that happiness is called sattvic. It seems like poison at first, but like nectar afterward."[1] In the coming pages, I look forward to sharing with you the wisdom of yoga and Ayurveda as a sacred and new relationship we must re-create within ourselves, a new approach to lifestyle to bring greater harmony into our lives. To attain victory in the battle of life, we must bring the sensory or material world into balance. As we have seen in both ancient and modern times, the bigger societies get, the faster they destroy themselves. The richer they get, the harder they fall.

It's a vicious cycle that never ends, but humanity never seems to learn the lesson. We keep coming back for more. Like blind fools, we live as if the body will last forever. We overstress ourselves with loads of work to buy more and more things that we often get bored of very quickly. We bury our emotions under the veil of blaming others for our misfortunes. Sadly, change eventually comes through suffering, as taught in Buddhism. Those periods in our life spur reflection and insight and gratitude for the obvious. The design of life seems so promising. We are born, play, go to school, work, and maybe marry and have kids. Then we watch others do the same. Over and over again, the patterns repeat themselves.

What about the mysterious question of why we are here? How do the events in our lives connect to one another? Where do I find complete fulfillment and satisfaction? Well, what we have been told is to live simply, love your neighbor

---

1   From *God Talks With Arjuna: The Bhagavad Gita* by Paramahansa Yogananda. (Self-Realization Fellowship, Los Angeles, Calif.)

like yourself, think positive, be in the moment, love yourself, listen to your inner guru, and the many other metaphysical stories that we have been told bring peace and wellness. These ideas all sound great, but they can easily become intellectual clutter in our mind that only makes sense as theoretical concepts with no practical application. I feel that the answer lies in nature and lifestyle. Lifestyle is the new religion that can carry us into the highest relationship of health, wellness, and spirituality. The way we live in this world is a reflection of who we are inside. As Gandhi said, "My life is my message."

Nature is what we are born from. The same elements that exist outside us exist inside of us, and influence our minds and all our physiological functions. As the sun warms our body and inspires us to enjoy the day, so it affects our metabolism and our capacity to reflect mentally. It is the sun's vibration that spurs us to search for the "One" love, and although most of humanity seeks to find it through human relationships, it also exists in all of nature.

What I am saying is that nature is constantly sharing with us the perennial intelligence to finding contentment, peace, and love. The wisdom of cosmic intelligence dwells within every atom and molecule, and through a living experience of life, everyone can find answers to every question. As the wind sings its song with various melodies, it also influences our physical movements, expression, and communication. Water in nature is beautifully attractive. It gives us a sense of an expanded awareness, a soothing comfort, and a feeling of being purified and healed. Internally, water is our cleanser and, through lymphatic function, sweat, urinary excretion, and tears, water allows things to flow. Earth is the landscape where all of life takes place.

The most important element is space. No matter where we are, the element of space is predominant, as sound, vibration, feeling, and the overall influence that any particular person, place or thing has, which is transferred or experienced through the collective energy predominant in any place. On a more esoteric level, this includes the quality of space in the field of our planetary mind. There are two perspectives to this. While we exist physically in one particular place, we also exist on a planetary level through the collective mind. This is precisely where lifestyle and environment factor into the quality of our life, and how we can bridge the gap to the unknown.

The tangible and etheric worlds transfuse into one present moment of awareness. Science has established that there are seasons or measures of time in nature, which demonstrate that time exists and that energy is measurable through the law of *karma*: for every action there is an equal reaction. All this can guide us back into relationship with the essence of all things.

Through proper lifestyle, we can regain the balance we are all seeking, but we must transcend the tangible and use nature as a doorway back towards the cosmic Self. All the troubling health issues the world faces can be healed through education on nature's wisdom, lifestyle, and practices that bring greater discipline to and between the mind and body. It is my hope that the profound wisdom of yoga and Ayurveda, interwoven with experiences of my personal life journey, will enhance the quality of your life.

Namaste,

Mas Vidal

April 2016

Background: The Sacred Relationship of Sun-Moon-Earth

The sun, moon, and earth have a special bond, much like that of a loving family. The moon reflects the qualities of the mind. With its waxing and waning qualities, the mind can ebb and flow from thought to thought, emotion to emotion, and thus in extreme cases gave birth to the term *luna*tic. The sun is the magnetic power of the soul and gives us physical vision, spiritual perception, and the inspiration to seek our deepest truths. The earth is like our house or apartment, or where we go to school and work. It is where we can explore and study ourselves, potentially discover the impermanence of life, and attain the realization of the place we can truly call home. Interestingly enough, the word "home" sounds like "Aum," the famous Vedic mantra and eternal vibration of creation that represents unity.

The great story of spirit and nature involves an eternal relationship that begins with the Soul and its relationship with creation. This eternal relationship has intrigued civilizations and humanity for thousands of years. It is the spark of every individualized soul's search for its original home, a higher place, a golden age, heaven, or even something beyond our imagination. This yearning is for something more than we presently have, materially speaking. In the grandest sense, this something is eternal love, but as we generally know it, and as it has been depicted in dramas, tales, and stories throughout history, it has failed to bring us what we are truly seeking.

The external world and its pleasures seem often times to leave us with a hint of discontent. We go from one desire to the next, only to see time, events, and aging move faster and faster. At the end of it all, the spirit must eventually find its way back to nature through the earth and the natural landscape. Through the many stories and fables told over spans of time, we may be encouraged to find what will satisfy us for all eternity.

Human beings also discover their relationship with the world through the dialogue we share with each other and the belief systems we follow over lifetimes. This learning process unfolds over time through the laws of karma and rebirth. The wisdom traditions of the East teach us that nothing just happens. Everything has a cause and an effect.

The ancient Vedic tradition has taught us that this is the essence of healing, the purpose of life, and why living a life in accordance to nature's laws is the complete way to creating a peaceful and sublime world. A great modern mystic, Sivaya Subramuniyaswami, speaking about Nature and Lord Shiva said:

One thing that science took away from us and has never given back is the knowledge that we are a part of ecology. Human beings are a vital part of ecology and not separate from it. With that in mind the whole mass thinking would change. I think it's very important for everyone to realize that whatever we do affects everything else. That's one of Lord Ganesha's great teachings and that's also a good thing that science has done is taught us that we make a movement like this and it affects something far out in the universe. Everything is connected to everything else.

In the mid-1800s, during the genesis of the American spiritual movement, Henry David Thoreau said, "There are a thousand hacking at the branches of evil to one who is striking at the root." This is something that still applies today, because it is not easy to change our habits, especially when societies imitate one another. Life is seemingly a gradual unraveling of our minds in hopes of discovering the true essence of our being and our most refined thoughts and aspirations.

Ultimately, to embrace this relationship of transformation requires an understanding of life's wisdom principles. These principles help us understand the miniature story of our manufactured, illusory world.[2] However, they can also give us an eternal awareness that we all live, partake, and share collectively, as distinct beings, in the whole. On a more personal level, this sacred relationship is symbolic of an individual probing into the true nature of who we really are. On another level, it extends into a responsibility for our relationships with each other, nature, and the planet we all temporarily share.

The wisdom of the yoga and Ayurveda traditions encompasses a broad scope of practices that enhance the quality of life on earth. They represent all aspects of life and, in the boldest sense, are founded on the principles of discipline (*sadhana*) and balance (*tri-dosha*), through a relationship with nature's laws. The wisdom of the ancients is necessary now more than ever, as we can see, in our current state of global affairs, that the purpose of life has been lost.

Yoga and Ayurveda are not concerned with modernization, commerce, or globalization, but are focused on balance and the evolutionary healing of mind and body and establishing soul union. One of the central themes of this book is that yoga and Ayurveda, as ancient sciences, are in essence inseparable, and demonstrate a complete way of life synchronized with natural or divine law. Any practice or wisdom rooted in nature's law is perennial and eternal, and

---

2   *Maya:* Law of duality that creates an illusionary effect on the planet so to bind humanity to the cycles of birth and death.

should therefore not be considered "ancient" or impractical. Human resistance to these practices and principles is superficial and requires personal change.

Typically, any process that leads to spiritual evolution begins with some type of revolution in belief, health practices, or lifestyle. Ancient systems such as these are based on laws not generally understood or accepted in the modern era. To embrace them often requires a shift in thinking. Integrating such practices into a modern lifestyle also requires time, a certain amount of surrender, and a faith that the greatest capacity any human being has is directly within oneself.

Both yoga and Ayurveda provide an approach to lifestyle that is practical and sensible when we are aligned with a higher purpose or *dharma,* that is: personal, according with our conscience; societal, involving awareness shared among individuals and communities; and spiritual, fostering the relationship between our own consciousness and the Divine. Self-discovery through yoga and learning to heal ourselves with Ayurveda are founded on the laws of nature (*dharma*).

Dharma, although very broad in scope, is the basis of life. It means that all beings have a duty or purpose and exist in a two-fold manner. Dharma, generally speaking, includes the laws that govern the planet and everything that lives on it. It also implies in a subtle way that we are born from one source of intelligence or consciousness. This is a massive womb of energy that produces sparks of life. Each person has an equal opportunity to remember from whence they were born.

On the personal side, every soul-being is distinct, with various physical, mental, and emotional qualities. The role of dharma in life is to require that each person find his or her unique purpose and attain balanced health and higher consciousness. As I mentioned earlier, adaptation to such practices in most instances requires various life-changing factors that produce the willingness to begin such a profound exploration. Once this process is in place, yoga provides an extensive teaching for understanding the nature of the mind and how to develop the right attitude for attaining the virtues of higher consciousness.

About Yoga and Ayurveda

Both yoga and Ayurveda are born from the same root of Vedic wisdom, dating back thousands of years in India. The term *yoga* first appears as *yuj* in the Vedic texts, meaning that which unites or holds the mind, body, and soul together. In the highest sense, it refers to union of the individual soul with cosmic consciousness. It stands for an expansive awareness or vision of life as arising from one source.

The term *Ayur* means way of life, and *Veda* means knowledge. Therefore Ayuvedic science gives us knowledge of the way to live naturally. When I first discovered the relationship between yoga and Ayurveda, I was overwhelmed but at the same time nourished by the fact that these two great sciences were rooted in one great ancient Indian tradition. These wisdom teachings (*vidyas*) are the gifts of gods and goddess and the highest representatives of life on this planet. They share common philosophical perspectives that help us understand how to apply them in practical ways, such as the social principle of nonviolence (*ahimsa*).

Yoga in the west has now become a common term associated with the use of physical postures, and is part of a cultural health phenomenon. The physical association with yoga is in stark contrast to the message of **universal oneness** expounded by the original messengers of yoga in the west. Swami Vivekananda, Swami Rama Tirtha, and Paramahansa Yogananda all shared the same message to an American audience that was seeking a more meaningful and purposeful life. By the early 1900s, America had already developed the reputation of being a land of opportunity and riches.

In India, the sacred yogic lifestyle is understood and practiced as a devotional spiritual attitude known as *Bhakti*. This message of oneness or non-duality comes from the philosophy of yoga known as *Vedanta*. Yoga can literally be interpreted to mean union with the Divine, but this will rarely be achieved through the practice of a few purely physical stretches. Yoga itself is part of a great "eternal tradition," known as *Sanatana Dharma* in Sanskrit, which some consider to be the original language of the human species.

I am proposing a return to the ancient principles that empower these teachings, but in a modern, practical, and adaptive manner. We might call this a sacred or spiritual-type lifestyle that could potentially replace religion. As cultures continue to recognize that harmonious and peaceful living is synonymous with the natural laws that Ayurveda and yoga are founded on, humanity may slowly begin to consider lifestyle as the new religion. There are many ways in which we can integrate the principles of oneness, non-violence, devotion, service, and simple living, while applying the yoga exercises that have become so popular throughout the world, but without diluting the essence of the teachings.

Yoga as a scientific practice is supported by its vast teachings, which have continued unbroken since the dawn of human history. The physical postures (*asanas*) primarily developed as part of the *Tantra* tradition specifically known as Hatha Yoga. The term *Hatha* literally means the balance of sun (*surya*) and moon (*chandra*) energies. The basis of yoga science can be explained as raising vibrational energy to increase our human potential. It calls all truth seekers to fulfill their quest for transformation as an experience that will transcend our current state of awareness into the true nature of our being.

Many of us are familiar with these vibrations in the body as the vortices of energy that run along the spine, known as *chakras*. The chakras reflect a much deeper aspect of our spiritual anatomy, which can help us understand the areas of our life that need healing and resolution. The yoga of mantras recognizes *Aum* as the eternal sound of the universe, which vibrates through every atom of existence. It cannot be heard through human ears, but yoga teaches us that its mystery is understood through the subtle faculties of intuition.

The message of yoga is consistent in that the source of our existence and happiness is to be discovered behind the fabric of our physical existence. All that we need lies within us, and this includes our ability to attain health and live peacefully in the world.

Ayurveda, as yoga's sister science, is just beginning to spread in popularity throughout the world. I don't think that Ayurveda's rise in popularity at this time is any coincidence. World cultures have evidently been quite negligent of health, the environment, and finding harmony with one another. After much ignorance and destruction in the world, both personal and social, Ayurveda gives humanity the knowledge to re-cultivate both a personal and divine relationship with our true nature and the world around us.

"How to live" was one of the strongest themes of Paramahansa Yogananda's teaching. Yogananda was the first Indian Swami to spend the majority of his life in the United States, in the first half of the 20th century. "How to Live" is precisely what Ayurveda teaches us: how to cultivate our health through divine purpose. The intention behind every aspect of Ayurvedic wisdom is to unite us with the force that sustains all life.

Ayurveda, when united with yoga, teaches us how to live in a way that expands our awareness beyond the little and limited ego self. By "little self," I refer to the ego concept that creates a false sense of who we are, as well as the conditions and emotions that individuals identify with over time. The ego is the crutch we carry in our lives.

The yoga system is divided into five branches. They are:

- Karma, which relates to our action
- Bhakti, which relates to giving love and devotion
- Jnana, which relates both to self-study and the need for introspection
- Raja, which ultimately is the practice of stilling the body and mind in meditation
- Hatha, which encompasses the physical postures and breathing techniques.

In this book, I explain how yoga, along with Ayurvedic principles, can be practiced as an integral system to improve the quality of life. My intention is not to portray myself as a guru or some higher being more advanced than those of you reading this book. I am an ordinary person who, like any human being, is seeking a greater sense of fulfillment from life, one that I hope is to some extent independent of the material world.

As a young boy, I found myself praying fervently for God's love and guidance, and that He might help others. In attracting yoga back into my life again, from where I last left off, I embarked on a new voyage of bridging the gap between my spirit and personal nature. In my youth, I had a fascination with trees. As I played in them, I felt a deeper connection to them as an extension of who I was at the time. This process of self-discovery today allows me to look at trees and nature in a way that enables my spirit to feel a true sense of freedom, a metaphysical freedom that transcends the boundaries of the mind and allows me to grow as trees do, slowly and gracefully. For me the tree now symbolizes the spine within the physical body, an inner tree that I must learn to climb as I did as a youth, but this time through the teachings of the higher ages and with the intention of realizing my unity with all of life.

Most American commercial "brands" of yoga misrepresent the teachings of classical yoga, and for the most part continue to cultivate an obsession with the physical body. Many students are being taught that physical ability is equal to spiritual capacity, when the two really don't have much in common except that the body is to be used as a vehicle for the journey of life and to lessen, so to speak, our karmic load. The reality is that the majority of people are in a "sleep-walking" mode of awareness. The concept of the "body as vehicle" is symbolized by the yoga tradition's many deities, who also have vehicles for transporting the energies each distinctly represents.

This book will also present research on the application of yoga as a therapeutic practice according to the Paramahansa Yogananda and Ghosh lineage of Bengal, as well as research on the beginnings of the Yoga Therapy movement, which apparently evolved in association with this physical culture movement. Although Yogananda and the Ghosh lineage did not specifically or in an obvious sense address Ayurveda, they clearly considered it from a scientific and spiritual perspective.

I have added my own specific commentary on asana yoga through the lens of Ayurveda, based on the influence of the early Bengali yoga movement and years of my own clinical experience. The application of asana as a precursor to deeper spiritual practices was strongly influenced by Yogananda, but is also linked to the entire line of gurus before him, as well as the influence of his father, Bhagabati Charan Ghosh. Yogananda subsequently passed on the proper spiritual use of asana to his youngest brother, Bishnu Ghosh, and to Buddha Bose, both of whom were influenced by the physical culture and anti-colonial movements.

I consider the teachings of Swami Sivananda of the Divine Life Society of equal importance. Although his approach differs somewhat from the Yogananda lineage, they both embrace an integral approach to enlightenment. I have integrated into this book much of my intimate study over the last ten years with Swami Jyotirmayananda, a jnani yogi who is one of the last living direct disciples of Sivananda.

The primary approach taken to postures is how they can be applied to impact the energy of our physiology to address common health issues. I will also present a distinct perspective on the *Ashtanga Yoga Sutras* of Patanjali, in order demonstrate how Ayurveda can be integrated into this model, and how they share clearly connected themes. Yoga can also be seen as providing a therapeutic path for balanced wellness, which can advance the practitioner towards spiritual freedom.

At the heart of the Ashtanga or eight-limbed yoga model, as compiled by the great sage Patanjali, there are a set of five sacred principles set forth in sutras 3-5 as the essential steps and procedures for practicing yoga. These five principles are what could be considered the *practical* and instrumental aspects of the whole eight-limbed system. Most practitioners of yoga will agree that the union of yoga and Ayurveda is common sense, but few have truly understood or learned how they can be practiced together.

What we are seeing now throughout the world, including the West, is a return to a complete system of lifestyle and practice. Vegetarianism has become more mainstream. Juicing, comfortable clothing, meditation, devotional music (*kirtan*), herbal medicine, and the importance of ecology are all clear signs of the impact that yoga is having on our global culture.

Early on, yoga was exposed to the West without Ayurveda, primarily because the British Raj undermined Ayurveda in India for over 150 years, and allopathic western medicine was riding a wave of popularity in colonial countries. By the late 1970s and '80s, the side effects of Western medical practices were surfacing, giving rise to what was to be called "alternative" medicine. At this time Ayurveda arrived on to American soil mainly through the Transcendental Meditation movement of Maharishi Mahesh Yogi, and its connection to yoga was apparent.

Ayurveda, like yoga, is founded on wholeness and recognizing the whole mind-body-soul trinity as necessary for any true healing to occur. An integrative yoga approach that includes meditation, lifestyle, and mind-body synergy can offer a more rewarding opportunity for many yoga practitioners who have only experienced physical postures or asanas. It can also bring balance to those who have enjoyed the benefits of meditation, but have not found a way to merge the physical with the spiritual.

For many who have stressed and abused their bodies in search of mental or emotional healing, the approach presented in this book is a practical solution. Americans have become obsessed with the material and physical culture at the price of spiritual deprivation. Many look for ways to heal themselves through the physical body or through outer sensory stimulation, without considering any form of self-analysis or introspection, which must come through the control of the mind. Seeking for the "One" person, place, or thing is a natural law and cannot be ignored. All must return whence they came.

I have learned that the body can be a very practical and powerful tool for transformation and transportation, but is certainly not the end of the process. An integral approach to yoga and Ayurveda considers beginning the journey with bodily health. Physical instruments and techniques, good action, devotion, and meditation can be used to help us transcend into the spiritual domain.

Such an approach realizes that *what is good for one person may not be good for another.* Therefore, all individuals develop a practice and a lifestyle specific to their constitutional type or *dosha*. The emphasis is placed on *how* we do things as opposed to *what* we do. Setting the right intention and having the right attitude are what bring success in the work of self-healing and improvement.

Both yoga and Ayurveda propound the importance of environment, community, and lifestyle in shaping the quality of the mind. Such factors gradually purify the mind, returning it to its original state of pure and peaceful awareness. Postures and breathing techniques can be practiced in many different ways and can be adapted to specific individual needs. The time of day and year must also be considered.

The same principles are applied to diet and all aspects of living. There must be an accord between the individual and nature's laws. It is wrong to reduce yoga to a physical exercise, considering its vastness and original purpose. Vedanta, the main philosophical perspective that yoga is aligned with, has never given much importance to the physical body. In fact, it is the antithesis of that, stating, "We are not the body!"

Some might view it as paradoxical that the teachings of Ayurveda expound the importance of aligning ourselves with nature, while Vedanta says you are not the body. But this is the magical essence of how these teachings become effective. We must comprehend the two juxtaposed perspectives of yogic and Ayurvedic teachings to extract their evolutionary power. Ayurveda is closely aligned with Samkhya philosophy, which explains the journey of consciousness into physical existence. It is therefore focused on how we manage the elements within the body. Simply put, Ayurvedic wisdom endorses connection to and relationship with the body and nature, while yoga encourages transformation through the vehicle of the body.

Many have incorrectly defined the Raja or "Royal" Yoga path as detachment or disconnection from the body, the senses, and their operations. This is a mistake. The Raja or integral system is a teaching of transcendence. Do we send a child to school only to learn mathematics, assuming that history or language should come at a different time, once the child has learned to add and subtract? No! The idea is that each subject or limb supports the other, while at the same time exposing our weaknesses in areas where we need to improve.

Swami Sivananda says, "You need not wait for ethical perfection before you start meditation." What changes over time is the depth of the practice and overall experience. Yoga and Ayurveda always work together to develop wholeness. Our depth of knowledge cannot be limited just to the body. While the physical postures are a doorway for many into the vast ocean of yoga, we should try not to fragment the practice only because a student may not yet be capable.

The best teaching anyone can receive comes through the process of uncovering the layers of ego which, once removed, reveal the sanctuary of the Soul. This process of shifting our awareness from the physical into the subtle is the highest intention of the Raja Yoga system, but also the least understood and practiced. It is my intention to explain this process in this book. The journey from the physical to the subtle realms is the *spiritual* healing that Ayurveda is founded upon, as it considers the three bodies, physical, astral, and causal, which reflect healing of the physical body, mind, and emotions. May we all practice yoga and live Ayurveda, and let Divine surrender take care of the rest.

Chapter ONE

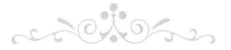

Yoga and Health in the World

In the end, it's not the years in your life that count. It's the life in your years.
Abraham Lincoln (1809 - 1865).

A Primitive Health Movement

If we take a perspective on the world at this time, we find that there is not much health present. When we consider the current size of the world population and the number of health-related issues we suffer from, the figures are daunting. These health issues are especially prevalent in the western world, where modern cities are sprawling left and right and all the most advanced concepts in medicine are being practiced.

It seems that humanity spends most of its time either spoiling the body or dealing with some physical discomfort. Current issues range from digestive disorders to sleep problems, chronic fatigue syndrome, and a gamut of musculoskeletal pain. There are also the five chronic diseases: heart disease and stroke, cancer, respiratory disease, diabetes, and obesity, which together account for at least 60% of deaths globally.

One core issue we struggle with in America is with the production, trade, and societal use of drugs. This all began with tobacco, which Columbus discovered being used by the Taino Indians, one of the indigenous peoples of the Caribbean. By the early 1600s, tobacco smoking, a tradition adopted from American Indians, had become widespread in England. Tobacco was cultivated at the early English colony of Jamestown, Virginia, where it became a cash crop.

The first coffee house in England was opened in 1652. The original word for rum, alcoholic liquor distilled from molasses or sugar-cane residue, made its first appearance in the English language the year before. By 1770, the two million people living in the thirteen colonies were consuming up to 7.5 million gallons of rum a year. As early as 1814, there were several commercial coffee roasters operating in New York City.

Such drugs as morphine and cocaine appeared in society in the early 1800s. By the mid-nineteenth century, addiction to morphine among Civil War veterans was so common it was called "the army disease." In 1884, the New York *Times* praised cocaine as a cure-all wonder drug that could be used for a variety of ailments: "The new uses to which cocaine has been applied with success in New York... include hayfever, catarrh and toothache and it is now being experimented with in cases of seasickness.... All will be given to understand that cocaine will cure the worst cold in the head ever heard of." This eventually led to the creation of Coca-Cola, which combined stimulants from the coca leaf and caffeine from the African kola nut.

By the twentieth century, cigarettes had become mainstream. Marijuana also became part of the counter-cultures of Bohemianism (1850-1910), the Beat Generation (1944- 1964) and the hippies in the 1960s. Prescription medications also became commonly used in western allopathic medicine.

The point I want to make with this short history of drug use in America is that, despite all its great ideals, the United States has had to contend with severe obstacles. The concept of individual freedom has led us into capitalistic greed and given birth to a culture addicted to stimulants, other drugs, and the promise of instant gratification and quick fixes.

If we consider the medical understanding of the nervous system as a network of sensitive impulses that operate on our entire physiology, influence our anatomy, and impact brain function and emotional wellness, shouldn't we be reevaluating the role stimulants play in our lives? Yes! I think so, and many more are beginning to think likewise.

Coffee misuse is more prevalent than we may realize and its effects are often overlooked. In 1895, health nut C.W. Post, founder of the Post cereal company, attacked coffee as containing a "poisonous drug, caffeine, which belongs in the same class of alkaloids with cocaine, morphine, nicotine...." According to the medical science of Ayurveda, stimulants of any kind are particularly cautioned against because of their capacity to disturb the endocrine system and the balance of subtle life-force energy (*prana*) in the body, especially if a person has a sensitive nature.

Stimulants also disturb the equanimity of the mind, which is the spiritual link to our inner, higher consciousness. As I see it, this hyper-stimulation is precisely where the process of disease begins to break down the body through the mind, leading to the gradual destruction of our health. Through the use of coffee, alcohol, and any other strong stimulant, the tissues (*dhatus*) can begin over time to become depleted or weak. In Ayurveda, this is an indication that the life sap (*ojas*), the energy that supports the physical heart, has been dried up or lost.

Historically in yoga, some stimulants have been traced to an elixir or tonic called *soma* used during the early Vedic era to revitalize the body for sacred practices. Later, during the Tantric period, other stimulants appeared and were used to hasten the awakening the special energies in the spine, although with only limited success.

What I have witnessed is: the faster the life, the faster the problems come. The body has a natural process for healing, fighting off disease, and recovering from injury. When we disrupt the natural balance of vital energy or prana, digestion is disturbed. This upsets the proper distribution of food nutrients and weakens the digestive strength (*jatharagni*) required to eliminate food waste properly.

According to Ayurveda, the basis for health is a strong and balanced digestive system. Diet is a critical factor in health, wellness, and inter-personal harmony. Food production requires a relationship to the earth. Natural elements should not be replaced with genetically modified foods, which is another current attempt at separating humanity from its natural origins.

I will discuss the sacred principles spirit shares with ecology in the last chapter of the book. The relationship between mankind and food is a sacred one and should not be disturbed or distorted. Otherwise, the body's energetic balance will struggle to connect with the source of nutrition. This topic is also further expanded on in a section entitled "Food as Medicine," which deals with how the energy in food is transferred into the consciousness of the person cultivating and eating it.

What Is Health?

Health is a term widely used today. It is considered the most important factor of life, although the lifestyle of modern urban societies strongly runs counter to the value of a healthy life. If you ask your typical person today what "health" is, they would say something like, "to have a long life free from disease," or maybe "having a lean body and being athletic."

Living a long life and establishing a higher quality of life are two very different concepts that require a deeper understanding of the scientific principles of creation. If one assumes the western religious view that we live only one life and are then sent either to heaven or hell, then it would make sense that we would want to extend our time in this sensory world.

In East Asian enlightenment traditions, such as the Vedic-Hindu, Buddhist, Jain, and Sikh, the laws of karma and rebirth teach us that the soul is eternally one with the universe. Through repeated embodiments, we experience what is called "life" on earth as a school and place to express free will and celebrate the gift of living.

How we define health is at the very core of the issues we face today as a global society. Today, and historically in the West, the understanding of what health actually consists of is based on the idea of mortality: longevity rather than quality of life. The Eastern spiritual traditions base health on very different measures: an immortal life or soul that temporarily inhabits a body.

According to the later Vedic traditions, life as we experience it operates under an illusionary force called **maya**.[3] This dualistic force relates to the magnetic one existing between the sun, moon and earth in planetary interchange. This bilateral, sun-moon, or dual force creates a living experience that seems very real, sensory and pleasurable. However, unanswered questions and mystery remain. History, as we think we know it, is a major part of our health problems.

Rising out of the very dark ages (**kali yuga**), we have now entered a new age of technology and communication. Instead of living with and simply trying to maintain prior knowledge, science and education are focusing on the advancement of new laws.[4] All history must be questioned and so-called "facts" or historical accounts that we read and hear about must be properly sourced and compared from various perspectives to decipher what the truth really is. The Buddha said, "Do not believe in anything simply because you have heard it. Do not believe in anything simply because it is spoken and rumored by many. Do not believe in anything simply because it is found written in your religious books. Do not believe in anything merely on the authority of your teachers and elders. Do not believe in traditions because they have been handed down

---

3   A central concept of the Vedanta tradition.

4   Neurobiology's recent discoveries of the nervous system and brain-body relationship; Isaac Newton's three physical laws of motion that laid the foundation of classical mechanics; Kepler's three laws of planetary motion; and Albert Einstein's theory of relativity.

for many generations. But after observation and analysis, when you find that anything agrees with reason and is conducive to the good and benefit of one and all, then accept it and live up to it."[5]

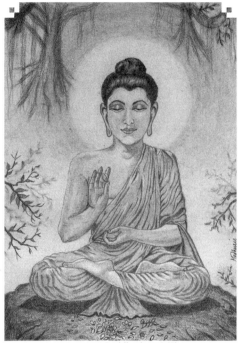

Gautama Buddha (500 BCE)

As a global traveler, one thing I have learned about truth is that what I have often read or heard about a certain society, country, person or even religion is often considerably different from my personal, direct experience. Sadly, much of the world lives and makes choices based on information from uninformed sources or ones that manufacture their own biased opinions. The Aryan Invasion Theory is one such example of this, and was concocted by the British Raj to justify their occupation of India from 1858 to 1947.

The British, led by archeologist Mortimer Wheeler, published the propaganda that the Indian sub-continent was invaded by nomadic dark-skinned people who killed the indigenous white man, based on excavations of the Indus Valley Civilization made during the 1920s. This was based on the interpretation of many unburied corpses found in the top levels of the Mohenjo-Daro excavation as victims of these dark-skinned invaders. Only recently has this theory been proven false, but it may be some time before the facts are widely accepted and corrected in history books.

---

5   Prince Gautama Siddharta, the founder of Buddhism, 563-483 B.C.

Without a scientific understanding of life, its purpose, and the laws governing this planet, an interpretation of what health is will be very limited. The world lives lost in a clutter of thoughts, religious identities, and dogmas, and is completely immersed in "I am the body" consciousness.

The myth of the "Fountain of Youth" has existed for almost two thousand years and across several cultures. Either drinking or bathing in its waters, one can attain eternal youthfulness and abundant health. This first appeared in the writings of the Greek historian Herodotus in the fifth century BC. During the Age of Exploration, it was extended to the indigenous peoples of the Caribbean, particularly around the island of Bimini in the Bahamas. The legend accompanied the collapse of the Western Roman Empire and eventually reached the Americas, entering Florida.

Those times, according to the Vedic teaching of epochs (*yugas*) and Plato's Great Year,[6] are periods when common sense and higher scientific knowledge were lost. Plato, along with his teacher, Socrates, and his most famous student, Aristotle, helped lay the foundations of Western philosophy, science, and thinking.

In a sense, as the New World was being "discovered," we developed concepts of health that were superficial and based on a fragmented concept of who we really are. As technology continues to advance, exercising the body will decrease, as the need for manual labor in farming, agriculture, and home-building is reduced.

There is something tremendously powerful when the mind and body are engaged equally in an activity. The Americas have, however, been overrun with the ideology of greed, a faster-is-better consumerism, and an egoistic attitude of entitlement. All this has destroyed our health.

Recently, the influence of yoga and Ayurveda has been felt in some way or another in most of the world. The principle of "oneness" set forth in Vedanta, the mystical yet practical system of yoga, and the common-sense principles of Ayurveda have affected many cultures and countries, all in a very short period of time, considering the traditions' antiquity.

Interestingly enough, the development of sacred spaces, such as temples and shrines, has fallen off. The spirituality that is replacing traditional religion and cultivates inner practices has become more portable. Looking on the positive side, changes in attitudes to health are occurring globally and have become

---

6   The period of one complete cycle of the equinoxes around the ecliptic, which takes 24,000 years. See Walter Cruttenden's *Lost Star of Myth and Time.*

noticeable in many areas of life. The concept of science is becoming more understood from a spiritual perspective. With globalization, economies are becoming more interdependent. Market cycles, government policies, and social trends are becoming cross-cultural and mainstream. The world is now a smaller place.

We are now all becoming more aware that the way in which we live as individuals can make a substantial impact on the global community and the world we live in. The potential of all individuals is becoming more apparent. Throughout history, individuals such as Lincoln, Gandhi, Einstein, and Jesus have been etched in our memory for their accomplishments, unique personalities, and the courage they had to follow their own paths. The power and potential of individuality have risen in the last few decades, but have yet to reach their culmination. This may reflect the changing paradigm of the quality of the relationships we have with ourselves, each other in partnership, our chosen God, and nature.

The Yoga Renaissance

The modern yoga revival began in the mid-1850s with the life and teachings of the great Hindu saint Sri Ramakrishna Paramahamsa in the eastern Indian state of Bengal. His motto was, "Paths are many, truth is one." To many, he was considered an incarnation of India's two great yogi kings, Rama and Krishna. He had a wide popular appeal, spoke in rustic Bengali, and made use of many stories and parables. He was married to Sri Sarada Devi, a great spiritual teacher in her own right and considered by many as the spiritual mother of the modern yoga movement.

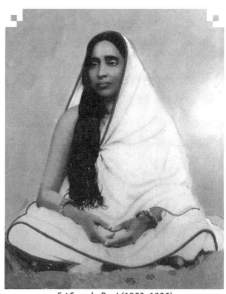

Though conventionally uneducated, and unable to read or write, Ramakrishna attracted attention among the Bengali intelligentsia and middle classes. By the mid-1870s, he had become the focal point of a resurgence of Hinduism, particularly among Westernized intellectuals. He gathered a group of followers, led by his chief disciple Swami Vivekananda, who continued his work as a monk following Ramakrishna's death in 1886.

Sri Sarada Devi (1853-1920)

It was Swami Vivekananda who first brought the message of yoga to the west in 1893, giving voice to the philosophical themes of Eastern mysticism in the United States. In an interesting synchronicity, Ralph Waldo Emerson's spiritual writings, as well as his friend Henry David Thoreau's *Walden,* began to gain popularity at that time, as did the influence of their contemporary Walt Whitman. These men spoke on important Eastern spiritual themes, such as solitude, love, nature, and self-reliance, often mentioned such scriptures such as the Bhagavad Gita, Vedas, and Upanishads.

Through them, these themes began to surface in opposition to mainstream society. They were the first American metaphysicians, who fed Western souls starving from years of literal interpretation of scripture and dogmatic practices that left many questions unanswered.

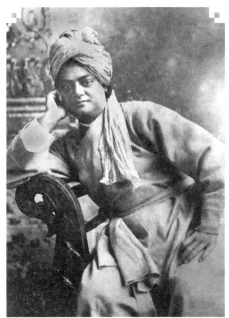

Sri Swami Vivekananda (1863 – 1902)

Earlier in the nineteenth century, Abraham Lincoln became president of the United States and, against much opposition, made the Emancipation Proclamation during the Civil War, emphasizing the war's crusade against slavery. Like Lincoln, Thoreau opposed slavery, and wrote and spoke publicly on the matter. These men were a voice for many that during those times opposed these practices and the limitations they placed on the potential of the individual.

It is important to remember that when Vivekananda appeared, our country (America) had recently experienced a Civil War in which the country was divided on the role government should play and the issue of slavery. America had to overcome fear just as it was riding a wave of new freedom and independence from Britain. At the same time, that same British Empire had just established its rule in India.

Many inventions, such as the photograph, steam engine, and automobile, also took place in the 19th and early 20th century. Did all of these major changes in thought and creativity occur by a stroke of luck? Hardly. The collective consciousness was changing. A major global shift that began in 1700 gave birth to individuals who become catalysts for freedom. This freedom was not limited to an exterior concept of space, but derived from new perspectives and a way of life that allowed us to think, speak, and act as individuals, beyond the limitations of the body, skin color, oppression, government, laws, and religious dogma.

In other words, in this new age people began to take greater responsibility for themselves. They recognized the power of their own minds, and this inspired a greater search for the meaning of life. This great shift was part of the transition from a dark and ignorant Iron Age period of almost tribal mentality and culture, to a Bronze Age. A new breed of thinkers began to question society and history, and seek out principles of character that had long been forgotten. When we deny our morality, we ignore our health. This shift is reflected in a new type of thinking and living that adheres to a "Higher Law" or dharma, an invisible truth that is the essence of our conscience.

This is the real meaning of the word "change," a concept that is poorly understood as an outer event independent of our will or action. Yoga teaches us that the faculty of intuition guides real change and creates transformation, which in itself is synonymous with the term yoga as an inner process that finds its source in every soul. The highest law is that of the individual who knows himself to be a part of the whole, but is at same time distinct. Anything else is a separation from the truth.

Humanity is now beginning to honor the true self, the self that can think and question, act and surrender to the calling of the real spirit nature. Such people and groups are often seen as renegades and anti-social. They are actually those on the path to truth.

Conformism and non-conformism now exist side by side. The current trend is to be spiritual as opposed to religious. Spiritual people are associated with ecology, diet, exercise, alternative medical care, and yoga. They are integrated in cross-cultural relationships and activities. Religions, on the other hand, bred a tribal identity that segregated communities and individuals.

We can see that much of society today is moving towards the "spiritual" or "natural," but not always by choice. In many cases, religious groups do not embrace new life choices such as yoga. However, certain religious and non-denominational organizations, and even corporations, in an effort to maintain themselves financially, are now offering alternative options and incentives to attract and maintain membership or appease their employees' new lifestyle demands. Even traditional restaurants now offer vegetarian options demanded by changes in lifestyle. Lifestyle reformation is becoming more pertinent in addressing the world's health care needs. Even the unwilling may slowly have to adapt to this growing new paradigm.

Ayurveda's Revival

When you look at the similarities and perfect relationship between yoga and Ayurveda, you may wonder why Ayurveda has only recently become a bit more popular. Yoga has been experiencing a renaissance for well over one hundred years now. Why is Ayurveda, yoga's sister science, just being recognized?

There are a number of reasons to explain their reunion. Originally, in ancient times, yoga and Ayurveda were unified practices, a lifestyle that was part of the greater Vedic culture of the Rig Veda.[7] Over time, they developed into separate sciences, each having its own schools and texts explaining their teachings.

The major formulation of Ayurveda took place between 1000 and 1500 B.C. Two great Ayurvedic physicians, Charaka and Sushruta, compiled what have become the main, classical Ayurvedic texts, the *Charaka Samhita* and *Sushruta Samhita*. Interestingly, the topic of yoga is also found in the *Charaka Samhita*, where it is described relative to the path of liberation (*moksha*). The text also describes the occult powers attained by yogis. Oddly, there is no mention of Hatha Yoga, the yoga of postures, or breathing techniques (*pranayama*). The various Vedic branches were fragmented during these times. In approximately 500 AD, Ayurveda was re-introduced in a more concise manner and simplified explanations in another classic text, Vagbhatta's *Ashtanga Hridaya*.

By the early 1500s, India had already been overcome by the domination of the Mughal Empire, what lasted until the 1850s, when the British Raj took over. When India gained independence in 1947, it did so through the practice of non-violence (*ahimsa*) and truthfulness (*satya*), under the leadership of the famous man of peace Mahatma Gandhi. During Islamic and British occupation, much of Ayurveda was destroyed, as a means of undermining the Indian people. Imperial rule over other countries is another characteristic typical of people and governments harboring dark-age consciousness. Sadly, the Indian people were downtrodden for many centuries due to the loss of their great Vedic knowledge.

Over the last fifty years or so, Ayurveda has grown substantially, not just in its motherland but internationally, with a strong presence in the Americas and

---

7   The oldest of the Vedic texts.

Europe. The term "yoga" is a household name and its popularity is serving to popularize Ayurveda, which is its ideal counterpart in terms of lifestyle, diet, health, and spirituality.

Much of yoga's popularity is associated with the practice of asanas as a form of exercise, garnished with some spiritual overtones. Although yoga is being stereotyped as a physical practice, asana has served as an entryway for many into the deeper side of the tradition. What Ayurveda brings to yoga is the idea that yoga is not just something that you practice a few hours a week in a room or resort, but a way of life that involves establishing daily and seasonal routines and understanding our personal relationship with nature as a divine aspect of life.

Yoga Today

Yoga in the West is found mainly in asana or fitness centers in most major cities throughout the US, Canada, Mexico, and Europe. It is estimated that some 36 million people practice yoga in the United States alone. That's quite a high percentage for a country with just over 300 million people. The majority of the practitioners are women, approximately 77%. The number of gyms and fitness centers offering yoga has increased to over 85%, up from 31% just ten years ago. The market for yoga has grown tremendously. It is estimated that Americans now spend $27 billion annually on yoga products.

In India, many of the well-known yoga organizations, such as Yogananda's Yogoda Satsanga Society, the Sivananda Ashrams, and Swami Ramdev's Patanjali Yogapeeth, all offer Ayurvedic services as a part of their mission. Yoga in India is mainly understood as a devotional path directed towards enlightenment, although the physical aspects of yoga and their therapeutic benefits are becoming popular because of western interests and globalization.

The number of Ayurvedic schools throughout India has grown substantially, with many now embracing yoga as part of a comprehensive education and an effective way to further expose Ayurveda. In 2006, I was asked to speak before a small group of Ayurvedic physicians in India about yoga and its role in propagating Ayurveda. They were all very enthusiastic about my concept of "yoga as the doorway" to Ayurveda. Afterwards, they were all encouraged to reach out to existing yoga schools and local centers to establish some type of working relationship with them. The same thing has taken place in the US, with Ayurveda connecting with yoga institutions, teachers, and related Vedic sciences such as astrology.

The growth of both yoga and Ayurveda should be no surprise, as much of our world continues to experience economic instability, growing health issues, and emotional bankruptcy. As we can see, much of the world and many people's lives are consumed with meaningless things that just keep repeating themselves, leaving us with no real progress. We acquire one new desire after another. We eventually realize that the "One" real need we have is not outside, but directly within us. Still, we keep ignoring it.

These Indian systems are a practical and common-sense approach to lifestyle. They are affordable and suitable to any of those willing to make the effort to improve themselves. Yoga and Ayurveda bring people together with a common language of health, peace, and love. They are rebuilding our communities and renewing our relationship with nature to one of appreciation and respect. They represent a balance between our inner and outer lives.

The Western Health System

When we see a physical body that has very little body fat and is perhaps muscular or athletic-looking, we assume that the person is healthy. The media, entertainment, and ego control are what drive our culture. One way or another, societies are driven by decisions based on what will attract the biggest audience and generate the most revenue. One trend spins others off, influencing people to believe that they must have this or that new pill, diet, or surgery to be healthy and accepted by society. Doctors make millions of dollars on surgeries and prescribing medications that often have greater side effects than benefits. Such measures are not always necessary, although they can have a place in improving the quality of health at the present time.

The health-care crisis in America, which has existed for some time but is only now being addressed, supports a pattern of spending unlike any other country in the world, as if that were the solution to improving health. Providing medical access to everyone and solving our health problems always seem to come down to needing and spending more money. Social and personal responsibility continues to be ignored. Education and prevention alone are too passive to curb the health issues we are now dealing with.

US health care expenditure is in the trillions of dollars annually, of which the majority is spent to treat illnesses caused by stress. This strongly indicates that our current way of living is out of order with the natural process of life. In the United States, much more is spent on health-related issues than any other industrialized country, but American life expectancy is far from the highest.

Stress levels are likely the main factor differentiating America life-expectancy rates from those of other countries where life expectancy is higher. This again indicates a lifestyle obviously not conducive to wellness. What we must realize is that it's not what we have attained but "how we live" that determines the quality of our lives. The intention behind our actions and the meaning of our life depend mostly on our relationship with the Divine.

For centuries, the Western world has been characterized as a place of material abundance, but not necessarily of health or spiritual wealth. So is it really our health care system that is failing or is it the intention behind the way Americans live? In considering what's wrong, we must look at the origins of any approach to healing born of materialism, co-dependence, instant gratification, and absence of individual responsibility.

Growing Epidemics of Mind-Body Fracturing

There is no question that obesity is a growing epidemic in America and around the world, particularly in the last thirty years. Obesity is the second leading cause of preventable death, after smoking. The United States leads the world in obesity, which affects over 30% of the population. Obesity among adolescents has tripled. This is not a disease brought on by an infection or foreign agent, but is attributed to lack of cardiovascular function or type-two diabetes. It is also a lifestyle issue of over-eating and large food portions.

Ayurvedic physician Sushruta correlated obesity to diabetes and heart disease thousands of years ago. The main causes of obesity relate directly to lifestyle, with people becoming more sedentary in addition to eating meat-based diets. When will Americans learn that fixed and strict diets don't work?

Everyone has to eat and the concept of one diet that works for everyone is another American dream. This is where the wisdom of Ayurveda's tri-dosha science is very effective. It is endorses eating a diet specifically attuned to our individual constitutional (*prakriti*) needs and nature's seasonal cycle.

What is American food? It's everything and anything we want to eat, as we do not have a staple food. Such variety plays havoc on our stomachs, the most sensitive organ in the body. The American diet is influenced by a diverse range of cultures and countries, as is also the case with large urban areas that attract a diverse population. These buffet-style diets disturb and over-burden the human digestive system, never really giving it a chance to get acclimated or habituated to a type of food. Such is the crux of the ever-expanding body and the weakening of the digestive fire or *jatharagni*.

These destructive dietary patterns are no longer limited to America, but are slowly developing in all major international cities, as globalization continues. Only the adoption of a natural system like Ayurveda can save us. Yoga preaches simple living, and Ayurveda preaches a simple diet and seasonal eating. Yoga recommends fasting occasionally on fresh juices and teas, and both sciences adhere to a vegetarian diet and cooking with herbs and spices. Even though vegetarianism is regarded as vital to purifying the mind and body, meat is eaten in Ayurveda in cases of specific medical conditions.

Food Consumerism

A plant-based or vegetarian diet has become a growing part of our mainstream culture. Many studies have proven it can lead to greater health. A greater number of people are choosing to eat vegetarian because it makes sense intellectually. Vegetarianism is also tied into the growing environmental or "green" movement. A community of people who are living more consciously is emerging as the voice of environmental issues, and their influence is also extending to medicine and politics.

Well-researched studies have proven that meat is difficult to digest, contains toxins present in the blood of the animals, and is high in fats that can promote diabetes and increase cholesterol and the incidence heart disease. According to yoga and Ayurvedic principles, meat is considered a low nutritional-grade, karma-increasing (*tamasic*) food that has many health implications and is contrary to the principle of non-violence.

A common problem with the standard American diet is **quantity**. Meals are simply too large and highly caloric. Large quantities of food consumed at a single meal bog down the digestive system. If the meal includes red meat, it slows the system even more, leading to increased weight and body fat.

Animals raised in feedlots, like 43% of the world's beef, accumulate omega-6 fatty acids,[8] a family of unsaturated fatty acids ("bad fats") that have been linked with cancer, diabetes, obesity, and immune disorders. Approximately 70% of all antibiotics in the United States are fed to pigs, poultry, and cattle, to increase growth and to counter sanitation issues caused by animals being confined to atrocious living conditions. The US is the largest consumer of beef

---

8   Some medical research suggests that excessive levels of n–6 fatty acids, relative to n–3 fatty acids, may increase the probability of a number of diseases and depression. Chronic excessive production of n–6 is associated with heart attacks, thrombotic stroke, arrhythmia, arthritis, osteoporosis, inflammation, mood disorders, and cancer.

in the world. In 2001, Eric Schlosser published his book *Fast Food Nation*, which gives a very raw account of today's factory-farm system.

There are many ecological drawbacks to producing meat as well. The amount of water and land required is enormous. Meat products have to be trucked great distances, as farms and slaughterhouses are located in less costly commercial and rural areas.

In a New York *Times* article, "Rethinking the Meat Guzzler," Mark Bittman writes, "Americans eat about the same amount of meat as we have for some time, about eight ounces a day, roughly twice the global average. At about 5 percent of the world's population, we 'process' (that is, grow and kill) nearly 10 billion animals a year, more than 15 percent of the world's total." Bittman is the author of a great book entitled *How to Cook Everything Vegetarian*, with many simple recipes for those looking for alternatives to a meat-based diet. The repercussions of America's approach to diet are clear and obviously a major cause of many chronic diseases and our dependence on a healthcare system with major disparities.

Changing the Diet Trend

There are many things we can do to begin to change our health and our society's habits. The first and foremost is to change your own diet and set an example for others to live by. Mahatma Gandhi famously said, "Be the change that you want to see in the world." Others will follow your example. I have seen how my own example has influenced many others to eat less meat, because, as a vegetarian, I excelled as a competitive athlete and was able to maintain sub-stantial muscle mass, disproving a common myth about a non-meat diet. The myth of needing a high-quantity protein diet will eventually be dispelled, but many Americans now have little education on where to find protein in non-meat foods like almonds, lentils, eggs, and many types of grains. Meat-eating societies have become fearful of not maintaining enough protein in their diets out of fear of losing muscle mass and strength—another huge myth. In fact, most Americans and meat-eaters in general eat more protein than they can actually digest, bogging the digestive organs down and stressing the liver and kidneys.

According to Ayurvedic principle,s each constitutional type (*dosha*) has different requirements in order to keep balance of the elements (air, fire, water, earth). The tri-dosha system is comprised of air (*vata*), fire (*pitta*), and water and earth (*kapha*), and each has its unique qualities that influence the body and mind. Vata types are influenced by the central nervous system and, having the lowest amount of body fat and muscular density, are delicate and can be sensitive and generally very lean. As a result, they can benefit most from bulking foods such as dairy products, pastas, oils, and nuts, which are higher in fat and calories. Vata types have a tendency to struggle when digesting large portions, or dry or cold foods, as their digestive fires can be a bit weak. Therefore, it is best if they eat warm, cooked, hearty foods.

Pitta types are hot. Being muscular and very focused, with strong digestive systems, they usually get away with eating anything they like. As their digestion is viscous, they usually fall prey to over-eating at meals. Fruits, vegetables, grains, and cooling green salads are good for these fire types.

Kapha types are stable, naturally hold more body fat and tend to eat more slowly and frequently. Their digestive systems are generally the most consistent, but in the evening they should try to eat foods that minimize dairy content, oil, salt, and most particularly starch, such as breads, pastas, potatoes, and so on.

There are specific foods from each food group—nuts, legumes, grains, fruits, vegetables, and dairy—that each dosha should be cautioned against during appropriate seasons and in certain locations Much of this can be found in Ayurvedic cookbooks, and is usually also included in consultations with practitioners.

"One-for-all" fixed diet plans don't work, because they force different body types with different metabolisms to adjust to the same foods. Much is compromised by forcing individuals to adhere to foods that do not accord with the elements and qualities of their dosha. One of Ayurveda's basic, essential dietary wisdom tenets is learning which foods are most beneficial to your system, according to the season, in order to attain balanced digestion. It is crucial to follow dietary rules that take a person's imbalances (*vikriti*) into account, in order not to create discomfort and disease.

There are a number of simple things that can help change current diet trends when purchasing food. Buying from local farmers at weekly markets or small independent stores insures that you are supporting smaller family-owned companies that place more attention on quality than quantity. Buying fresh, organic, seasonal foods is also important, as many larger food companies freeze and spray foods with wax-type preservatives to extend shelf life. The use of pesticides has become a prominent concern, as we now recognize how taste and nutritional value are compromised. As companies find more ways to make money, consumer health suffers.

When possible, we should avoid purchasing canned or packaged foods that have lost their life force *(prana)* and capacity to nourish the immune system *(ojas)*. I feel that one of main issues with health in the US and most large cities is immune-system depletion, largely as a result of poor diets that lack real nutrition or prana. Another fact previously discussed is the over-dependence on stimulants, such as coffee, that curb the appetite, and similarly on the many weight-loss products that tax the adrenals.

Shopping for food more frequently and purchasing it in smaller quantities insure that the food you eat is fresh and will not spoil. It is hard to imagine how much food is wasted in many households and the commercial restaurant industry, when approximately 35 million people in the United States, the wealthiest country in the world, live in poverty. The western mentality of over-sized over-abundance and over-accumulation will, I hope, gradually change in many respects, from diet to lifestyle. Westerners must learn to find contentment in simplicity and happiness from the inside out, as we continue to create new values that are based on intangibles and lifestyles that connect us to each other and nature.

When dining out, try to choose restaurants that are more *sattvic*, a Sanskrit word that means peaceful, and in this context refers to organic, vegetarian foods cooked by peaceful people in places owned by individuals who make an effort to live in an ethical and sustainable manner. The energetic value of food cannot be ignored on the path to higher consciousness. The great Saint Sri Ramakrishna once rejected food that was served to him because the energy it was infused with during preparation was impure and lacked balanced, positive vibrations. He could feel it, and so can we if we realign our mind-body relationship.

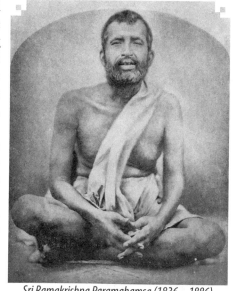

We must become more conscious buyers and take greater responsibility for the choices we make and the influence they may have upon others. Conscious food choices support sustainable agriculture and farms' ability to produce food for an indefinite period without causing severe damage to the ecosystem. Sustainability is

Sri Ramakrishna Paramahamsa (1836 – 1886)

vital with respect to health, poverty, and the future evolution of this planet. Sustainability's two key aspects are biophysical, long-term effects on the soil, and socio-economic, farmers' ability to manage their farms fairly and justly. Sustainable agriculture, a farming method that is growing rapidly worldwide, depends on replenishing the soil while minimizing the use of non-renewable resources.

The Solution

What I present in this book is the application of an education based on universal law and the wisdom of the Ancients. As taught in the yoga and Ayurveda traditions, this wisdom is founded on an integral relationship between the mind, body, and soul that reflects the grander relationship of the sun, moon, and earth. The blind can no longer lead the blind, unless we prefer self-denial and self-destruction. We must rely more on time-tested scientific methods not concocted by any particular individual, but which represent the truths the sun, moon, and earth demonstrate to us. We could say their relationship is the voice of the Divine.

Yoga and Ayurveda reflect the scientific truths and universal laws that govern the planet earth. They provide us with an innovative approach and insights that can help humanity solve the mystery of creation. Ancient wisdom encourages us to embark on a lifestyle revolution. The Vedas make the bold proclamation that all beings emancipate themselves to realize that Divinity is their birthright. This is about directing our energy back to ourselves so that each and every individual in this world will begin to take responsibility for his or her own life and partake in the burgeoning relationship between our spirit and nature.

We must take these steps with courage. Without great courage and social and personal independence, mankind will remain attached to the idea that solutions to health, strife, inequality, and peace can be attained through outer change, something outside of one's own mind-body-consciousness relationship. Vedic wisdom (*vidya*) is based on self-empowerment as the windows and doorways to discovering our Higher Self. Our minds must be clear, visionary, and embrace the power of the light to see through the "windows" of life's ever-changing experiences. The body serves us as a vehicle for personally responsible actions as we walk through the "doorways" of opportunity and growth to follow our highest dharma, self-realization.

It may seem that, as the demand for the magical, mystical wisdom of the East grows, the world seems to be regressing at the same time. There is some truth to this, as not everyone is evolving in a pure or sattvic direction equally.

It is clear that the greater majority of the world seeks to find peace and happiness in new ways that bring more abundance, consistency, and everlasting joy. The world is designed in such a way that we can learn through repeated effort. If we do not learn our lesson through a certain experience, there will always be another opportunity. We learn and change through pain and suffering. Positive discoveries arrive from having experienced the negative, and so the forces of nature provide the power to transcend the cycles of birth and death (*samsara*).

Yoga shows us the occult relationship these positive and negative energies share with the individual and the cosmos, while Ayurveda demonstrates their use in the practical relationship between our physiology and nature. Together, yoga and Ayurveda bridge the gap between mind and body, empowering us to experience freedom and enjoy life, while remaining aware of its true purpose.

To the lay person or outsider, these teachings seem to present a type of connection-separation, positive-negative, attraction-repulsion paradox. For devotees, yoga practices and lifestyle routines follow fixed instructions and conform to scriptural laws. Sri Ramakrishna says that one given the blessed insight of understanding the grander nature of Divinity in all things follows "…the process of negation and affirmation. First he negates the world, realizing that it is not Brahman;[9] but then he affirms the same world, seeing it as the manifestation of Brahman. To give an illustration: a man or women wanting to climb to the roof first negates the stairs as not being the roof, but on reaching the roof he or she finds that the stairs are made of the same materials as the roof. Then he or she can either move up and down the stairs or remain on the roof, as he or she pleases."

When our lessons are not resolved by way of truth or in accordance with dharmic law, catastrophic disaster can occur, as we have witnessed with the many wars throughout the world. Often, as we make efforts to stop external war, we seem to avoid its source and the realization that the battle is within us. All that we seek lies within us. The ancients lived in this manner and in complete harmony with nature's laws.

The lifestyle principles of yoga and Ayurveda redefine the role of the individual. This is a process of transforming the way that we think of ourselves and how we live in a world we share with others. Are we becoming more aware of our

---

9   The source of pure existence, consciousness, and bliss. Brahman is the term for the "creative" force, which is part of the Hindu trinity of life's existence. The word "God" is the English equivalent of Brahman.

thoughts, choices, decisions, and the environment we are creating? Are we fulfilling our highest purpose in life by honoring our truth? These are some of the questions we must ask ourselves.

The four ideals or Vedic dharmas of life provide us a platform for balanced and purposeful living through objective and subjective awareness and compassion for all living beings. This is represented in one of the great mantras of the Upanishads, "Aum Shanti, Shanti, Shanti," ("Aum, Peace, Peace, Peace"). In objective awareness, we remain uninfluenced by the traditions, belief systems, and opinions of others. We remain simply observers of the world as we exercise our own reason, will, and activity, and allow the grace and flow of the Divine to guide us.

In subjective awareness, we use our relationships with people, places, and things as opportunities for inner reflection and contemplation, seeing the Divine hand behind the things we can't always understand or make sense of. This type of awareness requires greater discipline, as the mind and body must partake of the world while at same time maintaining an objective attitude.

Lastly, through compassion for all life, we realize that, as we serve, give to, and love others, we provide the same back to ourselves. Through respect for others, we recognize that the Divine and sublime shine through all souls.

In Vedic astrology (*jyotish*), there are Four Dharmas or aims and ideals that bring us into balanced living. They are: *Kama*, the emotional, devotional and affectionate aspects that nurture us as sentient beings; *Artha*, the acquisition and use of tangible, material objects for practical needs; *Dharma* itself, which gives meaning to our endeavors to live a purposeful; fulfilling life; and *Moksha,* the movement towards enlightenment. These are various aspects of a life we all need to live holistically.

Education and Action as Means of Liberation

In April 2006, I learned about a commission of scientists, academic leaders, and humanitarian activists that had created a list of the top ten issues or critical problems the world would need to face in the near future. The ten items on this list were: *democracy, disease, education, environment, food, population, poverty, water, terrorism,* and *energy.* Then a group of Nobel Peace prizewinners was polled and asked which of these issues the world should focus on so as to best eradicate current challenges. The majority answered that almost all the issues could be resolved through education and new energy systems that are aligned with the sun as the source of power.

I'm not saying that Nobel Peace laureates are the highest authority on fixing the world, especially considering that the iconic man of world peace, M.K. Gandhi, was nominated five times and never awarded the prize. To some degree, education without the proper training of the mind becomes even more dangerous than humble ignorance. However, the education I am referring to is that of mysticism, the principles that synthesize the fundamental laws uniting both science and religion. Both Eastern and Western mystical traditions are most valuable, teaching us to use yoga meditation tools to develop mastery over the nervous system and experience the spiritual dimensions of expanded consciousness. Ayurvedic teachings provide the proper education for balancing the nervous system for greater health and wellness in the physical realm.

Also, both yoga and Ayurveda enable us to exercise right action and discipline over the senses, to further us on the spiritual path, and to undertake lifestyle regimens that keep the doshas in balance in accord with nature's laws. Whether for physical or mental benefit, both wisdom and action are necessary aspects on the journey towards higher consciousness. The Bhagavad Gita extolls these two paths towards enlightenment. Krishna, the Cosmic Lord says, "O Sinless One, at the onset of creation, a twofold way of salvation was given by Me to this world: for the wise, divine union through wisdom; for the yogis, divine union through active meditation."[10]

Paramahansa Yogananda's commentary in his translation of the Gita gives insight into this profound stanza. Essentially, *Jnana Yoga*, the path of wisdom and discrimination or Samkhya, and *Karma Yoga*, the path of responsible and conscious spiritual and meditative action, "are really one twofold highway (meditative activity, and not just ordinary activity, is implicit in Krishna's reference to *Karma Yoga*.)"

The point I am trying to make is that education is not enough. We must also practice right action according to nature's laws and include active meditation. The conscious healing practices taught in Ayurveda—cooking, eating, herbs, spices, stretching poses, body oil massage, etc.—are touted to having a calming and "meditative" quality, because they require active engagement of the mind-body relationship. However, such lifestyle disciplines should also lead the practitioner to attain an active meditative seat (asana) in stillness, uniting mind (jnana), body (karma), and spirit.

---

10 From *God Talks With Arjuna: The Bhagavad Gita* by Paramahansa Yogananda (Self-Realization Fellowship, Los Angeles, Calif.) From Bhagavad Gita Chapter III, verse 3: *Sribhagavan uvaca: loke 'smin dvividha nistha pura prokta mayanagha jnanayogena samkhyanam karmayogena yoginam*

Yogananda goes on to say, "many devotees falsely imagine that a theoretical knowledge of scriptures (divine laws) without meditation will lead to ultimate freedom."[11] Over years as director of the Dancing Shiva center, I hosted many workshops on a variety of topics. I found many fixed on the intellectual side of things, repeatedly making an effort to improve their lives through attaining greater wisdom or finding some answer through astrology, but without making the effort to meditate. They remained stuck in their heads, trying to think through a way to finding peace.

A balanced lifestyle must include education and study of the Divine laws as taught in the mystical traditions, alongside the practice of active meditation. Ayurveda is the most vital and mystical education system the world can use for natural care of the body and mind and the prevention of disease. It aligns with Jnana Yoga and the Samkhya philosophy system of the 24 principles of creation to help us understand the mystery of human existence and how we might all live in harmony with nature and enjoy our planet as one global family. Greater access to the vast wisdom of yoga and Ayurveda, and education on living a responsible, active lifestyle that includes meditation, are our world's direst needs. Both yoga and Ayurveda provide us with great wisdom tools to guide us through life and achieve balance between the material and spiritual realms and the true mystical unification of science and religion.

It is the birthright of every living being to access this knowledge, the cosmic intelligence hidden behind the portals of our hearts. The teachings of yoga and Ayurveda are not limited to old books and intellectual jargon, but are the truths of our conscience and the real power of the awakened mind. These traditions teach us the importance of developing a divine relationship within ourselves, aligned with nature and her beauty. It is a new way of living that is beyond individual thinking. It is an understanding that our thoughts, words, and actions create the world we live in and influence the world around us. The sun can be symbolized as the "One" union of the transformative process of yoga and Veda. It brings rays of wisdom to our life, changing us into ideal human beings living in harmony and peace with one another and Divine Mother's natural world. All living things are chasing the sun on a quest for higher meaning and the purpose of life. May the rays of light continue to guide us, protect us, heal us, and inspire us to live in the highest place, giving our best always.

---

11   Ibid.

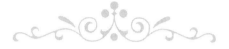

Chapter TWO

Creation and Nature

The combined study of yoga and Ayurveda is of great importance for
each discipline and for helping us understand the whole of life.
David Frawley (Author, Vedic Scholar)

Consciousness Becoming Matter

When we speak of the idea of creation, we are referring to the manifest world and the life that exists on planet earth. According to Vedic wisdom, there are three worlds of existence: the physical (including the five elements), subtle (mind), and causal (soul). The Creator of these worlds or vibratory fields remains invisible although the continuous process of the unraveling of consciousness is described in various cosmic principles *(tattvas)*.

Samkhya, one of the six Vedic philosophies, calls this journey of consciousness into matter *prakriti,* and the unmanifest state of both pure consciousness and creation is called Brahman or *purusha*. From these, we have the birth of the law of duality or *maya*.[12] One side remains silent, unseen and mysterious, and is intangible. The other is the embodiment of an all-pervasive cosmic intelligence that transmutes atoms[13] and sound into the various frequencies of the five elements of life. In this material world, we manufacture karma, create and fulfill desires, and experience the dual nature of life.

---

12   Vedantic concept, which means "illusion," also known as the "mother of the universe."
13   Consisting of a nucleus of protons and neutrons surrounded by a cloud of negatively charged electrons. The three units of the atom are bound together by an electromagnetic force that reflects the three-fold nature of existence. Protons and neutrons mimic the vibrational quality of the planetary sun and earth relationship, and the moon can be related to the negative electron cloud around the nucleus.

The world is essentially energy that has become gross matter and, depending on the quality or measure (**guna**[14]) of our thoughts, which leads to certain actions, we either become more attached or rebellious, or alternately find peace and freedom in life. The five elements, ether, air, fire, water, and earth, are the reasons for the creation of the five senses (hearing, touch, vision, taste, and smell) and the five actions of these elements correlate to speech, touch, walking, procreation, and elimination.

Study of the five great elements helps us understand the design of the body and its operations. The five elements are also composed from nature and what we experience in the living world. The qualities of each element are also very valuable in applying the common-sense practices of yoga and Ayurveda, which aim at maintaining the balance of these elements and the connection between mind and body. Essentially, the elements are forces of nature, which sustain all living organisms, operate within the daily cycle, and give distinct characteristics to the seasons.

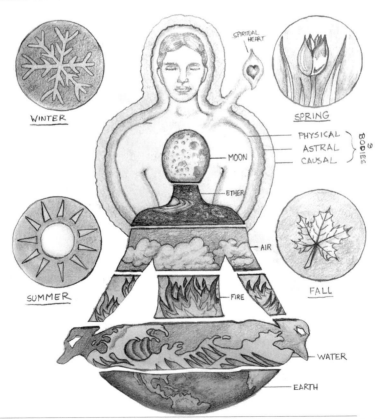

14 Three qualities of consciousness in the mind; namely *sattva* (peacefulness), *rajas* (activity), and *tamas* (lethargy).

On a mental level, the elements rule the sensory mind (*manas*). Our senses operate through the element's energy or vibratory cord, which sends signals back and forth to neurons or nerve cells in our brain. Physically, the elements govern all physiological functions. In Ayurvedic medicine, the elements function more specifically as doshas in the three main digestive organs. In Ayurveda, the five elements are simplified into the three main forces of vata (ether & air), pitta (fire), and kapha (water & earth). This approach aligns the elements with the threefold principle of the Vedic-Hindu cosmology, which originates from the sun-moon-earth relationship and extends into the popular concept of mind-body-soul.

Law of Karma

We now arrive at the law of cause and effect, which explains that for every action there is an equal reaction. Karma is based on the law of the energy of will, which encompasses understanding our minds and taking responsibility for our thoughts and speech as well as actions. All karma begins with expression of volition, or the act of exercising or acting on the energy whose source is the will or the power to initiate and manifest what we need in our lives. The same energy that causes the earth, moon, and sun to move through their respective cycles also creates a will powerful enough to send forth and fulfill desires. Every voluntary action creates a mental groove that remains etched in the ether of our mind as a patterned behavior (*samskara*), whether good and bad. For this exact reason, the spiritual path begins with purification of previous tendencies created in past lives and with developing the right attitude through good associations (*satsanga*) and lifestyle.

Karma is based on good conduct (*sadachara*) and is developed through the four virtues of purity, devotion, humility, and charity. A type of subtle purification occurs when we perform actions that consider the benefit of all. Purity must be supported with a consistent effort to live selflessly in our family life, friendships, and societal relationships. Devotion is first and foremost love for God, Goddess, and guru, and learning to see the Divine in all living things. Humility is a form of humbleness, and involves exercising effort to observe and learn from our experiences, rather than reacting, blaming, or criticizing others. When we give, we receive, and good conduct includes giving to others and practicing some type of charitable service to improve humanity.

Ayurvedic health services that also educate are a great charity, because they not only improve health, but also empower people to learn how to heal themselves. Education and empowerment are essential to reforming health care in the modern age, and the law of karma is one of the most valuable and powerful concepts in understanding and improving lifestyle quality. Understanding the law of karma improves health and well-being, because it instills the importance of personal responsibility. Every person creates their own patterns and is the architect of their destiny. Where we leave off in one life is where we begin in the next. This is the basis of rebirth and reincarnation.

With this in mind, it makes more and more sense that we take complete responsibility for our health, because only we can heal the physical body. Only greater awareness of who we really are can heal us. We must learn to reconnect the mind and body and embrace the power of the soul within us as a pure reflection of the Divine.

Karma teaches us that things do not just happen by good or bad luck. Things happen because of energy patterns set in motion days, months, years, and lifetimes before. Over many years, I have seen countless numbers of people with health issues that just suddenly arose, with no trace of a genetic family pattern, or even a health habit, that might contribute to the disorder.

Many people come to find themselves with health issues and can't seem to understand where they came from, Often times, health issues or diseases have little to do with what we are currently doing, and more to do with what we were doing in the past, during early childhood, or in a previous life. Modern medicine has no clue how many diseases originate. At best, it can list some factors, such as vitamin deficiencies, or some pathology, but the real answer is still missing.

What is the cause? It has to come back to our thoughts, words, and actions, and our relationship with nature. Any disharmony, disease, disorder, dysfunction, or neurosis must be created from some lack of accord with the elements and their natural balance. This is what makes Ayurveda such a profound healing system. It strongly considers the sources and causes of disease and disorder, whether they be environmental, psycho-spiritual, or derived from the soul or a past life.

Ultimately, real healing must include factoring in the mind and working on clearing it in order to truly heal the body. As the body and mind grow more harmonious, life becomes simpler, and we actually begin to feel peace. Peace is something we experience within, and is a product of the soul.

The law of karma and the principle of dharma, that is, duty or purpose, demonstrate that the relationship between mind and body and the guna or quality of consciousness being distributed between the two are of prime importance. The mind and body share energy pathways that distribute conscious thought waves from a place of awareness back and forth between them. Even more subtle, sub-conscious, and usually hidden waves of thought are also exchanged in this mind-body link, giving birth to many of the health issues commonly categorized as "mysterious." Such psychological patterning is difficult to deconstruct, especially when it has been deeply impressed into the mind and has been part of a lifestyle. The physical body exists to serve the mind as a vehicle for exploration, recreation, and as a temple to house the occult and Divine energies. This is precisely the view of Tantra Yoga. Today, the body has become more of a burden and an obstacle to life than a sacred sanctuary.

People try to find the easiest way to keep the physical body functioning, perpetuate its existence, and seek instant gratification for the five senses. The relationship between mind and body has been severed in recent times. This is one reason why overly stimulating yoga leads nowhere, because it supplies the same thing that we already have in our culture, constant stimulation.

Many Western schools of asana yoga and their teachings have re-constructed their approach to be more appealing to the distracted minds of our times. However, the magic of yoga lies in its simplicity and ability to slow the mind so as to help us gain greater awareness of our thought processes and patterns. In this way, the law of karma becomes an asset rather than a mysterious concept. Understanding our thoughts, words, and actions can create greater abundance in our lives and instill real wellness, not just continued cycles of destruction, pain, and suffering.

Laws of Nature

The foremost principle for living a spiritual life is ahimsa or non-harming. Vedic sages said that in order to live in harmony with nature, one must practice ahimsa in order to achieve compassion within ourselves. The greatest modern hero of ahimsa was Mahatma Gandhi, who once said "Fearlessness is requisite to spirituality. Cowards can never be moral." Fear must be uprooted in order for us to act in a moral way, and this is demonstrated through compassion, calmness, and awareness. Non-violence is not simply the absence of being violent, but is actually rooted in being fearless.

If the mind is restless like the wind, it creates an amplitude of thoughts that increase anxiety, restlessness, and, worst of all, fear. Excess thought creates ripples of disturbance in the mind,[15] which blurs the reflective quality of discerning between right and wrong, and between healthy and toxic or harming thoughts that can lead to harsh words and violent actions.

Self-preservation is the strongest instinct in all life. This is a fact in both human beings and the animal kingdom. If we can shift our mind away from fear to compassion, the practice of ahimsa will be much easier. This is easier said than done, and, later in the book, I will share with you some ways to attract these inborn qualities.

It is also important not to make practical decisions from a place of fear. In the higher ages, when animals were not threatened by attack from humans, they were able to share a common space without any fear of being harmed, and vice versa. It is all in the attitude of the mind and state of consciousness. A young monk named Swami Rama Tirtha shared instances when he would directly confront tigers and bears in the wild Himalayan foothills and stare at them directly without being attacked. Unlike in the golden ages of higher consciousness, animals today stay hidden and keep an eye out for human predators. Humanity should learn to coexist with nature and cherish life in all forms, including plants, trees, and land and sea animals, and enjoy the beautiful landscape of this Divine soil we call earth.

Emotionally, fear of being hurt, exposed, or unsettled produces anger. Anger is simply an emotional defense mechanism created to avoid the experience of feeling fear. It is through anger that retaliation or violence arises. The sense of being separate from humanity and other living things is said to be the inner root of violence. This idea of embracing a unified consciousness comes from the ancient wisdom of Non-Dual (*Advaita*) Vedanta. When we support dualistic thinking, we separate ourselves from the essence of our existence.

Societies, families, and our circle of friends breed certain beliefs that mold our attitudes. If we are conditioned to believe we are separate, better, or above others, this attitude can lead to violence. It justifies hurting others because they are different, "not me." On the other hand, when we embrace the observer in us and recognize that consciousness exists in all life, then we understand that when we hurt another, we are injuring ourselves.

A broken consciousness leads to broken bones and broken hearts. To repair a separated awareness, one should spend more time in nature, giving the mind space to breathe and witness the beauty of the environment. Natural living

---

15   This powerful point is found in the second of Patanjali's *Ashtanga Yoga Sutras* 1:2, which says yoga is the calming or fixing (*nirodha*) of the activities and fluctuations (*vrittis*) of the mind (*chitta*).

can be a beginner's form of meditation and a powerful means for slowing the mind and creating more mindfulness. This is not an intellectual process, but one of understanding our feelings, which can lead us toward attaining more insight into the nature of our existence.

> *The very best method of spreading the Vedantic Philosophy is to live it. There is no other royal road. –Swami Rama Tirtha*

Truth (*satya*) is another pillar of life, with the entire universe resting upon it. In the yoga teachings of the sage Patanjali, truth is a foundation principle for beginning the practice of yoga. This includes the practical concept of speaking your truth unless it is hurtful to others. In that case, you do not lie, but you withhold the truth. As the great yogi Baba Hari Dass once said, "Silence speaks." This was a motto he lived by, literally.

Truth might be considered relying on what is tangible or that which is experienced through the senses. My point is that truth is born of faith and trusting that the Divine hand of higher consciousness is guiding us. When we are living our truth, we are in our dharma and our individual consciousness abides in accordance with natural laws. The beauty of the Vedanta tradition is that it always affirms there is one truth, although there are many paths to reaching it and ways of living and feeling it.

The word "God" is the Judeo-Christian term for what in Hinduism is called Brahman, the creator of our world and the one truth of infinite intelligence in the field of consciousness. Whatever the term is does not matter so much as that we are listening to our conscience. Divine intelligence guides us through our awareness, and often tells us whether we are living or speaking in truth. Lack of truth reflects a fragmentation of our individual thinking from the source of wisdom and eternal realm of spirit. Our true spirit is a part of the Divine. Truth allows us to make choices between what is right and wrong, and how we, as distinct beings, are attracted to the Divine.

Cycles of Time and Space

All creation is based on cycles, various rhythms that are consistently changing and produce what humanity calls *evolution*. Understanding the grander cycles of the *sun, moon, and earth* can help bring us into living a practical and natural lifestyle. It is the relationship between these three planets that gives rise to the creation of the mind-body and soul. The law of karma exercises its force through the planetary movements we witness in the sky. These cyclical patterns also manage the five elements, ether, air, fire, water, and earth, which make up creation.

Three main cycles have the greatest influence on life and the relationship of humanity and nature. The first is the relationship the moon shares with the earth, as it orbits the earth in 27.32, rounded to 28, days. It imposes the strongest energy of any planet, as it is the closest to the earth. The earth-moon relationship is a binary system and, of all the major planets, they share the strongest relationship with each other. The moon is like a partner to the earth as it accompanies it in rotating around the sun in an approximately 365-day period.

In Vedic astrology, the moon's many moods within this 27-day cycle are known as *Nakshatras*. These qualities represent the main indicators determining a person's personality, temperament, and overall psychology. The moon affects the rise and fall of sea levels with respect to land, because of its magnetic attraction to the earth. Similarly, this bond can be compared to the magnetic and almost intuitive attraction a mother shares with her children. Each day, there are two high tides and two low tides, because the earth is rotating while the moon is orbiting around it. These varying degrees of tides are known as spring and neap. The strongest gravitational forces occur when the *sun, moon, and earth* are aligned, and this is called spring. When the three planets are not in alignment, in quarter phases of the moon, the tides are neutralized, and this is called neap.

Women's menstrual cycles are mimicked in these various cycles or phases of the moon. As Christiane Northrup, MD, beautifully states in her book, *Women's Bodies, Women's Wisdom*, "The macrocosmic cycles of nature, the waxing and waning, the ebb and flow of the tides and the changes of the seasons, are reflected on a smaller scale in the menstrual cycle of the individual female body. The monthly ripening of an egg and subsequent pregnancy or release of menstrual blood mirror the process of creation as it occurs not only in nature, unconsciously, but in human endeavor. In many cultures, the menstrual cycle has been viewed as sacred."

The moon also symbolizes the quality of romance for its capacity to enhance fertility and ovulation, which naturally attracts men, and can be likened to the magnetic current between the moon and the earth. Dr. Northrup goes on to say, "Specifically, the moon and tides interact with the electromagnetic fields of our bodies, subsequently affecting our internal physiological processes." In a way, the moon is the mother of nature and all humanity, who ebb and flow with her cycle. The moon is like our subtle or intuitive mind, like a mother's mind that feels everything. The moon's energy is what connects us to nature and each other.

The moon can probably be considered the most spiritual planet, because it provides us with the capacity to love and attract everything we need to fulfill our greatest desires. The moon's sacred energy in ancient India was called *soma* for its nectar-like quality of restoring and replenishing us mentally, physically, and emotionally if we are attuned with its cycle. Our relationship with the moon cannot be ignored if we want to evolve as a species. In order for our consciousness to expand, we must develop a new lifestyle that intimately embraces the moon. The month represents a completion of the moon's very unique cycle and its very distinct and dynamic qualities.

The second very influential, somewhat slower cycle is the earth-moon's orbit around the sun, which creates the twelve months or moons of the zodiac. Within this twelvefold division of the zodiac, we have the four major seasons. The seasons can be looked at as phases, with winter being destructive, the dark season when all things die, so to speak. Summer is when all things live, and spring and fall are transitional phases that shift us out of one season or mood and guide us towards transformation.

I think that we all can recall many of life's experiences by the time or season they occurred. Seasons also seem to instill in us a particular feeling that influences our behavior, the choices we make, and our attitudes. When we begin a new year, we create resolutions and aspirations, and therefore each new year represents another sacred period in our lives. When we reflect, we often look back to the overall accomplishments and events of years past and categorize them as either positive or negative experiences.

This is another example of how our micro-life experiences are measured against the macro-movements of the sun-moon-earth relationship. The twelve months of the calendar year allow us to experience the seven rays of light distributed from the galactic sun (*vishnunabhi*), this being the center of the creative force (Brahma) that produces life on the planet earth. The twelve months are like a living replica of the twelve constellations of the zodiac.

I follow David Frawley's[16] view that the zodiac is oriented to this galactic center, through the sign of Sagittarius, because in the sidereal zodiac it is located

---

16   Vedic scholar, also known as Pandit Vamadeva Shastri , one of the foremost authors on Vedic literature, including works in yoga, Tantra, Ayurveda, jyotish and Indic cultural history. He is internationally recognized.. I was greatly influenced by his teachings and studied closely with him for many years.

at the beginning of this constellation. My point is that the planet earth and its consort the moon maintain a very consistent relationship with the creative force within the galactic center. I feel that we as human beings inherit this creative energy. It inspires us and keeps us searching for truth and the purpose of life. It is this magnetic force that is constantly pulling us to find our way back to the pure source of consciousness.

The third cycle is little-known and has long been a great mystery in the field of astronomy and astrology. This is the cycle of the sun. There is much evidence that the ancients, like the Vedic Indians, Egyptians, Greeks, and Mayans, knew of the sun's binary cycle. It seems that the sun's celestial motion had been forgotten, like the earth's spinning, which creates the 24-hour day, and its orbiting motion, which creates the 365-day year, had also been forgotten. To this day, modern humanity does not have an acceptable measure for the sun's repeating cycle of time relative to the stars. In other words, we have not had a clear and consistent view of how to measure the sun's cycle like the days, months, and years of the earth and moon, which allow us to create a measure of time in our lives. One view is that this partly has to do with the current level of collective consciousness on the earth. Modern calendars have lost their connection to larger celestial motion. This means that the count of days of the year will continue forever, with no end.

In some ways, this may not seem important to know, because it obviously is quite a long cycle, and would seem to have little relevance to our short lifespans of 100 years or less. On the contrary, however, it could help humanity understand that we live in accordance with a grander force that influences all aspects of life. Most particularly, knowledge of such a cycle could empower humanity to live with greater detachment (*vairgya*) to the ever-changing nature of life.

This long cycle is called the Precession of the Equinoxes. It is the slow shifting of the equinoxes[17] in relationship to the fixed stars. Currently, at a rate of about 50 arc-seconds per year, it takes about 26,000 years to precess or move backwards through the twelve signs of the zodiac. Currently, we are in the sign of Pisces.

In 1894, Mahavatar Babaji, the immortal siddha yogi, commissioned Swami Sri Yukteswar, Paramahansa Yogananda's guru, to reveal the wisdom of the yugas,[18] so as to explain the reasons for the loss of human intelligence and compassion, and to anchor the rebirth of Vedic astrology in the modern era. One obvious reason that Babaji asked Sri Yukteswar to write such a book was

---

17 Meaning "equal night," the two days of the year, the first day of spring, the vernal equinox, and the first day of fall, the autumnal equinox, when day and night or of equal length.

18 Cycles or stages of human consciousness that shift over a 24,000-year period.

because he was both an astrologer and had attained self-realization or enlightenment. There had also been obvious errors made by astrologers and scholars in the current age that placed the current period (*yuga*) in a very long dark cycle known as Kali Yuga.

If the idea of living in such a 432,000-year long, dismal cycle had prevailed for much longer, it would have precipitated mankind into even greater self-destruction, loss of purpose, and hopelessness, further delaying human evolution. The timing of Sri Yuktewar's scripture, titled *The Holy Science,* coincides with current technological developments, globalization, and the propagation of the Vedic sciences of yoga, Ayurveda, and jyotish in all parts of the world.

Not only did Sri Yukteswar introduce the yuga concept to the western world, but he corrected the mistake made about the actual age we are currently in by stating that the global shift towards higher consciousness took place at 500 AD, and then more prominently in 1700, with the advent of the electrical and atomic energies. This was critical to hastening humanity's spiritual evolution. The yuga system was probably first introduced to the western world through Yogananda's famous *Autobiography of a Yogi*, published in 1946. These four periods of time actually reflect stages of development in human consciousness, each being one-quarter of mankind's capacity for conscious awareness.

These cycles are depicted in an arc of rising and falling ages. In 500 AD, we began the ascent upwards from the lowest point in human history. If we look at the quality of life and the historical events during these times, it seems to make sense that "Kali" predisposed the ignorance or darkness displayed by most of humanity through acts of brutality, conquest, and the urge to rediscover the geographical world.

Keep in mind that Christopher Columbus, proposing that the world was flat, sailed off to the Americas to make the Taino "Indians" prisoners, raping and eventually killing them. This brutality was typical of the Western world and Spain, and demonstrates the mentality and behavior of the 1400s.

The *Kali Yuga* is 1,200 years in duration. The next yuga cycle is the *Dwapara,* and is the electrical age that began in the year 1700. At that time, we began the first major shift towards greater interest in subtle or spiritual concepts, although residual materialistic mental qualities still exist today. On the positive side, it is refreshing to see how prevalent health, wellness, and spirituality have become with the expansion of Vedic traditions from India, reaching all continents across the globe.

The third cycle, *Treta Yuga*, will bring greater advancement and efficiency in lifestyle and mental powers such as telepathy. This yuga cycle will begin in the year 4099 and last for 3,600 years. This will eventually lead us into the *Satya* period, or age of truth and highest level of consciousness, where collective human consciousness will be double what it is now. Sri Yukteswar stated that the total yuga cycle has a duration of 24,000 years, the time it takes for the sun to orbit its partner star, and for the Precession of the Equinoxes to complete the cycle through the twelve constellations.

Today, with some Kali Yuga residual consciousness still in the ether, astronomers and astrologers have calculated a current rate of precession of 50 arc-seconds per year. This produces a Maha Yuga cycle of 26,000 years, thereby asserting that Sri Yukteswar's teachings were incorrect. The reason why I think it is vital to understand these cycles is based in the idea Sri Yukteswar introduced in 1894 in his book *The Holy Science*, which is that human cycles are not as much tied to the Precession of the Equinoxes, but more to the forgotten cosmic motion our sun shares with another star. He was endorsing the importance of "relationship" and the capacity we have as humans to heal ourselves by cultivating a relationship with the Divine. This is the "forgotten cosmic motion." It is about cultivating a new living relationship with the Divine through the unseen or formless. Nature in the form of trees, water, animals, etc., can be a powerful vehicle for shifting our awareness into the subtler domain of spirit.

Meditating on the thought-free state of consciousness was also one of the central tenants of Sri Yukteswar's guru Lahiri Mahasaya's teachings. What he extolled was one of the key themes of the Bhagavad Gita. In brief, in holding to the state of eternal consciousness, the pure tranquility of God exists where the sun, moon, and earth are all dissolved in the light of eternity. This establishes my key point in this book, that all life is based on a cyclical relationship that shifts through various periods of energy or consciousness. This binary cycle between the sun and some distant star is the basis for a balanced life as proclaimed in the dharmic yoga system, in Ayurveda's concept of spirit and nature, and even in modern mind-body medicine.

What we have forgotten is that the things of this world are not separate from some grander force. Albert Einstein once said, "The Ancients knew something, which we seem to have forgotten." The trend of an accelerating rate of precession is clearly evident in the measurements taken in the last hundred years. As the sun began its return from the furthest point from its companion star in 500 AD, there has been an increase in consciousness on the planet. Fortunately, there has been much research done to bring greater validity to the scientific points made by Sri Yukteswar on the complex subject of astrology.[19] Interestingly, if we take the average rate of the Precession of the Equinoxes from its slowest to fastest points, we get a 24,000 year period. Therefore the rate of precession is a variable speed and also depends on what Sri Yukteswar says: "The Sun also has another motion by which it revolves round a grand center called Vishnunabhi...the universal magnetism...When the Sun in its revolution round its dual comes to the place nearest to the grand center... (when the Autumnal Equinox comes to the first point of Aries)....the mental virtue, becomes so much developed that man can easily comprehend all, even the mysteries of Spirit."[20]

24,000 YEAR YUGA CYCLE
The rise and fall of consciousness on planet Earth

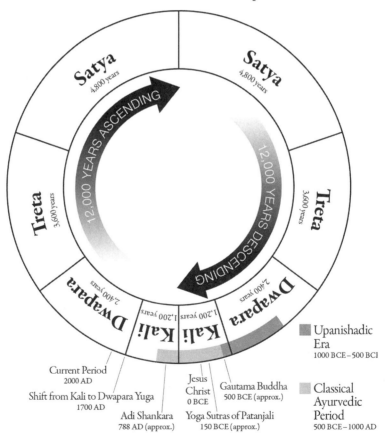

19 I have found the most profound and concise explanations of these astrological concepts in Walter Cruttenden's remarkable *Lost Star of Myth and Time.*

20 From *The Holy Science* by Sri Yukteswar (Self-Realization Fellowship, Los Angeles).

The seven rays of light emitted from the seven major planets account for the seven chakras that bring us into physical existence and support the five great elements (*pancha maha bhutas*) of which they are created. Characteristics of the sun-moon-earth cycles reflect different aspects of our being. The earth-moon binary system influences physiology, procreative energy, and the entire emotional body in general. The earth-moon orbit around the sun influences the mind and enhances its reflective qualities. When we plan ahead for the coming new year, it encourages us to take up a perspective and fosters an opportunity for introspection and expansion of our thinking through creative visualization.

The Sun's binary relationship penetrates to the deepest level of our being, that of the soul. Over the 24,000-year big-clock cycle, the consciousness of souls taking embodiment fluctuates, with higher awareness existing in the golden (*satya*) and silver (*Treta Yuga*) ages, and lower forms of consciousness taking birth in the lower ages. The very primitive law of energy, where *like attracts like*, applies here. In the lower ages like the bronze (*dwapara*) and iron (*kali*), humanity has little regard for nature and ecology, as we have seen in recent times. Simply put, how we behave internally is reflected externally.

I hope we can all gain some insight into life's higher purpose through the sacred sun, moon, and earth relationship. My point is that they are directly linked to influence human behavior, the attraction we share with one another, and the capacity humans have to enjoy the grandeur of impermanent existence. The fact is the living world has inherited the energetic coding of the sun-moon-earth paradigm, which appears to mankind as hidden and mysterious.

The scriptures of the great yogis, sages, and saints claim that looking within and spiritual experience can solve this enigma. The body (earth) merges into the mind (moon) and transcends into the soul (sun) through the process we call "yoga." The first requirement is balancing the doshas of the physical body. Then, through the development of mind-body synergy, the elements consolidate, with earth moving into water, water into fire, fire into air, and air expanding into space. This psycho-spiritual process requires a shifting of consciousness, from an attitude of being self-centered into a self-less awareness.

In speaking of the gunas or qualities of the mind, it is said that, by taking action (*rajas*), we exercise the will power to overcome inertia (*tamas*) or patterns of unconscious behavior, and then aspire to feel the sublime state of perennial calmness, gratitude, and stillness (*sattva*). The final step towards liberation (*moksha*) entails going beyond the mind stuff (*chitta*) to discover our existence in an ever-deepening stillness that reveals the Soul beyond name and fame, brand, or form. This is the true yoga!

As we move through life, we can find deeper ways to experience our relationship with the seasons and the longer cycle of life in one particular physical body. The magnetic pull between the earth and moon, which they share with the sun, gives birth to the power of attraction we experience in our lives. It is this natural force that keeps us relating to things outside ourselves, as we continue to deal with a perpetual yearning for greater understanding and fulfillment from life as we know it.

On the most subtle level, the law of karma manages the five elements through planetary forces and the relationship of the seven major planets with one another. Simply put, the 24-hour clock is like a miniature yuga cycle, with the sun appearing, or rising, and disappearing, or setting, from the sky.

The twelve-month calendar year takes us through a miniature version of the twelve constellations to enhance our reflective qualities. The 28 lunar days are the creative cycle of activity, fertility, and sensual expression. These planetary cycles explain the nature of relationship in our lives. Understanding these cycles and principles allows us to use them in a practical manner to enhance our connection to broader aspects of creation. They help us cultivate a more unified field of consciousness. Education can help us think outside of our little lives for a moment. We may realize there is an expansive universe we are not separate from, but are actually an integral part of. This is the very nature of our existence.

A Renaissance of the Vedic Era

There is no doubt that if we stand back and take a perspective on the entire world process in recent times, we can all agree that the world is becoming smaller and smaller. Technology has had a substantial impact on global communications and continues to advance, making everything faster and bringing East and West in closer contact each day. One thing we often hear is the idea of history repeating itself. As we look back in history, we discover new things and ideas that perhaps existed before, but in a different way. The calendar date of human existence gets pushed back ever further.

Traces of the ancient Vedic tradition clearly exist today and we could in fact say the tradition is undergoing a renaissance. But is this simply because history is just repeating itself coincidentally? Or is there some other reason? In recent years, yoga has become a globally recognized term, mostly understood in its physical aspects. This is even somewhat the case in India, where Hatha

Yoga only represents a small but popular portion of the Vedic religion, which remains enmeshed in festivals, rituals, and special ceremonies called *pujas*, all of which fall under the umbrella of an eternal tradition.

Most Americans imagine that India, like America, is filled with yoga centers, and may even contain a broader collective of yoga brands than we see here in the West. Not at all! Yoga is virtually unseen with regards to asana, and remains secluded in ashrams, some elementary schools, and universities. Auspicious planetary alignments elicit large celebratory gatherings called Kumbh Mela, where yogis from all over assemble at different places in northern India.

What you certainly will not find in India are the same brand names of yoga representing the styles we practice in the Western world. These yoga "styles" are essentially products of America and the culture of consumerism that thrives on spending, advertising, and branding. The truth is that all this physical yoga comes under the branch of Hatha Yoga. The only good thing these "names" or "brands" do for yoga is to distinguish the particular influence of a specific teacher or guru.

The term "hatha" is derived from the Sanskrit terms "ha" and "tha," which mean "sun" and "moon" This implies a system centered on balancing these energies in the body and mind. To clarify, over ninety percent of what you find in commercialized yoga places no emphasis on and has no structure or capacity to balance the left and right energy channels in the body.

So, where does that leave this approach? Well, the answer is nowhere, except exhausted, stretched out, and with a sweaty body. So, under the yoga asana umbrella, we could create two types of path. One is the fitness or externalized, stretch-and-sweat yoga. The other is the system of Hatha Yoga that includes asanas or postures held for proper lengths of time, pranayama or breathing techniques, *bandhas* or energy locks, and *mudras* or subtle gestures using the body, hands and other body parts. All these are used as preparation for purifying the body of imbalances from the doshas to enhance the practice of meditation.

It seems that many paths now exist for yoga, and participation in both paths is simultaneously increasing around the world. It is obvious that postural, asana, or Hatha Yoga is gaining more momentum each year, with magazines and newsletters pumping out articles boasting about yoga's therapeutic value in relieving stress, increasing flexibility, and enhancing athletic performance. Some professional sports organizations now include yoga asana as part of their training camps. Elementary and high schools, and even universities, are now offering classes. Privately owned yoga centers can be found in every major city across the globe, and now suburbs and rural towns in the United States also have yoga asana centers.

Sadly, on occasion, some yoga guru or asana teacher is mentioned in a sex scandal that shocks the community and hurts the greater yoga movement. But this has existed as long as yoga has been in the West,[21] for the past 120 years or so. Part of the injustice is owing to the media, which gains revenue through propaganda. The other has to do with the perils of practicing yoga's ancient wisdom in societies that seek materialistic aggrandizement.

The second side of yoga is more religious and spiritual. It silently continues growing through lineage-based organizations that came from India to expand their outreach in the West. Today, these organizations have international members and affiliations and are focused mostly on the higher purpose of yoga or the dharma of finding happiness and creating peace among societies, teaching us how to live a balanced life as we strive towards enlightenment. Typically, these organizations, such as the Art of Living Foundation, the Sivananda Yoga Centers, the Self-Realization Fellowship, Integral Yoga, Patanjali Yogapeeth, and many others, choose a name that represents their approach and distinguishes it in the context of the broader yoga teaching as being led by a living guru or an initiated representative of the lineage.

Each of these lineages generally adheres to one or several traditional yoga forms. Some follow a devotional, Bhakti Yoga approach, which includes such practices as mantra and music or kirtan. Other organizations are more focused on meditation or Raja Yoga, and teach specific forms of stilling the mind and approaching the Divine. Others provide a simple integral approach to yoga, wellness, and lifestyle that embraces physical asana yoga, breathing, mantra, and meditation.

Regardless of the path, all of these traditional India-based organizations embrace the path of Karma Yoga and venerate the practice of selfless service to humanity *(seva)*. They operate as non-profit organizations and provide extensive community services, build hospitals, offer medical healing camps, and create food drives to feed the poor. They persistently find new ways to promote the Vedic wisdom or Jnana Yoga of the higher ages through public-speaking tours, humble satsangas or spiritual gatherings, and annual conferences. In lineage-based yoga organizations, the leader or guru does not say, "Follow me." Rather, devotee-students are encouraged to follow the dharma or teachings,

---

21   See Robert Love's book on Dr. Pierre Bernard, *The Great OOM: The Improbable Birth of Yoga in America.*

their tenants and principles, so that we can recognize that this wisdom is all born of universal law. In other words, these teachers do not lay claim to being special beings who possess supernatural powers and the ability to entice followers to believe in them.

There are some current concerns about the divisiveness within yoga and its obsession with physicality. I have an example I'd like to share about this important point. There are perils to placing too much attention on the body. My spiritual counselor of many years once cautioned me about the use of asana. Brother Bhaktananda was one of Yoganandas early disicples and I sat with him regularly for a period of almost ten years.

One afternoon he shared the following with me: "Guruji[22] said we must be careful with Hatha Yoga, because when we do too much of it, placing much attention on the body, we become associated with the physical form and attached to it." I continued to listen very humbly as his cosmic blue eyes illuminated my intellect. "Master taught the system of energization[23] as a higher form of mind-body connection that goes beyond the senses and prepares you for meditation." In short, the clear message was to use a limited amount of yoga asana. The higher purpose of yoga is to transcend the senses and draw the consciousness inward, beyond body identification. The approach to asana I am presenting in this book reflects this higher intention set out by the great yogis of India. The asanas become vehicles to distribute the prana throughout the body and eventually transcend beyond it.

In this regard, there are a few points I have learned that may potentially bridge the gap and bring these two paths together. One is that yoga has always been first and foremost practiced as an entire lifestyle founded on ethical and moral principles known as *yama* and *niyama,* as described in the classical Yoga Sutras of Patanjali. Integrating such principles as non-violence, truthfulness, non-stealing, and surrender to the Divine into yoga asana centers can give them a proper backbone to rest on, a foundation to promote lifestyle change.

22 Paramahansa Yogananda was often referred to "Guruji" or "Master," but never because of the wisdom or powers he attained. He often stated the importance of following a guru or "preceptor," one who acts as a conduit of Divine energy, wisdom, and sublime qualities. The suffix "ji" is commonly added to express endearment.

23 *Energization* is a specialized series of exercises that integrates tensing and releasing of muscles along with deeply focused concentration to promote the balance of life-force energy or prana throughout the body. The concept of tensing muscles as a bridge to the mind also seems to have influenced the eighty-four asanas referred to in Hatha Yoga texts. Paramahamsa Yogananda formulated this mind-body-muscle tensing approach at his first school in India, which influenced his brother Bishnu Ghosh, Buddha Bose, and others, during his pre-America years in the north-eastern states of Bengal and Bihar, India.

The other consideration is that asana can also be used as a preparation for meditation, not such a bad idea considering that this is its original intention. Ending asana classes with meditation, or even including meditation as a separate class offering, can elevate asana's virtues. Asana or Hatha Yoga is a more recent expression of a more ancient Vedic Yoga, which corresponds to a three-fold approach of Mantra Yoga as the power of speech or *vak*, Prana Yoga, connected to the breath and the atmosphere, and Dhyana Yoga, which relates to the mind, meditation, and heaven. However, there are traces of asana being used during early Vedic periods. A Vedic type of yoga is certainly less physical but represents aspects of yoga that can be practiced in either ritualistic arrangements or find more practical expressions in our daily lives.

These three forms of yoga also relate to the three bodies, the physical, astral or pranic, and causal or soul. While asana is a great system for the physical body, its tissues or dhatus, and systemic balance, it does not penetrate into the more subtle aspects of our existence. The new age of technology has blessed the world with the disbursement of Vedic wisdom throughout the world, whether it be a physical practice at a yoga center, or as part of a lineage-based yoga organization. We have much to choose from and little excuse for not creating more peace and harmony in our lives.

Chapter THREE

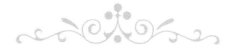

The Birth of Nature's Wisdom

Mind, self and body, these three make a tripod on which the living word stands.
That (living body) is itself Purusha (fully conscious being),
sentient and is where this Veda (wisdom) Ayurveda can be found.
For him alone, this Veda is brought to light.
Charaka Samhita Sutrasthana 1.46-47

Nature's Lifestyle

Ayurveda is a wisdom-based tradition that integrates scientific principles, derived from the five elements, into a practical living dynamic. Ayurveda is an integral part of the Vedic tradition of India, and many of its principles are woven into the culture. Its concepts have been embedded into this vast culture for millennia. As a medical system, it focuses mainly on issues related to the physical body, and emphasizes a synchronistic relationship with nature, the elements, the seasons, and their fluctuating qualities.

While Ayurveda, like its counterpart, yoga, recognizes the five elements taught in Samkhya philosophy, it also acknowledges a three-fold aspect of existence, which is manifested in the functionality of the human body. It is from this perspective that the tri-dosha system developed.

Other forces, such as the sun and life-force or prana, underlie the elements and are primarily responsible for their function. Prana is not part of our consciousness and remains inert without awareness, although it is linked to it. Our mental states influence our prana, and shape our karma, as influenced by our minds. The functionality of the doshas is the last in the chain, along with prana karma, to be affected by the mind.

It is important to understand that prana enters the body at birth and it leaves it at death. Management of prana and its fluctuations is one of the key concepts of yoga, both spiritually and therapeutically. This concept is also important in Ayurveda. It is understood that balancing vata depends on working with prana and the mind. As our life follows in accordance with natural law, we can develop a more balanced state. Ayurvedic wisdom is based on our capacity to realize that the prana that sustains your physical body and influences the nature of our minds is also the prana that provides cosmic vitality and sustains the entire universe. In other words, there is a direct link between the individual self and the cosmos.

It may seem that Ayurveda, being an ancient teaching with profound connections to the elements and cosmic forces of nature, is very far from the idea of living simply. We might, however, consider that "simple living," as a collective and broad principle in Vedic teaching, is a metaphor for the deeper relationship we share with the true nature of existence. It is simple in the sense that we are removing extra layers of thought from the mind. This allows us to enjoy the qualities of the soul.

What defines a "simple" way of living is when one adheres to natural laws and does not transgress them. It is essentially the truth of living in alignment with your inner conscience. How righteous can a law be that constricts a person to a specific standard of living that is fabricated, rigid, and based on generic societal conditioning and historical events? Each person must adjust their life according to their own consciousness.

Ayurveda is wisdom that is based on scientific principles extracted from the universal laws that govern this planet. As a vast and broad system of practical principles, its basis is aligning the physical spirit being with nature, as represented in the cycles of the sun, moon, and earth. Life is made simple when we adhere and surrender. Its complexity lies mainly in the denial or ignorance of our true self. When we embrace our divinity, we are practicing yoga in its purest essence. The separation of the soul from nature fractures the individual from the very core of being.

When I was first introduced to Ayurvedic practice, I remember realizing it was all about the relationship I was having with that practice and the task at hand. In my particular situation, it was about learning that mild spices and sweet-tasting foods balanced my constitution during the summertime. I realized that this required a conscious understanding of what I was doing and why it was beneficial. I had to feel that what I was doing made sense to my constitution and where I was at in that time of my life. I needed to know that I was not taking herbs and changing my diet just for my body, but that this was something for my whole being to digest.

Ayurveda's Three Energies

According to the science of Ayurveda there are three major forces or elements that constitute the entire body-mind complex. These are known as doshas, and they are vata, pitta, and kapha. These are derived from the five great elements, but reflect a simplified view that combines the five elements into three main forces.

Ayurveda follows the practical teachings of the Samkhya philosophy as set forth in Ishwara Krishna's *Samkhya Karika*, Samkhya literally means "to enumerate." Its twenty-four principles are called tattvas and provide a structure that explains the mystery of the world and human existence. They are the building blocks that explain the universe as it transforms us into living, individual human beings.

The last five of these twenty-four cosmic principles are called the *pancha maha bhutas* or five great elements. The five elements are earth, water, fire, air and ether. All are derived from ether—space and sound—itself. Three of the five great elements are classified as the main energetic forces or doshas. Vata relates to the ether and air combination; pitta relates mostly to fire; and kapha relates to the water and earth combination. A dosha is simply the negative aspect of the element, which has the capacity for creating disease when the three are not kept in balance. When the doshas are in balance, their effects are neutralized.

Ayurvedic Dosha	Element	Force in Nature	Planet	Life
Vata	Air	Wind	Moon	Mind
Pitta	Fire	Sunlight	Sun	Soul
Kapha	Water	Rain	Earth	Body

Ayurveda is a science of laws representative of mother nature herself. Ayurveda classifies the function of the different bodily organs and tissues according to the elements. The doshas have specific anatomical sites where they tend to accumulate and create complications for the body and mind. Yoga in a therapeutic context can only be effectively practiced on an Ayurvedic basis. Ayurveda gives yoga a therapeutic capacity, and a measure of accuracy and adaptability that the Western medical system cannot provide.

The purpose of Ayurveda is to teach us that we are not separate from nature, but that we are nature herself. Nature is the womb of all living things, and separation from her energies creates disharmonies in life. Nature reflects an ever-changing process of transformation that mirrors our own being. Various times of day and seasons influence the choices we make and ultimately the way we live our lives.

Ayurveda and yoga teach us that the sun is the father of our universe and gives life to all in the form of conception, direction, inspiration, and the will to live. The moon is the energy of the mother, which nurtures us and brings us the love that sustains all life. Both the sun and moon are major concepts in the Hatha[24] Yoga tradition, as they represent the two aspects of our being, the masculine and feminine.

Traditionally, Kapila was the founder of the Samkhya system and Hiranyagarbha of the yoga tradition, and both are related to the sun as Brahma, the creative force of the universe. Krishna himself gives credit to Hiranyagarbha as the original source of knowledge, beautifully expressed through Samkhya philosophy.

The intention of Ayurveda is to teach us how we can maintain a balance of the doshas, so that with yoga we raise the energies of the sun and moon as the unified force of prana. What this unified force equates to, practically speaking, is an ability to access an aspect of the mind that sustains a tremendous equanimity, regardless of the external situation or condition. The balancing of these energies is not for the mere attainment of occult powers, but to better enjoy this world without becoming entangled in its affairs. This should be the primary intention of a yoga practice, as attaining this energy balance is requisite to the higher aspects of yoga practice, such as concentration and meditation.

Ayurveda is the solution for a world enslaved by physical limitations. The physical world is of a dual nature: as we have day, so there is night; as we have positive, we have negative; and as we have male, we have female. Ayurvedic principles can guide us to find balance among these dualities. The mystical power of yoga also comes in its ability to bring balance to these two aspects, which gives us a unified vision of the world and the universe that sustains it. The highest potential for harnessing these forces comes in two forms, the first

---

24   Hatha is a sub-branch of the broader yoga system and has an association with Tantrism. It has a dual personification, one that uses the body in occult gestures, and the other that involves rejuvenative (*rasayana*) healing, which restores us during the dark ages of the Kali and Dwapara yugas. Its deeper esoteric meaning is represented by its two syllables *ha* and *tha*, the sun (Surya) and moon (Chandra) respectively. The clear intention of Hatha Yoga is balancing the energies of reason and feeling. In India, these aspects are commonly symbolized as Shiva and Shakti.

of which is the practice of *pranayama* or breath control. Various breathing exercises are one of the central tenets of the yoga system.

Pranayama in an Ayurvedic context is a practical means for balancing the element of air or vata dosha. This teaching of energy mastery is strongly present in the great yogic scriptures, the Bhagavad Gita and Patanjali's *Ashtanga Yoga Sutras*. Controlling the mind, as taught in Raja Yoga, can be equated to the control or balance of vata in Ayurveda.

Secondly, Ayurveda looks to a positive, healthy, and natural environment to balance one's prana. Healthy living (*vihara chikitsa*) consists of various principles that, in accordance with a natural, daily, and seasonal, lifestyle, produce a therapeutic effect on the mind-body relationship. Natural lifestyle allows us to purify the senses.

Ayurveda also considers subtle energies (*tanmatra chikitsa*) to play an important role in refining the balance and quality of the mind. Such therapies include sound, mantra, and gem stones (*marma*), all of which act as agents for moving prana. Power over prana does not come from the independent practice of pranayama, but is attained when combined with the yoga asanas or postures and relaxation techniques (*pratyahara*) described in the integral Raja Yoga system and the "how to live" principles of Ayurveda, which complement one another. Swami Sivananda of Rishikesh, India, was among the most influential teachers of the integral approach to yoga, and his lineage has been propagating yoga and Ayurvedic teachings for the last century. Paramahansa Yogananda coined the term "how to live" as an integral approach certain to uplift human consciousness and improve the quality of life.

Constitution and Imbalance: A Common Confusion

The two main aspects of identifying how the elements create our physical body and how they fluctuate as we move about on our life journey are called prakriti and vikriti. Both are the key factors in how we should approach our yoga sadhana, live a balanced lifestyle, and integrate clinical treatments and protocols to achieve a harmonious body-mind relationship.

Prakriti is your distinct mind-body type or constitution. It is partially influenced by one's karma from prior lives, as well as by parental genes and one's astrological sign. All these factors play roles in determining the mind-body type one is born into in this life. Also, a mother's action during the three trimesters of pregnancy and at time of birth, including her relationship with her partner or husband, diet, and lifestyle, all influence the newborn's constitution physically and psychologically.

Prakriti also refers to nature and is a term used to describe the creative capacity of Divine intelligence. For this reason, we refer to Nature as motherly. This wisdom was expressed in sacred Indian Samkhya philosophy and represents the core principles influencing the scientific view of Ayurveda.

When the term prakriti is used to describe a mind-body type, it infers which aspects of creation's five elements are most predominant in us. It identifies which elements exist in the greatest abundance in the operation of our body and mind. This does not suggest that certain elements are absent in us. It simply implies, as Charaka[25] says, "All mind-body types (constitutions) are always prone to some imbalance (due to a predominance of one or two doshas), and therefore the body cannot enjoy total health or balance." This gives rise to the secondary factor of vikriti or imbalance that we are all prone to.

Vikriti is evident in the fact that no two bodies are exactly alike. The timing of each birth is different, planetary positions are constantly changing, and so the elements change like weather and the seasons. The body is an ever-fluctuating entity that is not meant to have perfect balance. It is an illusion to think this is attainable and it would be a poor intention to set this as a measure for health and wellness. The precise moment of conception (*janma*) is when the prakriti is determined. As the sperm and the egg unite (*samyoga*), a particular genetic code is produced.

Basically, Ayurveda is a science that teaches us how to manage the predominant elements in our body type or prakriti by the most natural and direct means. Because prakriti is determined by predominant elements, it also indicates what is most susceptible to becoming imbalanced. Many factors can influence these imbalances, such as diet, yoga practice, environment, seasons, work, and lifestyle. Depending on the strength of the immune system or ojas, the doshas can shift from being part of the general constitution to determining a specific disease or acute disorder, otherwise known as vikriti.

Many people commonly make the error of trying to determine their dosha type without proper study or through the superficial means of taking a questionnaire, without truly understanding the difference between mind-body type and disorder. When we experience symptoms of physical discomfort or mental unrest,

---

25   *Charka Samhita*: Chapter 7, verse 40. He was one of Ayurveda's main teachers and assembled its wisdom in one of the tradition's earliest texts.

these are signs of vikriti. What this means is that one or more of the doshas has gone out of balance and has become more prominent than the others.

A sound mind-body relationship supports establishment of a balanced, tri-dosha state. This comes about when the elements share their respective responsibilities equally, and the mind is able to sustain focus, calmness, and a level of awareness. When the mind-body connection shows symptoms of imbalance, we must look for some lack of accord with nature's laws. This is what happens when we oppose nature's rules, like not eating properly according to what the body needs during a certain season, or if we stress the mind to the point that excessive vibrations affect our physiology.

The basis for this teaching is that our psychology governs our biology. This is the core principle that teaches us the importance of personal responsibility. Diseases do not just appear. Imbalances in the body are created by choices, thoughts, and actions. Any time we are in a vikriti state, it becomes the primary focus of treatment until balance is restored.

This is not to say that, in trying to regain balance of our doshas, we ignore the prakriti or mind-body type. The prakriti does not change but is fixed. The vikriti involves variability in the elements, which we must work with throughout our lives.

The most effective way to get an assessment is with an Ayurvedic practitioner or doctor, as many factors exist in determining a person's type, and even more particulars are involved in dosha imbalances. In this regard, treatment can be a process of experimentation. I specifically use the term "experimentation," because Ayurveda is not a standardized practice. What is prescribed for one person may affect another person with the same prakriti or vikriti in a very different manner.

Ayurveda is not a fixed-formula approach. It is a system of adaptation and cultivating a more profound relationship with the forces of nature within and all around us. I have seen this with the practice of different asanas, diets, or treatments, with many different people having their own unique reactions to how these affected the body or mind. This has taught me never to try to fix a person in a single yoga class or consultation, and to work with each person distinctly and slowly.

Vata Dosha: Master or Disaster

The Upanishads say, "O Vayu. You indeed, are the immediate Brahman. You alone I shall call righteousness. I shall call you truth. May he protect me. May he protect the teacher." Vayu is another word for the wind as the vital force of prana. It is directly cognized by the witness or Self, It is more closely linked to the Self or true source of our existence than that which is perceived by the sense organs. Brahman heals us through the power of transformation. Ayurveda is born of prana, the life force, and has the power to heal the body when it is linked to the unlimited power of creation. The word Brahman is derivative of that which nourishes. Prana nourishes the body, so with respect to the body, it is Brahman.[26] Vata is that aspect of the air element that is directly linked to prana, which sustains the physical body.

Our connection to the body as creation itself is vitally expressed in scripture as the potential for attaining the pure consciousness that is creation. The mind (moon-awareness) and body (earth-creation) are linked through prana and give us existence.

This again is one of the central themes I am emphasizing in this book with respect to how healing can begin to take place. Prana is what supports our body and gives vitality to our consciousness, if properly directed. In Ayurveda, prana has the primary role in wellness. This link between the mind-body and breath is a foundation of healing and core to asana or Hatha Yoga teaching.

In the second limb of Patanjali's eight classical principles, the niyamas, or personal virtues, we find *brahmacharya*. This term is derived from two words, *Brahma*, creation or creative life force, and *acharya*, meaning teacher or mastery over that force. Typically, it is defined as abstinence, but it means much more than that, reflecting the importance of the subtle mind-body relationship and the fine thread woven between these two aspects of our life.

Thoughts govern our body and all the energies contained within it, including the life-force. According to Ayurvedic wisdom, vata is the master dosha, due to its similarity to prana. If vata can be kept in balance, so can pitta and kapha, and more easily. In general, balance of health depends on balance of vata. In order to experience sound vata dosha, societies will need to change their ways. Few in this world understand what a balanced state truly is and what changes are required to experience it. Balance and fortitude of the body depend solely on the mastery of vata and its forces.

Classical Ayurveda, as expounded in the *Charka Samhita*, Ayurveda's hallmark scripture, describes the importance of the five pranas as the directional influ-

---

26   As described by Swami Gambhirananda in Volume One, *Taittiriya Upanishad*.

ences[27] that vata has on all systemic functions. Health is primarily based on the body's capacity to eliminate physical waste, sustain a strong digestive metabolism, and rid the mind of worry and fear, all of which correlate to balance the force of excretion (*apana vayu*). *Apana* is the natural gravitational force that influences all physiological functions and allows us to stay consciously connected to the earth. Feeling grounded and calm requires a sound mind-body relationship and vata, being directly linked to prana, is the master energy that we need to pay attention to in this regard.

We must pay homage to this force, spiritually speaking, for it is the core power of propulsion. It is what moves things into action and inspires us to stay on the continuum of life. Primarily, vata dosha rules the mind, nervous system, spine and skeletal system, and digestive elimination. When vata is out of balance, it can have the most disastrous effect on our lives. The majority of health issues today are due to not understanding this Ayurvedic concept.

In order to learn how to master our prana, we must understand it and how it operates. Education and study are required to understand the true nature of our existence, and unfortunately this wisdom is not taught in the modern school system. Then, daily, seasonal, and yearly routines incorporated in various health regimens should be in place to keep us connected to the body, as I will discuss further in later chapters. Yogic discipline (*sadhana*) plays a key role in empowering us to work with the subtle energies within us. These pranic and occult forces can invoke a devotional and meditative mood that enhances calmness and intuition. A natural lifestyle supports all these factors: each supports the others.

> *Good discipline without knowledge leads to nowhere, leaving us lost in mindless action. Knowledge with no discipline leaves us trapped in the intellect. Unless the two are united and integrated with natural living, we shall never gain mastery over the life force or our life for that matter. Spirit and Nature must come together for the evolution of man to occur.*

Vata will always remain to blame for the endless fluctuations of our body and mind. There is no one single way to manage and balance vata. This is done through an integral approach to healing and wellness.

---

27 In Ayurveda the five pranas are *udana, prana, samana, apana,* and *vyana*. (See Chapter 8 for more on the five pranas.) On the more subtle level, these energies are reflections of the light of pure awareness. The unitary or maha prana is a manifestation of primal sound or *pranava*. As an outer physical form, the prana is dualistic, encompassing inhalation (lunar) and exhalation (solar). The aim of yoga is to balance these forces and return them inward to the spine. As the lord of yoga, Shiva represents the pure light of healing in life, and the capacity to expand our awareness and the power of evolution.

Ayurveda and Therapy

Ayurveda is founded on the principle of maintaining a balance of the elements in the three main forces or doshas that rule the mind and body. The word dosha is a negative term in the sense that any element has the propensity to become imbalanced when it becomes excessive or more concentrated than the others. The most common issue in the modern urban era is an excess of vata, as I have just explained. This is because vata controls movement and is a sensitive element disturbed by noise and any sensory stimulation, especially visual.

The other reason the term dosha is used to characterize a person's bodily constitution is due to the fact that we, the soul, exist in a body because there is karma to be worked through. So, by nature's design, the body is faulty and has variability we must contend with on our path to wellness and greater awareness.

What aligns Ayurveda with the concept of treatment (*chikitsa*) is its connection to repetitive lifestyle routines. The "practice" (*abhyasa*) of doing any action repeatedly is what determines the quality of our habits. This is why daily lifestyle routines constitute the largest factor in reversing disease and changing the state of our awareness. This principle is particularly important in cases of mental unrest and emotional imbalance. The thoughts in our minds must be accounted for, and the overall environment a person is exposed to is a major influence here.

There are several types of chikitsa, and this topic in Ayurveda can be divided into two aspects: clinical and lifestyle. The latter represents a large body of Ayurvedic teaching called *svastha vritta,* which mainly deals with various health and dietary regimens, and relates to individual behaviors. Clinical chikitsa focuses on the prescription of herbal medicines, and application of oils, along with various uses of steam, enemas, and other very ancient and sometimes odd types of treatment. The principle of abhyasa basically states that yogic habits, done repeatedly, can heal us by calming the mind and establishing a deep state of concentration that eventually leads to great peace.

Abhyasa simply equates to a continuity of inner and outer efforts, and is particularly important in vata types, because their minds tend to disperse prana in many directions. Outer abhyasa efforts include Hatha Yoga, pranayama, and any austerity done with persistent concentration. Inner yogic practices like mantra and various forms of meditation also serve to produce therapeutic effects that can help manage vata dosha.

A vata person's mind is much like the wind, which likes to move, as is commonly the case with people living a fast urban lifestyle, where the mind can easily become over-stimulated. So their key practice is slow and steady application of abhyasa. The Buddhist teaching of mindfulness is developed through the simple yet profound principle of abhyasa.

Pitta types can run into a trap when exercising abhaysa in yoga because of fire's sharp and hot quality. They can over-do it and even create addictive patterns, believing they need to do more. One of the most important lessons for pitta types, which should also be an American cultural lesson, is the practice of moderation. Consistency is important, no doubt, but so is knowing when you are over-doing it.

Over many years in clinical Ayurveda practice, I have seen many women who have become trapped in yoga asana or some other fitness exercise. They do it excessively, with the "I can't get enough" attitude. One could almost say this is an addictive approach that completely depletes them without their even knowing it. Most suffer from adrenal fatigue, severe muscle loss, and, in some cases, infertility. They could not correlate this to their approach or attitude to wellness.

There is a great story that I have enjoyed telling for many years, which involves an important lesson and therapeutic practice for those of a fire or pitta constitution. Astrologically speaking, those with Aries, Scorpio, or Leo rising signs can also fall into this category.

There once were two wood-choppers. They were neighbors and used to observe each other chopping wood from their yards. Especially during the fall, they spent much time outside chopping enough wood for the fast-approaching winter.

One morning wood-chopper Peter noticed his neighbor Freddy was starting to chop wood at the same time, early in the morning. They both began chopping away as usual, although today Peter decided to check on how much wood Freddy had chopped. Every time Peter checked on Freddy's woodpile, he noticed how much more wood Freddy had. Peter could not understand this, because he did not stop chopping the whole time and noticed that Freddy had stopped several times.

Somewhat baffled, Peter decided to chop more and more. He had to live up to his pitta nature! Steady Freddy kept coming back to his woodpile and it kept growing larger and larger as the day went on, while pitta Peter was getting more and more exhausted, and his pile remained much smaller. Finally, pitta Peter reached a point of complete exhaustion and bewilderment and went over to talk to steady Freddy to see how this was possible.

Peter asked, "How come, Freddy, your woodpile is so much larger than mine and on top of it you seem so calm and relaxed?" Freddy responded, "While you were chopping away, I was taking little breaks to sharpen my blade." Suddenly, pitta Peter had a realization about his forceful approach to doing things. Thoughts began to pour into his head about how he seemed to act this way in many aspects of his life.

So the journey of self-discovery continues. Much of our lives lie in the certain ways we keep doing things, rarely realizing that we create our own health and do not always do things in the most efficient manner. Ayurvedic wisdom teaches us to live in the most efficient manner that can afford us the greatest health. Our lifestyle and the way we approach our lives can either be very therapeutic or very depleting and unhealthy. It is simply a matter cultivating the right attitude and having the right understanding and awareness of our own inherent tendencies. In order for Ayurveda to heal us, we must understand that therapy or chikitsa is not limited to the act of getting treated, but is reflected in how we treat ourselves and apply nature's wisdom in our daily lives. Many fall into the trap of practicing Ayurvedic "therapy" to the exclusion of simply being practical. This only leads us right back where we started.

A branch of Ayurveda called *kaya chikitsa* or internal medicine deals with treating the body. It is very important for treating disease and provides a thorough understanding of how imbalances can lead to severe disorders. It enumerates six stages of how a disease comes into manifestation: aggravation, accumulation, overflow, relocation, build-up in a new site, and manifestation into a recognizable disease.

Ayurveda teaches us two things: First, diseases don't just appear. They must go through various stages, which take time to develop. Second, Ayurveda gives us the opportunity not only to remedy the symptoms but to remove the original causes of the disease.

One of the main methods used in Ayurveda to remove excess dosha from different sites in the body is called *pancha karma* (five actions), a powerful system of purification of the entire body. Another foundational branch of Ayurveda is called *svasta vritta*, which is a practical code for wellness. These include diet and lifestyle practices that harmonize with the seasons. When done consistently, these practices support maintenance of a good mind-body relationship through a healthy, tri-dosha balance of the five elements, and by strengthening of the body's tissues (dhatus) on a holistic level.

The key component in applying these vital branches of Ayurveda are lifestyle and treatment according to your distinct nature, as mentioned earlier. What you do is not as important as how you do it. This is the foundation of Ayurvedic wisdom. This becomes a powerful metaphor that has practical application in any aspect of our lives. In this way, individuals begin to understand the impulses and intentions behind their actions.

Ayurvedic wisdom is perennial and not limited to Indians or those who like spicy food and chai. I believe that it should be taught first in a metaphorical sense, in order to have a universal effect on humanity. The world has become too academic and intellectual, and operates more from the head than the heart. The law of karma operates and manages the five elements through the instrument of the mind, but begins with planetary forces.

As nature yields her Divine powers through the daily, seasonal, and life-long cycles of life, humanity can experience them as powerful forces to be reckoned with. They influence and impact our lives in ways we can ignore no longer. In a way, this is Divine mother's way of calling her children to listen and learn from her, so that she can guide us into healing and bring us back home to the heart of being One.

When we understand how energy works, it can help us to reprogram our brains to re-create a new mind-body relationship. This new dynamic relationship will instill responsibility in the mind for what the body is experiencing. The mind is responsible for the body and its functions. So, what the mind thinks, the body will experience. In order to heal the body, we must learn to understand the nature of our actions and impulses, and see how they impact our body. This is the real Ayurveda therapy.

Ultimately, the most profound healing in this regard must begin by accessing the field of infinite consciousness, rather than depending on the diluted and polluted, sensory-driven aspects of mind, which send signals to the body from a conditioned brain that manifests unconscious behaviors. Healing is a long and sometimes arduous process of rediscovering who we are, where we came from, and the direction we are headed.[28]

28　"What lies behind us and what lies before us are tiny matters compared to what lies within us." Ralph Waldo Emerson

Characteristics of the Dosha Type

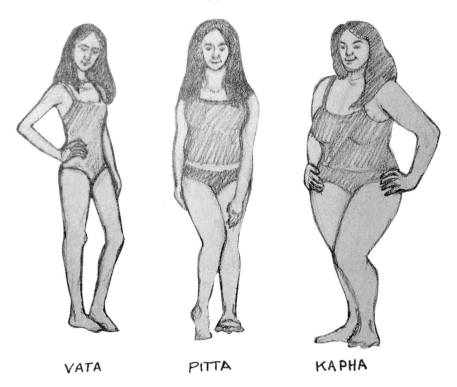

VATA   PITTA   KAPHA

Vata *(Air Element)*

Physical: Tall or short, long or condensed torso, thin overall, muscular defi-nition, thin face, small beady eyes, thin lips and flat buttocks, but overall very vascular. Vatas can move very fluidly, are athletic, enjoy staying active, and have minimal perspiration. <u>Imbalanced,</u> they can be weak, struggle to maintain body weight and fat, and have fragile bones, with such diseases as osteoporosis and arthritis. Dry skin, nervous and sensitive to touch, temperature, and environ-ment. Can be very tight, especially in the lower hips and back and hamstrings.

Mental: <u>Balanced</u>, they are fast thinkers, creative, reactive, and responsive, enjoy multi-tasking, speak quickly, and often chatter excessively. They are spontaneous, unpredictable, and excitable. <u>Imbalanced</u>, they can be forgetful, over-thinking, anxious and fearful, sensitive, indecisive, and lack consistency in completing tasks.

In Yoga Practice: Generally, vata types are good with asana but are challenged by holding postures for long periods. They excel in a fluid-sequence *(vinyasa)* approach, but benefit from slower combinations of posture followed by short rests. Often, they move into postures too quickly, and have a tendency to over-adjust or fidget while in a pose. Physical shaking is common, especially in postures that require strength, and often this can lead to losing balance or having to pause for a rest. In breathing exercises, they do best with shorter intervals and benefit from complete expansion of the diaphragm. Meditation is probably the most challenging of yogic practices, but in the long term is very beneficial for keeping vata in balance.

Pitta *(Fire Element)*

Physically: <u>Balanced</u>, they are very symmetrical, lean, muscular, strong and somewhat flexible, medium in height, weight, and overall structure. They excel in many physical exercises, martial arts, and sports, as the body demonstrates bursts of strength and speed combined with agility, and are quick to sweat profusely. Pitta-predominant bodies are the most adaptable and practical. <u>Imbalanced</u>, they can overheat, sweat very easily, have skin redness, develop rashes, and are prone to inflammatory conditions. They have a tendency to exercise or do things excessively, can have strong sexual desires, and often over-eat.

Mentally: <u>Balanced</u>, they are focused, have strong concentration, and are great at accomplishing tasks. They are driven and goal-orientated, enjoy debating, and have sharp memories. <u>Imbalanced</u>, they are competitive, aggressive, and can be argumentative, angry, and short-tempered, taking on large tasks and then becoming overwhelmed or exploding from taking on too much at one time.

In Yoga Practice: Fire seems to be very beneficial to all aspects of yoga. Physically, pitta is reflected in the ability to develop a strong, balanced body. Mentally, it is reflected in great discipline and motivation to practice, and emotionally by the ability to transform and overcome adversity. As yoga postures are very forceful stances and positions, pitta types often fall into the habit into pushing through postures rather than embracing them and surrendering, especially if there is any hint of an imbalance or vikriti. They have good alignment and can hold the postures well. They enjoy using the body as a vehicle for the mind, but often do more than is really necessary. This is why they are usually the best athletes or yogis. In breathing techniques, the breath is strong, but can get too forced or pushy. Initially, in meditation, a pitta type's breathing can remain a bit proactive or voluntary. They may require more time in corpse pose *(Savasana)* to disengage the mind's grip from the body.

Kapha *(Water Element)*

Physically: <u>Balanced</u>, they are tall or short, but generally sturdy, and have thick, dense bones and joints. Strength and stamina are very good, as is immunity or ojas. Water gives the body great endurance and support in varied climates. The kapha body is usually higher in fat, has moist skin, and experiences enduring sweats. They can have large features, such as attractive eyes, big lips, and a round head. <u>Imbalanced</u>, they can become obese, hold excess water, and have slow metabolism. They can have a tendency to tire quickly, especially during exercise or physically laborious activities.

Mentally: <u>Balanced</u>, they are calm, slow, thoughtful, stable, consistent, loyal, and make good partners in all types of relationships. They are soft and gentle, but can be strong when they need to be. <u>Imbalanced,</u> they become lethargic, attached, depressed, hesitant, intellectual, and often complacent.

In Yoga Practice: Depending on individual body structure, generally kapha types tend to move slowly and are usually challenged by yoga postures, especially standing or balancing poses. Flexibility is usually not an issue, but managing the body is, particularly with transitions in dynamic sequences. Inversions can be difficult without support, but very beneficial, as they help increase heat and promote sweat. Breathing is usually good, deep, and slow, and this is helpful, especially when practicing meditation.

Chapter FOUR

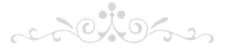

One Yoga

Do not bother about spiritual experiences. Go ahead with your Sadhana.
Knowledge dawns of its own accord.
Sri Swami Sivananda (1887 - 1963)

The Meaning of Yoga

Yoga is a term that means to unite or bring the mind, body, and soul together. I have often asked what it might mean when the mind-body and soul are united. What I have learned is that it means there is no division or separation between yourself and all living things. It is the ultimate realization: that you, as a miniature living universe, are fully absorbed into the grander cosmic reality. Yoga is an ancient Indian tradition that combines many different practices and rituals, and affords mankind salvation from the ever-fluctuating and treacherous physical world. It has existed for millennia precisely for this reason. Yoga exists as a "soul-solution" for life on the planet earth. It is the "sol" or "sunlight" that brings the soul into harmony with the universe and the laws that sustain it.

Yoga itself is derived from the Indian Hindu-Vedic religions. It is not considered a separate system, although many maintain an attitude of blindness to this connection. Yoga in India is related to a path of renunciation (*sanyas*) and based on lifestyle principles of non-violence (*ahimsa*) and truthfulness (*satya*). Those who practice yoga in its many aspects are called "yogis" and adhere to different austerities. As the great ambassador of peace Mahatma Gandhi once said, "I have nothing new to teach the world. Truth and nonviolence are as old as the hills." Austerities such as silence and solitude are practiced to develop a witnessing awareness, a type of detachment from the five senses and the world's ongoing fluctuations. This is not to be confused with aloofness or carelessness. It has to do with sustaining an attitude of mind beyond external triggers. Probably the greatest difficulty lies in just that: enjoying the world, but at the same time remaining unshaken by it. Keeping a witnessing attitude is like attending the theater. We go to the show, we watch and enjoy it, but we do not become the drama in it.

In the most practical sense, yoga is about erasing a relationship to something or someone who is not who we really are. It instead teaches us how to create a new understanding of who we really are. We all have to relate to something called the "ego," but at the same time we need to learn when the ego can be useful in our lives and when it is getting in the way.

The ego is what usually creates obstacles to our emotional balance and spiritual progress. I think one reason yoga is so popular in the Western world is that our society is emotionally bankrupt, as explained in chapter one. The "American dream," both the idea and the lifestyle, have fractured the core bond of family. We are taught to value our lives solely from an external perspective. Everything appears to be in place if money is coming in and the house, toys, and achievements are all there. We are not taught to look within for anything, especially not our feelings or emotions.

Yoga is healing our young culture from narcissism[29] and showing us that love has nothing to do with an idealized picture of our selves or what our lives are supposed to look like. In the original Greek myth, Narcissus was a beautiful youth who hears the calls of a mountain nymph named Echo. After being in nature for some time, Narcissus had become tired and hot, and decided to rest by a pond. Seeing his own reflection, he falls in love with it. He rejects the nymph Echo's call for love and becomes infatuated with his own face reflected in the pond. Ultimately, his own reflection deceives him as well, because it shows only his external beauty and hides his inner world of pain, fear, and chaos.

Our passion for the false self or ego makes it impossible to love others truly. Worst of all, we cannot actually love and accept our own true Self. Yoga teaches us a new meaning of the word love and how to experience it. Yoga actually teaches us how to experience and feel love from within ourselves.

The idea of having a relationship with who we really are and not something we thought we were may not make much sense. It can be rather confusing. Yoga is about developing a new relationship with the source, the power of who

---

29   The legend of Narcissus in Greek mythology is the origin of the term narcissism, a fixation with oneself.

CHAPTER FOUR: *One Yoga*

we really are, and not what we have been told or conditioned to believe. Yoga teaches us how to reorient our mind so that it operates according to a new paradigm that brings freedom from identity, name, and pride.

The most recent discoveries in neuroscience on how the brain functions are similar to the ancient scientific truths that seers and rishis have known of for ages. However, they used the mind, not technology, to discover these truths. We now have brain-imaging technology, known as the functional MRI, which can tell us what part of the brain is operating in relation to a specific thought or activity. Joy Hirsch, who directs the fMRI Research Laboratories at Columbia University Medical Center, refers to it as a "mindscope": "...because it allows us to connect the intangibles of conscious experience with the structure and function of the brain." I find this interesting because it can help us understand, medically, "how" the brain functions with respect to certain thoughts, emotions, and sensory images. We may then be able to produce therapeutic methods for healing the mind.

Yoga has long understood that "why" we experience pain and suffering, and how much we can change the brain, have mostly to do with time, karma, and environment. We spoke of time, karma, and the cyclical nature of life in the previous chapter. How yoga works with the environment to enhance the power of the mind is fascinating. One of the main intentions of a yoga practice is to develop the power of attention or concentration, known as *dharana*. Patanjali, a great sage of the yoga tradition, stated in his *Ashtanga Yoga Sutras* that one of the intentions of yoga is to reduce the mental discussions and debates that go on in our minds. In other words, it is about removing the excess clutter of thoughts. Yoga's other intention is to reduce negative stimulation to the brain or mind, so we can reveal an abundance of peace and sensitive feeling to ourselves. Yoga guides us to experience realms of consciousness beyond the mind.

The Three Pillars of Yoga

Living simply is at the core of going beyond the mind. Yoga provides three great pillars for healing the mind and attaining soul-realization. *Sadhana* is the personal discipline or practice we do in yoga, and includes postures, pranayama, mantra, meditation, and study. Then come the *sangha* or good associations, which support constructive thought and well-being. Spiritual associations are an important part of yoga, but are often overlooked.

After leaving my guru's ashram in the East Indian state of Bengal, I arrived late one afternoon in Delhi. As I was walking, I came across a billboard that read

"Rather than spending so much time trying to make yourself happy, dedicate some time to helping others feel happy," a quote from Yogananda. I instantly understood this to mean *seva* or serving others. It's about shifting the attention off our little self or ego. By serving others, we can have powerful experiences that destroy the clinging of the ego. In service to others, we recognize that the spirit that exists within us is the same as the one we are serving. Serving others takes us out of our heads and into our hearts. Medical science now believes that there are hidden secrets to healing our mind, which can remove depression and fear, and reduce the amount of prescription medications taken for mental disorders. I say to you, however, that these discoveries are not secrets but have been alive and thriving in the yoga tradition for thousands of years. Healing our mind is something we have to do for ourselves and yogic Vedanta gives us great tools to do this.

Certainly, yoga has much to do with the powers of the sun and moon. We learn to surrender to that which we have no control of. We not only learn to surrender, but in doing so become able to relate to what we can't control in some crazy way. The world is a crazy place. It has no constant, reliable message except that we cannot look anywhere else for answers but within ourselves. The adage "simple living and high thinking" is a wonderful way to approach the world's craziness. I think the world's "craziness" was meant to be, because it keeps encouraging us to turn inwards for answers, love, and peace. It's all within us. This is the underlying message of yoga, and this wisdom can be found either in tangible or abstract fashion.

Yoga has become known in the west as using, stretching, and contorting the body. However, it really has much more to do with the mind. America has given many names to yoga, identifying it with a specific person or approach. But this can only segregate it from its true essence: There is <u>no one way</u>!

Many different forms of yoga can co-exist as long as two things are maintained. One is that we always recognize that yoga, along with its counterpart Ayurveda, represents a complete lifestyle. Secondly, when we practice yoga, we should do so with the right attitude and intention. Yoga is not something we do when things are good or when we are wealthy and have everything in the right place. In fact, quite the contrary. Yoga should be practiced when we resist it the most. The best time for yoga is when there is struggle and adversity.

Some time ago, during a particularly emotionally challenging period, I struggled with adhering to my sadhana. I had lost the motivation and energy and could not seem to get certain emotions out of the way. One afternoon, my spiritual counselor said something that struck clear into my conscience: "Yoga is a lifelong commitment and there will be many small things that come across your journey, but never lose sight of the goal. It's a practice to the end of your life." When we look at yoga this way, we surrender to a continuous process of unfolding the mystery of life. In this way, our purpose or dharma becomes clearer. When we find greater security within ourselves, we have a peace of mind that stays with us more of the time.

Yoga in India is mostly practiced as a form of devotion. Prayers and mantras are used for celebrations of specific calendar days associated with planetary alignments. This honors the relationship between human beings and the Divine. *Maha Shivaratri* or the great night of Lord Shiva is one of the most auspicious days of the year and marks the convergence of Shiva and Shakti, the day when Shiva married Parvati. It honors the sacredness of the male-female or sun and moon relationship. Another festival is *Guru Purnima,* a day to honor and thank our teachers as an indelible part of our lives. The word guru is derived from two words, "Gu" and "Ru." The Sanskrit root "Gu" means darkness or cave. "Ru" denotes the remover of that darkness. This particular day lands on the full moon (*purnima*) in the month of June or July. Yoga teaches us to give love and respect to our teachers, another sacred relationship for ascending into Divine consciousness.

Just prior to Guru Purnima, on the eleventh lunar day of the bright fortnight,[30] is *Shayani Ekadashi.* The myth tells us that Lord Vishnu, symbol of water, fertility, and the power of preservation, fell asleep in a cosmic ocean of milk or *Ksheersagar* for four months until the period that aligns with the rainy season in October – November.[31] In the scripture Bhavishyottara Purana, the God Krishna tells the story of King Mandata. The king's country had faced a serious drought for three years. King Mandata took the advice of the great sage Angiras and began to observe vows to the Goddess Lakshmi on this day. By the grace of Lord Vishnu, rain began to fall on the kingdom. The vow or austerity of fasting on this day is an obeisance to the sacred primal energy that sustains our hearts and gives us life, abundance, and prosperity. The Goddess Lakshmi, Vishnu's consort, is prayed to.

In Ayurveda, fasting is done during various periods in these four months, according to the constitution, and to strengthen the digestive fire or *jatharagni* during the dampness of the heavy monsoons. Alternately, during nature's acidic rains, pitta types need to be cautious by reducing nightshade foods and eating

---

30   The first fortnight between New Moon Day and Full Moon Day is called *Shukla Paksha*. This holy day is of special significance to Vaishnavas, followers of Hindu preserver god Vishnu.
31   This period is known as *Chaturmas*.

foods that are more bitter and sweet-tasting, to avoid heat-related symptoms that may arise.

Another such culmination celebration is *Diwali*, also known as the "festival of lights." It signifies victory of the light over darkness, as set forth in the Vedas. The light of positivity, love, and transformation enables us to acquire all we are seeking. These are not just events, but are actually "holy" days that connect us to subtle forces inside us, which operate as universal laws.

We can see there is great power in myth. Having myths to live by is crucial to realigning with the purpose of life. Yoga reminds us that life must have purpose and a balanced relationship to all things. America and the world that follows our lead have forgotten the truths of the sun and moon. Through yoga, these sacred stories can guide us to a safe haven in our hearts. Yoga can help dissolve the mind of worry into the heart of knowledge. In this way, yoga is more than a practice of postures. It becomes a sacred lifestyle that encourages us to have the "One" relationship we long for. Each one of us is born with the capacity to discover how we can best experience the evolution of our soul's destiny. Yoga gracefully gives us many paths to experience truth. "The paths vary, but the goal remains the same. Harmony of religions is not uniformity; it is unity in diversity."[32]

Yoga and Ayurveda for Transcendence

The essence of the yoga teachings was shaped through an environment of intense practice over centuries. Yoga is presented through a voluminous number of texts and described with great beauty and insight, Scriptures such as the Mahabharata, which contains the Bhagavad Gita, the Ramayana, and the Yoga Sutras contain the boldest themes of yoga: *dharma, karma, chitta* (mind stuff), *samskaras* (mental patterns), and *pranayama* (energy control). They continue to bring yoga's core messages into the modern era, thousands of years later.

Krishna, who was a king and divine incarnation (*avatara*), is considered the original teacher of yoga. He is connected to the sun.[33] In the Yoga Sutras, God is referred to as Ishvara, the original teacher. As discussed earlier, yoga currently exists in two distinct paths, one physical, Hatha Yoga physical culture, and the other more spiritual, led by lineage-based organizations. This also reflects the

---

32 Swami Adiswarananda of the Ramakrishna-Vivekananda Center of New York.

33 "I taught this eternal Yoga to the Sun God Vivasvan. Vivasvan taught this to Manu, the first king, who taught it to Ikshvaku, the founder of the great solar dynasty." Bhagavad Gita IV.1 as translated by Pandit David Frawley.

two main types of yoga described in the Gita, Karma Yoga, the Yoga of Action, and Jnana Yoga, the Yoga of Knowledge.

As Krishna shares his Divine counsel with his warrior disciple Arjuna, he goes on to explain that he created two main paths of yoga, one for those that are more of a "contemplative mind," and the other for those of an "active bent of mind." Krishna states, "He who follows one *completely* also gets the fruit of the other."[34] In this stanza, when Krishna refers to the Yoga of Action, he clearly suggests an integral approach, as defined in the Yoga Sutras. According to Patanjali, right behavior, study and aspiration to know God or Ishvara,[35] define the Yoga of Action or Kriya Yoga.

This three-fold process constitutes complete transformation into the higher Self. Right behavior, known as *tapasya*, is a form of discipline and implies the heat or fire that creates a mind-body synergy. Study of scriptures also includes self-analysis, and produces the fire of knowledge that reveals the Real Soul. When we aspire to know God, to realize a higher purpose in our existence, we can surrender all our actions to Him. All our efforts are dissolved in the One. We recognize He is the doer. It is not us that sustains our body, nor food, but God as the formless sound of the universe or Aum, the vibration of life we know as mind, body, and spirit.

The Bhagavad Gita defines yoga as a type of sacrifice or *yajna*, which activates the sacred fire or agni of the mind, using it to transcend all things. In simple terms, yoga is a way of moving beyond the fluctuations of life by offering our actions and experiences to the ever-changing process of the world. Ayurveda is similarly focused on transforming our health through the fire of digestion or *jatharagni*, removing the doshas (excesses) that create toxins in the digestive tract.

While yoga is concerned with empowerment through union of the mind-body relationship by following the path of wisdom or action, Ayurveda is centered on the balance (tri-dosha) and health of the body from the inside out. Health, according to Ayurveda, begins internally and is reflected externally. Yoga and Ayurveda both consistently embrace transcendence of ego consciousness through the control of prana. In yogic thought, "prana" is directly linked to the mind, but "apana," the descending force, another form of prana, connects us to our body, helping bridge the mind-body gap. However, the essential motive of practice or sadhana is in merging these two pranas to dissolve them into the heart of our being. This is done through pranayama. Proper breathing

---

34   Bhagavad Gita V.5.
35   *On the Practice of Yoga; Yoga Sutras of Patanjali* with commentary by Vyasa, chapter 2, verse 1.

produces peace by erasing disturbances in the mind, and promotes physical longevity by calming the heart.

"Others offer Prana into Apana as a sacrifice and Apana into Prana. Controlling the movement of Prana and Apana, they are devoted to Pranayama."[36] In the Yoga Sutras, Patanjali states, "Yoga is the restraint of mental operations."[37] Ayurveda similarly considers vata the master dosha because of its link to prana. Without management, it becomes unruly and destructive to health. In order for transcendence of consciousness to occur, we must first learn to balance the mind and body. This means following basic rules of lifestyle and diet and practices mentioned later in the book for keeping the body fit.

The majority of the world either abuses health by living against natural laws, or neglects the fact that health must be maintained, until they too must struggle to regain their health. Nobody gets away with neglecting health, even though at times it may seem that way. In some cases, the loss of health can awaken a person to change their ways, although at some point we must move beyond physical identity either by taking the path of action, disciplining the body, senses, and mind, or by taking the path of knowledge that gives us the capacity to surrender ourselves to Divine will. May His will be done. May His will be clear to all.

The Importance of Lineage in Yoga

In the yoga tradition, there are many lineages or *sampradayas* that have carried the wisdom teachings of yoga through several millennia of global evolution. The lineage originated with the sun, the giver of life and the brightest symbol of the Soul in man. Much of what we see in yoga today is all part of the *Natha* (Knower of the Self) theological traditions: Hatha Yoga asanas (postures), pranayama (breathing), sadhana, tapas (discipline), Patanjali's *Ashtanga Yoga Sutras*, Tantra, mantra, and meditation. All acknowledge Shiva as the Lord of all Yogis, and Shakti, the Divine power of the Goddess, as not something distinct or separate from the manifest-unmanifest world, but as direct expressions of the One Reality.

A sampradaya bestows wisdom, rituals, and practices that come from an enlightened being (*satguru*) to his disciple (*sishya*) with sincerity and compassion, so all may benefit. Lineages provide a sacred transmission of Divine energies that flow "from one to another" (*parampara*). In the higher ages, these

---

36   Bhagavad Gita IV.29
37   Yoga Sutras 1.2

transmissions were oral and never written, but now we acquire them through books and compilations.

All lineages can be linked back to the Vedas and follow a succession of kings, gurus, and ritualistic practices that have always honored the symbolic relationship mankind has with the sun, moon, and earth. The doctrine of lineage is not limited to yoga, but can also be seen in other ancient civilizations, like the Egyptian and such Central and South American cultures as the Mayan and Inca, as well as in the religious and cultural groups connected to Buddhism, Jainism, and Sikhism. Although many of these have perished, as much does during the dark ages (Kali Yuga), yoga has endured and continues to thrive in the modern era.

The lineage thread is very different today, given how commercial yoga has developed, with asana schools producing "teachings" and "teachers" with no connection to a living lineage. In order for yoga teachings to endure, they must be aligned to a living sampradya that carries the shakti of transformation leading to moksha or inner freedom. This is a message for those already practicing yoga: without a true lineage, yoga styles become boring and unfulfilling, leaving one seeking other solutions for happiness and contentment.

All yoga lineages embrace many yogic paths to one truth, whether they be Hatha (technique), Karma (service), Bhakti (devotion), Jnana (knowledge), or Raja (integral knowledge, discipline, and surrender). Alignment with a lineage is a sacred relationship that can guide us towards higher consciousness as spiritual beings, as opposed to remaining physical beings striving for greater longevity. Commitment to a lineage can teach us how to become even-minded while living in the material world, by developing inner peace and compassion.

Commitment to a lineage should only produce favorable qualities in the mind and should not give rise to a sanctimonious attitude about others and other traditions. Commitment requires loyalty and increases the power of sadhana by enhancing discipline and mind-body synergy. When at times I have found myself resisting practicing yoga meditation, or even questioning the yogic path, I take a few moments to study some of my guru's teachings or read a story about another of the great gurus in my lineage. Moments later, I begin to feel inspired with greater fervor to stay the course towards realization of the Self.

The Kriya Yoga lineage, which uses the force of kundalini to purify karma, as revived by Babaji and passed on through a succession of other enlightened gurus, such as Lahiri Mahashaya and Swami Sri Yukteswar, was eventually handed over to Paramahansa Yogananda, who became well-known in the West for his book *Autobiography of a Yogi*. He and others of the Bengali Yoga tradition, like Ramakrishna, Vivekananda, Aurobindo, Anandamayi Ma, and Narendranath, all brought about a renaissance of yoga in the modern era. The lineage of Swami Sivananda of Rishekesh and his many disciples also helped spread yoga globally, and was exemplary for passing the wisdom their guru imparted to them on to more people. Lineages not only teach us to honor and respect the teacher-student relationship, but impart the deeper meaning of loyalty. In order for us to be loyal to our teacher, guru, or lineage, we must be committed to the path of natural living and spiritual liberation.

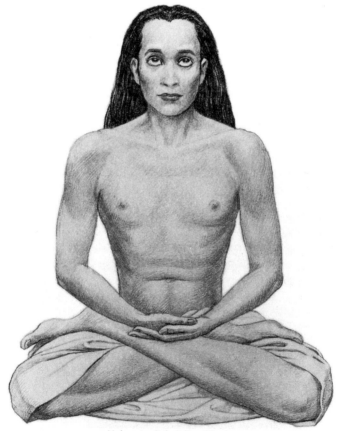

Mahavatar Babaji (Deathless)

The Nath lineage teaches us how the body can effectively use asanas and breath-work (pranayama) to ignite the sacred fire (kundalini) within us, so the mind can expand prana (life-force energy) into greater awareness, compassion, and love. The Bhakti lineages teach us how to use mantras, kirtan, service, and compassion as direct paths to God. The Jnani lineages teach us the value of studying the great scriptures to gain knowledge of self-realization, and the Raja yogis emphasize meditation and its methods of discrimination (*viveka*), witnessing (*sakshi*), and concentration (*dharana*) as the integral path to the Divine. Lineage is a colorful display of spiritually conscious lifestyles and rituals that can serve our intention of reaching the highest place. It's about fulfilling the secret need of humanity through wisdom traditions that align us with the purpose of life. When we become linked to a lineage, we attain a pow-

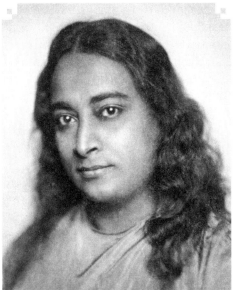

Paramahansa Yogananda 1893-1952

er beyond the mere mechanical practice of yoga. It elevates the entire process of evolution.

Original Forms of Yoga

The words **veda** or wisdom and **sadhana** or practice go hand-in-hand and represent the main principles of a balanced lifestyle. The yoga tradition remains one of the most comprehensive lifestyle systems, based on a routine of spiritual disciplines that maintains and enhances the mind-body relationship. Yogic practices include physical postures and various sequences, gestures, and movements that gradually build upon one another. Breathing exercises or pranayama and mantra techniques are used to prepare the mind for meditation and other rituals for cultivating devotion and intimacy with the Divine. Similar to Ayurveda, Hatha Yoga also includes cleansing actions for purification of toxins (*shat karmas)* from the body. All aspects of Hatha Yoga require action or Karma Yoga, and involve active participation of the mind and body. The intention behind such practices is to unite the individual self with cosmic consciousness.

The *Ashtanga* (eight-limbed) *Yoga Sutras* of Sage Patanjali are an extension of the four main branches of yoga, Karma, Bhakti, Jnana, and Raja Yoga. These traditional forms comprise the main paths that can be taken to cultivate integral and holistic healing. Technically speaking, the term "holistic," coming from root word *holos,* is characterized by the treatment of the "whole" person.

This takes into account mental, emotional, and environmental factors, rather than just treating the external, physical symptoms of a disease. For example, emotional people find great healing and balance through devotional practices like chanting and kirtan, part of the bhakti tradition. Such persons typically demonstrate a good connection between the moon and its sign Cancer in the Vedic astrology natal chart.

The *Ashtanga Yoga Sutras* contain what are called social (*yamas*) and personal (*niyamas)* moral and ethical codes of conduct, which are considered precursors to beginning a yoga practice. This is an area of training that has been largely excluded from western yoga schools due to the lack of training and access to the ashrams where this is taught. The path of yoga begins with Karma Yoga. As Swami Sivananda said, "The first step in the spiritual path is the selfless service of humanity." Seva or selfless service is a core part of Karma Yoga and is a primary means of purifying the mind of **vasanas** or subliminal desires. Mahatma Gandhi and Mother Theresa were examples of Karma Yoga in society, always there to help clothe and cook for others. Good friendship in many ways is an expression of Karma Yoga. Karma Yoga is an important model for modern yoga centers to consider, reestablishing themselves as service and educational centers rather than yoga businesses.

For thousands of years, yoga has existed to serve and educate humanity on how to live and attain self-realization. Now, in the last century, America has converted yoga into a billion-dollar business industry.

The Four Branches of Yoga

Bhakti Yoga is the path of love, compassion, and devotion. Bhakti is the essence of who we are. Bhakti Yoga cultivates feeling and the various moods or *bhavas* that attract us to recognition of the Divine. The path of Bhakti Yoga is connected to the vast Sanskrit tradition of Mantra Yoga or primal sound, and integrates the use of various seed sounds (*bijas*) to unleash powerful energies (*shaktis*). Mantra Yoga is the largest and oldest of the yoga practices: life itself and mysticism began with "the Word." Mantra Yoga is rooted in sound or *Shabdha Yoga,* as a vibration connected to the supreme Reality or Brahman. Generally in yoga, all mantras are born of the AUM vibration. Mantra yoga begins always by acknowledging the One source of all living things. From this place, we attain the capacity for action, creation, and transformation.

Mantra seems to be the fastest growing area of yoga, as people are drawn to it through the popularity and attraction of music. Sounds or songs carry energy, feeling, love, and power or shakti. While popular mainstream music focuses on songs about the drama of life, Sanskrit mantras aim to take us beyond this. Mantras have a transformational quality that is unexplainable and may be considered a type of Divine revelation. Insights are pathways to healing and unifying our consciousness with a grander force connected to our souls. Sanskrit mantras are currents of energy that can link us to the Divine.

Ayurveda as a system of self-care reflects devotion to healing that leads us towards the true Self. We must learn to keep our bodily temples pure and clean, as sacred spaces where the soul temporarily resides. Bhakti Yoga is mostly connected to practicing the chanting of *bhajans* (devotional songs) or mantras. Kirtan and even ancient temple dance rituals are artistic expressions of devotion. All music, as presented in the Gandharva Veda,[38] was performed with devotional intention and for clearing the subtle pranic pathways or *nadis*. In India, the seven musical notes were discovered as sounds in nature also connected to animal sounds. These can also be correlated to the vibrational sounds or frequencies of the seven chakras.

The practice of Bhakti Yoga transforms us from physical to spiritual beings. In the beginning, it is a common experience for some who are new to devotional practices like chanting to become self-conscious, because the ego is trained like a good dog to stay attached. This makes us aware of the idea that "I am chanting" and removes us from falling in love with the Divine. Pure chanting removes the "I" consciousness and slows the mind down. There is also much benefit to simply listening and feeling the energy of the mantra when others are chanting, as this also serves as an entry into the spiritual heart. I usually recommend that anyone new to Mantra or Bhakti Yoga just listen. Music becomes another formidable path to connect us to nature, promoting healing and balanced wellness. Love keeps us all searching for more than what we know, and keeps us open and receptive to a grander possibility.

Jnana Yoga is the cultivation of Divine knowledge through study of the scriptures. It also includes self-inquiry and analysis as a path of personal growth and self-improvement. Jnana Yoga types retain information well, are wise, are good writers, make for good astrologers, and enjoy discussions on scriptures and saints. Jnana Yoga requires powers of mind and develops discernment. In a mainstream sense, we could say these people are often professors and teachers.

Raja Yoga culminates in the practice of meditation, which is the culmination of both yoga and Ayurveda. The themes of Raja Yoga are very consistent with those

---

38   A section of the Sama Veda, one of the four books of the Indian Vedic wisdom traditions.

of Ayurvedic healing. In fact, the connection between Patanjali and Ayurveda is clearly noted in various scriptures and Sanskrit teachings. As an integral path, Raja Yoga shows how the same energies that can raise consciousness are also powerful forces for balancing and healing our physiology. In yoga and Ayurveda, psychology and biology are not separated.

Raja or the royal path, best elucidated by Patanjali, also consists of sadhana as an integral approach to enlightenment. It is well known in the yoga community that yoga is an ancient science dating back thousands of years and somehow connected to India. It was strongly influenced by the work of a great sage named Patanjali who lived in the fifth century AD. The depth and intention of Patanjali's teachings has been misunderstood and has incorrectly been focused around bodily postures. Patanjali has also inaccurately been considered the creator of yoga, rather than a compiler of yoga's main tenets.

Patanjali is connected to Shiva, the Lord of all yogis, but was also influenced by the teachings of Bhagavan Krishna (3,200 BC). Patanjali is known to have taken *diksha*[39] from Mahavatar Babaji, the immortal siddha of the Kriya Yoga lineage, who shared similar teachings with Jesus Christ, who was in India for a period of eighteen years. Patanjali essentially reformulated the vast yoga teachings into several compilations known as Padas, which include 196 aphorisms. In this simple yet profound model, he presents an outline describing Raja Yoga in eight *(ashtanga)* steps. These seem to be the origins of the Kriya Yoga lineage revived by Babaji during those particular yugas to begin a shift to the awakening that has recently taken place.

Various lineages share a common thread to the yoga of action (kriya, kundalini, karma), which are powerful systems for purifying the residual seeds (samskaras) of the Kali Yuga. Raja Yoga as the royal path encompasses various practices that lead towards the purification of the mind of all vasanas or desires and karmas, as well as development of psychic powers or siddhis. Raja Yoga explains that final liberation *(kaivalya)* must be accessed through the mind alone. Thus, liberation is achieved through *samyama*, the unification of concentration, meditation and *samadhi* or contemplative trance. This state is the light of all wisdom and can be applied to all planes of consciousness: physical, mental or astral, and so forth. It gradually eliminates all karma.

When I first came across these teachings, they seemed very esoteric and out of reach of the life and times of today. Like any great truths, they must be adapted and made practical for the individual and the times. This is the secret to success

---

39   Spiritual initiation.

in yoga and Ayurveda. We must learn how to personalize them, adapt them into our lives, and use them to the best of our ability. The rest involves Divine intervention and the guidance of a guru, according to our individual karmic cycle. In trying to practice Raja Yoga, I am not suggesting that it be reinvented, but that we find a path on our journey on which to live it.

During the early Vedic period, yoga or Ayurveda were not formulated into separate branches or teachings, as was eventually the case with yoga in the Bhagavad Gita.[40] The Gita was authored by Sage Vyasa, who is also given credit for authoring some of the four Vedas and some of the Puranas, which are another, later series of sacred texts. Krishna and Arjuna are the main characters. Vyasa refers to the four main branches of yoga, karma, jnana, bhakti, and raja, in critical sections of this timeless story filled with allegory and metaphor.

I think Patanjali's intention, influenced by Babaji, was to re-compile the broad scope of yoga from the perspective of both the Vedanta and Samkhya philosophies, and produce a practical, step-by-step formula for attaining complete enlightenment. I feel to a large degree the Ashtanga Yoga Sutras are still far beyond our time. We are still dealing with an infant consciousness trying to comprehend the fundamental laws of how to live in accordance with nature and maintain respect and reverence for the Divine in all things.

The first two of the eight limbs of the Yoga Sutras are known as the *yamas* and *niyamas*, which reflect social and personal principles for conduct, and provide the foundation for an effective yoga practice and balanced lifestyle. The yama principles develop ways to interact with others that are in accordance with natural law. As I mentioned earlier, this begins with the practice of non-violence. It is an immense statement to say that in essence non-violence is a fundamental requirement to achieving success on the yogic path.

The niyamas are the principles essential for personal and spiritual development. Yogananda compared these ten principles to the biblical Ten Commandments, as a support system for living in accord with the true nature of the soul. Traditionally, the student of yoga would begin at the age of seven by learning how to apply each of the yama and niyama principles in an ashram and in various circumstances, as guided by the guru or teacher. These were fundamental steps in spiritual development. In the modern era, we discover yoga largely through the physical postures, as a form of exercise. So, many of us who find yoga as

---

40 The most revered scripture of India, which is found in the sixth of the eighteen books of the Mahabharata, India's epic poem, considered the longest in the world. The book contains the original teachings of Krishna as given to his disciple Arjuna, and was written in allegory and metaphor. It is considered the yogi's bible.

young adults or in middle age end up having to learn some basic ethics, morals, and principles of right living later in life, after much struggle and suffering.

We should be propagating the importance of how we are living in accordance with the actual practice of yoga. This begins with teaching children the disciplines and guidelines of simple and natural living. Such principles include purity and cleanliness, discipline or austerity, being content on the inside, self-analysis and the study of sacred books, non-possessiveness and surrendering to God. These are innate qualities of the soul or pure being that reside in all humans.

Patanjali, having been exposed to the very Buddhist India of his time, seems to have been influenced by the eight-fold path philosophy of the Buddha. There is much similarity between the traditions, and both endorse the practice of meditation. Many Buddhist practices are predominantly based on meditation. There is much merit to its simple approaches to stilling the mind and cultivating compassion. However, it can be confining to those who need a more comprehensive mind-body-spirit experience.

Here are the ten principles that make up the first two sutras of the eight-step system:

Yama - *the principles of social behavior and discipline:*

    A. Ahimsa (Non-violence)
    B. Satya (Truth)
    C. Brahmacharya (Abstinence)
    D. Asteya (Non-stealing)
    E. Aparigraha (Non-possessiveness)

The yamas provide a basic outline of the efficient development of moral behavior. These bring moral balance and serve to deepen our relationship with our true self, the spirit dwelling within us beyond the ego.

Niyama - *the principles for personal behavior and discipline:*

    A. Santosha (Contentment)
    B. Shaucha (Purity)
    C. Svadhyaya (Self-study)
    D. Tapas (Self-discipline)
    E. Ishvara Pranidhana (Surrender to God)

The first two principles of the niyamas help us maintain our daily routine and give us a perspective on how to approach life. The last three, self-study, discipline, and surrender to God, are the foundation for the internal processes or actions toward reaching higher consciousness. They are also key components of Kriya Yoga. These three should be considered very important steps in enhancing the power and potential of meditation.

The yogi-aspirant (*sadhaka*) must always be consistent in the process of self-analysis in three aspects: thought (*chitta*), speech (*vak*), and action (*karma*). These three aspects of integrating sacred principles support the integral balance of each limb. The practice of self-study must be an ongoing process throughout life in order to move to the end goal of liberation or *moksha*. Healing the mind begins with observing our thoughts. The variety of thoughts in the mind can lead to a variety of challenges. The mind is our most powerful instrument, but can also be our greatest enemy, especially if thoughts are not controlled. Thoughts have their place in life, but thoughts must also be kept in their place in order to have a balanced life.

As yoga aims to establish control of the mind, similarly Ayurveda aims at managing vata dosha or the balance of prana in the body and mind. Therefore, in working with the yamas and niyamas, we must first learn to be observant what goes in and out of and passes through the mind, in order to remove the samskaras or habitual tendencies that bring us great suffering.

With control of the mind, we produce a higher quality of thought, which then brings clear and proper speech. Without value or meaning in our choice of words, we fall prey to gossip and worthless chatter. Our words should be sprayed with the sweet fragrance of kindness and clarity, so as to penetrate the heart of every being. But when words are tarnished with emotional swings, they can create the cruelest of wars between individuals.

The power of speech can extend into the reciting of mantras as sacred incantations to the divine, although it is important to understand the mantra, as well as the devotion behind the words. Otherwise, we become nothing more than a parrot.

Our actions are the third component in practicing the primary, yama and niyama, sutra principles, and hold the greatest consequence. Our actions bear a substantial impact on our own lives, our society, and the environment we live in.

What Is An Integral Yoga?

The use of the term "integral" was coined by the Bengali guru Aurobindo, and has much broader implications than referring to a yoga of completeness or wholeness. Aurobindo's use of the word integral[41] has more to do with the complete reformation of man and the integration of the human being into the nature of existence. Aurobindo's view is much more than a mechanical synthesis of principles and techniques. It involves synthesizing the fabric of human identity into nature and the grander universe. This metaphor is reflected in one of this book's central points, expressed in the use of the term "mind-body synergy" as a microcosmic perspective on the sun, moon, and earth archetype. This integral vision can also be found in the practical principles of classical yoga, although this requires insight and the lens of soul awareness.

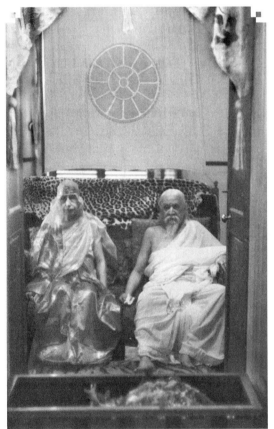

Sri Aurobindo (1872 – 1950)

Alternatively, we can see the eight limbs of yoga in the *Ashtanga Yoga Sutras* boldly transition from lifestyle principles in the yamas and niyamas to specific technical practices in steps three through seven. This begins with asana or postures that prepare the spine and hips for the "seat" of meditation. Of all the possible and sometimes contorted body positions, the lotus or seated position is the most sacred, as this how meditation is practiced. In its highest intention, the term asana is used to define the "seat of stillness" in meditation.

The next step is pranayama. Although this is usually described as "breathing techniques," it can more appropriately be defined as practices for "energy control." It is through the breath and the mechanism of the lungs

---

41 Purna Yoga is the Sanskrit term for Sri Aurobindo's Integral Yoga, which exists as a merging of the Self, or Spirit into the material or sensory domain as a practical manner of transmuting the life force energy.

and heart that we can affect the prana or subtle life force energy that rules all operations of the body and dictates the state of the mind. It is said that breath control is equal to self-control.

Pratyahara can be described as a feeling or state of deep inner relaxation. It has a neuromuscular effect on the body that shifts mental energy or prana away from the senses. It is the least understood of these specific yoga steps mentioned by Patanjali, and the most important. Without it, the body cannot properly rest and restore itself, and the mind will never experience its natural state of equanimity and peace.[42]

The complete system of yoga aims at improving our capacity to concentrate, known as *dharana*. Concentration is needed for the practice of meditation or *dhyana*. As the sixth step in the yoga sutras, concentration and focus are not something acquired later on the spiritual path, but developed as an integral part of the mind-body relationship.

Developing a higher quality of mind is an integral part of the complete lifestyle system of yoga and Ayurveda. This is overlooked today, as we continue trying to fix the body without giving much attention to what is going on in our minds. The example I often use is the Western idea of fitness where people stand or sit on machines, moving their bodies, while their minds are fixed on a TV screen, a magazine, or loud music. Meanwhile, an air-conditioning system pumps cold air into the room to control the amount of perspiration. The Western approach to wellness fragments the mind-body connection and does not recognize the importance of having the mind focused on what the body is doing and how it feels.

Dharana or focused attention is enhanced through proper asana, especially balancing postures, as well as pranayama and mantra. An Ayurvedic lifestyle fully enhances our power to hold attention and be more mindful. Walking meditation and T'ai Chi are practices in the Buddhist and martial arts traditions that are very good for establishing a focused mind. Patanjali explains in Yoga Sutra 3.4 that dharana (concentration) and dhyana (meditation) actually become united or *samyama*, along with *samadhi* or self-realization. The last three steps or sutras in the eight-limbed system become a single experience when one reaches a high level of mastery.

All these limbs are essential and should be completely interwoven in an integral yoga practice. They are not to be practiced one at a time until each one is mastered, as some confusedly believe. The contrast between lifestyle (yama &

---

42   "The Forgotten Limb" in David Frawley's book titled *Yoga & Ayurveda.*

niyama) and enlightenment (samadhi) in these principles must be understood and taken in the proper perspective. Working with them takes time. Lifestyle represents a proactive approach to life, while meditation is a contemplative practice. One involves becoming fully responsible and establishing a sound mind-body connection, while samyama (concentration, meditation, and enlightenment) is established by separation from or negation of the body and shifting the mind into a witnessing mode.

The gradual shift in consciousness that occurs on the yogic path is like vision that transitions from the lens of our human eyes to glimpsing life through a large set of binoculars. We not only see but comprehend more. We feel more connected to all living things. Our perspective on life shifts and we begin to recognize the impermanence of life more clearly. Through yoga, our depth of vision becomes more based on feeling or intuition and less limited by the tangible. The term "seeing" or "seer" is synonymous with cultivating or having intuition, and its development requires a deeper understanding, through discrimination, of who we are, that is, Jnana Yoga.

I have found when practicing yoga as a fully integrated system that it creates a deeply unifying experience both internally and externally. The senses develop more acuity in their daily function, becoming more efficient externally, while internally our awareness enters the greater field of consciousness with less resistance from the mind. Yoga practiced with the intention of working towards an inner experience brings a cleansing effect to the senses, which are usually bombarded by the media, urban living, and attachments. In the current age, the media and capitalism continue to over-impress our minds at an ever-increasing pace. This creates an over-stimulated brain that attaches to the senses and outward functioning.

Nothing is more detrimental to our health than the inner denial of who we truly are. We are souls having a temporary human experience. Yoga can teach us to experience the inner side of the mind because, scientifically, it is aligned with the soul. Yoga is a guiding light back to our soul nature. However, when the yoga system is practiced in a fragmented manner, it provides only a limited capacity for psycho-spiritual transformation. The effects of a purely physical asana practice or fitness workout are immediate but short-lasting. The effects of an integral approach to yoga and wellness require more time and deeper study, but have an enduring therapeutic benefit.

For the most part, when we practice asanas, we usually experience immediate results in the muscles, and the overall bodily structure becomes more aligned.

Through asana, the mind does get some release from its agitation and emotional swings. This is usually experienced as a physical sensation and does not penetrate as deeply as pranayama, mantra, and meditation, which are inner devices for attaining soul contact.

An integral approach to yoga begins with the physical and transcends to the level of the mind and its deeper dimensions. This energetic shift from the physical to the more subtle is clearly explained in the Bhagavad Gita as the two aspects of the mind known as *manas* (outer/lower) and *buddhi* (inner/higher). I will cover these two aspects of the mind further when discussing pratyahara or sensory control.

The advice I continually give to those new to yoga practice is to be "consistent and persistent," and embrace patience along the way. It takes time to feel the profound benefits of the more subtle aspects of yoga like pranayama (breathing), pratyahara (inner relaxation), dharana (concentration), and dhyana (meditation). The effects of a consistent yoga practice are not measured by the capacities of your physical body, but through inner qualities of the mind. Are we more peaceful, adaptable, tolerant, and patient? Do we feel greater compassion for each other and nature's kingdoms? Do we "feel" more attuned rather than "think" ourselves to be attuned? Do we experience sensitivities of the mind and are we enjoying having greater discipline over our emotional moods? Such mental qualities begin to purify the nadis (channels of subtle energy) and then the central nervous system, creating greater balance and harmony systemically between our various physical operations.

Without a sense of dharma, our entire sadhana (spiritual practice) becomes much harder. Our dharma is not based on something tangible. Having dharma gives the sadhana a subtle shakti (energy) that propels us forward, regardless of the hurdles we face. At first, the practice of subtle yogic techniques can feel somewhat mechanical. Gradually, with continuity of effort, the very sweet feeling of peace begins to seep into our consciousness. We must remember, as we make our continued effort in sadhana, that peace, love, and contentment are within us. What we really seek, consciously or unconsciously, is the discovery that all we need lies within us. "What lies behind us and what lies before us are tiny matters compared to what lies within us."[43]

The other form of yoga of which Hatha Yoga is part is Tantra. The term "Tantra" is synonymous with another Sanskrit word, *shastra* or book. It is a specific approach to reaching enlightenment that involves worship of Shiva and Shakti

---

43   Ralph Waldo Emerson.

as the sun and moon or male and female energies. Most tantric practices involve awakening the kundalini (serpent) energy and rely on somewhat occult efforts for transcending the ego-mind.

To clarify: Tantra, as a powerful form of yoga, does not focus on sexual performance, but does include the importance of sexual symmetry and transmutation of the procreative force towards compassion, love, and emotional healing. Each chakra or subtle energy center can be correlated to various anatomical and physiological functions of the body. There are inner forms of tantric practices that include meditation, the use of mantras, particularly to the devi or goddess, and yantras, geometric figures meant to rearrange the landscape of our minds.

Several yogi saints in the recent renaissance of yoga both in India and America were worshipers of the Divine Goddess Kali, who is probably the most recognized of all Tantric symbols. The Goddess in Tantra is active and sublime, and becomes a power-filled vehicle for the transformation of our consciousness. All such practices purify the mind and subtle channels or nadis, and increase the vibration in the chakras so as to expand our awareness.

The outer forms of Tantra are the popular Hatha Yoga practices that have spread throughout the world. Tantra is considered by some teachers and lineages as a way to expand creativity and promote expression of prana, while Raja Yoga withdraws prana from the senses to enter into stillness. Many great yogis like Yogananda warned of the perils of excessive attention on the body through asana, because this engages the ego and creates attachment to our physical form. Equally many agree that asana serves an important role as a preparation for meditation, especially when practiced in an integral manner along with pranayama (breathing) and pratyahara (inner relaxation). Sadly, much of this integral approach to yoga has been lost in commercial yoga.

Hatha Yoga serves as a powerful physical, mental, and emotional preparation for higher meditation, and really has much more to do with uniting the energy and establishing the mind in a calm and centered space. The four branches of yoga follow the sutras and allow practitioners (*sadhaka*) a chance to develop themselves in the path that suits them most. We are drawn towards a path depending on our nature or constitution and the quality of our personality, as reflected mainly in the rising sign and moon sign. If we practice the path we are most drawn towards in this way, the other aspects will develop equally. For example, if a person is more drawn towards devotional practices (Bhakti Yoga) and focuses most of their energy on that path, to a certain degree that particular path will also increase their knowledge and desire to perform good actions (Karma Yoga) and even produce a predilection for meditation (Raja Yoga) and the study of scriptures (Jnana Yoga).

Each path is considered to develop the "whole" being equally, as explained in the Bhagavad Gita, India's classic spiritual text. Therapeutically, an integral approach to yoga can also lower blood pressure, as it lowers the resting heart rate. This occurs as a result of holding inverted positions like headstand (*Sirsasana*) or shoulder stand (*Sarvangasana*) or very therapeutic positions like spinal twisting (*Ardha Matsyendrasana*) and floor postures, like the bow pose (*Urdhva Danurasana*). It takes more time to see the benefit of the subtler practices of pranayama, body locks (bandhas), mantras, and meditation. They slowly cleanse and purify the body's subtle nerve channels within the deeper layers of the tissues and cells.

Practitioners must persevere in pranayama, mantra, and meditation to win the light of higher consciousness. As I have mentioned, Hatha Yoga primarily works on the physical body's dhatus[44] (tissues) of muscle, fat, and bone. However, specialized breathing techniques transcend the ego mind to heal us inwardly by awakening prana, the life force, as a type of inner medicine. When we awaken this dormant life-force energy, it removes the obstacles to internal health physically, mentally, and emotionally. We can then truly begin our quest for soul realization. Let's remember the word yoga itself is derived from the root word **yug**, which means to unite or merge together. The term yoga also implies a system of transformation and transcendence. Practicing yoga in its true form is about wholeness and unity. It is the dissolution of the "I," "me," and "mine," and creates an expanded understanding of life and its mysteries through selfless action and detachment from outcome (vairagya). Patanjali states that yoga develops human potentials internally through the settling and control of the mind's thought fluctuations (vrittis).

In the modern field of neurobiology, the term neuroplasticity is used to describe the brain's capacity for reprogramming itself when new neurons are created in response to experience. This means a person can change the manner in which they respond to experience, overcoming emotional conditioning. This seems to have great similarity to how Patanjali defines yoga as the ending of mental disturbances (nirodha).

Yoga aims at clearing the mind through the management of prana and adherence to a vata-balancing lifestyle program. The more disturbed and stimulated

---

44   According to Ayurvedic anatomy, there are seven supporting tissue layers that make up the entire body: *rasa* (plasma), *rakta* (blood), *mamsa* (muscle), *medas* (fat), *asthi* (bone), *majja* (nerves), and *shukra* (reproductive fluid). These tissues are the secondary sites where the doshas accumulate.

a mind becomes, the more susceptible a person is to their emotional history. It is important to understand that the vast majority of humanity utilizes a very small portion of the brain. The main organ able to expand the power of the mind and consciousness becomes limited to just firing off emotional history stored in the amygdala.[45] What I mean by small portion of the brain has to do with the aspect of mind that operates only on the sensory-emotional level. This is mainly the limbic area or mammalian brain, which works closely with the brain stem.[46] This part of our brain evaluates experiences, so we can decide whether something is good or bad. It creates emotions that encourage us to act in accordance with the meaning we have assigned to whatever it is we are experiencing at that moment.

The expression of having "no brains" is equivalent to the level of consciousness we are currently living with. Most people's minds function primarily on the sensory level. Because the mind-body relationship has fractured, we are dealing with a world living in emotional deficit. We search outside ourselves to balance our emotions, but can only do so superficially.

fMRI studies of monks and other meditators show they have the capacity to modulate the amygdala and related parts of the brain, like the insulae, which are believed to be involved in consciousness and play a role in diverse functions usually linked to emotion and regulation of bodily homeostasis or balance. It seems clear that the ancient yoga sutras can play a prominent role in healing the modern mind. What medical science will continue to do is validate the importance of a great wisdom we used to know and practice, but have obviously lost for some time.

According to yogic teaching the sensing mind or manas, which operates through the five senses, is the smallest aspect of the mind as a whole. As just explained, it relies predominantly on the limbic system, which is the basis of stored memories and experiences, and limited in its access to pure, untainted, unreactive consciousness. Integral yoga aims at awakening the higher dimensions of the mind, which allow us to be more attuned to the universal intelligence perceived through the intuitive function of our higher mind or buddhi.

The material world continues to advance in endless technological ways, such as gadgets and sense-attracting instruments. The spiritual world seeks to develop

---

45 Performs a primary role in the processing of memory, decision-making, and emotional reactions, which are part of the limbic system.

46 Consists of the medulla oblongata, pons, and midbrain, and continues downward to form the spinal cord.

its own telepathic radio that far exceeds the capabilities of any instrument created by the intellect. The intention of yoga is to turn the energies of our senses inward. The essence of a real yoga practice lies in our capacity to redirect the five energies of the senses from their usual outward flow into the material world, inward to the realm of Spirit. The outer or physical world under the direction of maya has a very strong current that is delusive in nature and gilds the lily, so to speak.[47] The great yogis have suggested that the practice of yoga must become a way of life, as taught in Ayurveda, which consists of a collective array of healthy habits all working towards the same goal. Simple living is the secret strategy that great yogis have said can help us outwit the outward pull of the material world. Simple also means natural, staying connected to nature and her elements.

The eighth limb of the Ashtanga Yoga Sutras is samadhi, the highest state of consciousness. It was described by the Buddha as nirvana and by Jesus as the kingdom of heaven. In common English, we know it as enlightenment. Samadhi translates as the ultimate state of being. Call it whatever you like, attaining samadhi requires a clear understanding that the purpose of human existence is to know God. The longer I continue on this path, the greater my desire to experience the Divine mystery from within. When one is afire with such a desire, the search for its Source never ceases. We then realize that nothing in this world will ever fulfill us until our consciousness is one with this Source. Few are the blessed who have this rare opportunity, Krishna said, "Out of one thousand, one seeks me; and out of one thousand that seek me, one knows me."

All humanity is seeking the one experience that will transcend their consciousness to a state of joy and everlasting bliss, but only a few are truly aware of making a conscious effort to reach this state. The quest for happiness in yoga can be expressed through the chanting of various mantras and soulful songs, by practicing meditation, and serving others. In our daily activities, we must maintain the consciousness that we are divine beings first and foremost. Once the commitment to yoga has been made with strong determination, which includes concentration and continuity of practice, the yogi or sadhaka (practitioner) will arrive gradually at the highest place.

There are so many variables to be considered in reaching this blissful consciousness. Most important is to consider one aspect of our sadhana at a time, and then mold the different aspects together into one practice, one life. Yoga is so broad in scope that trying to learn everything at one time is not possible.

---

47 Having a pleasing or showy appearance that conceals something of little worth can also be a synonym for maya, the delusory energy present in creation.

Trying to apply all these ancient principles to our modern understanding of life may not be very easy, practical, or even necessary. But I have learned that as I continue on the path, what is next for me on the journey appears in my consciousness and daily activities. Such realizations usually come during moments of daily introspection and meditation. As an observer, I am able to view myself and my actions from an objective, discriminating perspective, and intuitive guidance then becomes clear and concise. We are often misguided when the mind is dependent on the senses, but divinely lighted when we can discern or distinguish between the ego and soul.

Our state of happiness is often determined by how much pleasure we are able to give the physical body and its commanders, the senses. Another reason for the popularity of asana fitness yoga is that learning the more subtle limbs, four through seven, breathing, relaxation, concentration, and meditation, requires substantially more time and personal practice. Unlike the physical postures, which give quite immediate results, it takes more time to feel the actual transformational benefit of limbs four through seven, which, being subtle, address the more profound spiritual aspects of the energy body. How can we be receptive to the subtle aspects of yoga when the majority of our life is involved with bathing the senses and the body? The senses are a necessary part of living and learning, but, if used improperly, they can strangle our capacity for transformation and create bad habits and mental ruts.

American culture operates from the idea of individuality and opportunity, which gives birth to capitalism, something very far from being democratic, because it feeds the hunger for greed. Yoga is a system of sustaining wellness in anyone regardless of who they are or their income. When we improve ourselves, we do our part in changing the world around us. Personal transformation enhances the vibration in our soul so that we can attract abundance and have success in whatever we choose. When we look at yoga as a business venture, we ignore the selfless intentions it was founded upon. The devotional essence that has sustained these traditions for millennia becomes veiled behind gestures like "namaste" and a good hug. Perhaps the Hollywood expression "fake it 'til you make it" may actually influence those involved in yoga to find the meaning of devotion within themselves.

In summary, the eight limbs of yoga can be divided into three parts: **lifestyle** (yama and niyama), **practice** (limbs three though seven) and **Being** in bliss consciousness (limb eight, samadhi). Lifestyle is the principle of *Sat*, a life in pursuit of truth. *Chit* includes the practices we perform that can enlighten and expand our vision and understanding of truth. *Ananda* is the principle of love and bliss consciousness sourced from the soul. As we can see, there is much to understanding yoga, its history, practice, and connection to a lifestyle system like Ayurveda.

Physical Culture Era and Yoga

Yoga fitness in several instances ignores the ethics and morals of traditional yoga teachings and dedicates much of its time to physical sensation. Living ethically and morally is a cornerstone of the principles of yoga and Ayurveda and imbues them with valor and sacredness. In some ways, the modern approach to health and fitness has become like an art form reflecting our culture's consciousness. Spiritually speaking, too much attention on the body is one of the perils of over-indulgence in the senses. Excessive movement becomes disconnected from the sacred.

There are several reasons why instruction beyond the physical postures is generally lacking in the modern yoga asana movement, although the situation is slowly changing. This is primarily because we live in a physical culture, an age obsessed with the physical body and anything experienced on the sensory level. Nevertheless, the physical body can be a powerful and creative artistic vehicle for expression, which can be inspirational and transformative in its own right, mystically speaking,

Yoga can serve as a great system for connecting us with the energies that lie within the body without being focused on the body alone. In fact, the physical culture movement has interesting connections to the yoga that developed in northern India. Yoga in southern India was influenced by gymnastics and wrestling.

During the late nineteenth century, German-born Eugen Sandow became the father of modern bodybuilding. With his great strength and muscular features, he was a fitness phenomenon who lived mostly in London but gained popularity throughout the world. Sandow launched a periodical called *Physical Culture,* and opened a Physical Culture Studio in London. Audiences who saw him perform were more fascinated by his chiseled muscular appearance than by his strength.

Sandow went to America to perform at the 1893 World's Columbian Exposition in Chicago. Interestingly enough, this was the same year that Swami Vivekanada spoke on Vedanta at the World Parliament of Religions in the same city. Sandow also visited Calcutta, India, in 1904-05, during British rule, and was a sensation, with thousands visiting him. He traveled throughout India with a large tent that could hold up to 6,000 people during his popular demonstrations. He became the leader of a powerful crusade that was bringing people in touch with their bodies. He was a showman who knew how to display his body and earn a good living doing so.

It is probable and somewhat coincidental that Sandow was not only one of the earliest pioneers of the mind-body relationship, but also helped shape the rebirth of the asana movement. A Bengali newspaper editorial states: "The essence of his system [is] to concentrate the mind upon the physical effort, so that mind and body may both work together to produce muscular development…. It is the cooperation of the mind with the body that makes the system so unique and explains the great results which have been attained." Sandow was undoubtedly exposed to yoga during his visit to India, and became very fond of the country and its oppressed people.

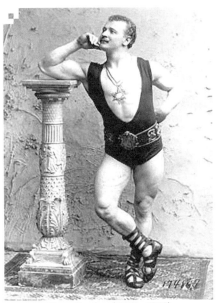

Eugen Sandow (1867 – 1925)

Maxick, a strong man, was also influential in the physical culture era. He wrote a seminal book explaining the mind-body relationship, which gave more credit to the mental aspects than Sandow did. "The serious student of muscle-control will soon become aware of the fact that his willpower had become greater, and his mental faculties clearer and capable of increased concentration. Thus it will be observed that the controlling of the muscles reacts upon the mind and strengthens the mental powers in exactly the same proportion that the control of the muscles strengthens the body and limbs."

Swami Vivekananda responded to the question of why India was under colonial rule by saying India needed to pay more attention to the three Bs: beef, biceps, and the Bhagavad Gita. Other great yogis and philosophers, like Nagendra Nath, Aurobindo, and Rabindranath Tagore, endorsed Vivekananda's prescription for overcoming colonialism. All promoted physical culture for the building of both body and morale.

A monk from Bengal whom I have delighted in sharing dialogue with over the years candidly related his sentiments about the challenges of colonial times in India. "Bengal was then the hot seat of anti-British revolutionary guerilla warfare, with youth and teenagers getting more and more inspired to 'fight the British out of India.' Indian type gyms were overtly and covertly sprouting all over, where the youth and teenagers went not for a work-out merely to keep fit, but to grow in strength to fight the British, and to happily die for the cause. They wished to gain strength and agility. That the indigenous system of yoga asanas offered greater strength, endurance and agility (even among the poor who could barely afford a square meal a day), and which was now being scientifically explained by Kuvalayananda and Yogendra (both of whom were themselves great nationalists), was the principal motivation behind the growing interest in asanas during this period."

Part of the reason that Calcutta became the hub for the growth of the physical culture was because it was originally the nation's capital[48] and the East India Company and later the British Raj used it as their headquarters As a karma yogi, I don't think Vivekananda was suggesting eating meat, but was endorsing the country's need to stand up and reconnect their mind and body as an instrument for overcoming colonial rule. Obviously, Vivekananda diverted a bit from his priestly guru Ramakrishna, who never really left his Bengal neighborhood and spent much of his time at the Dakshineswar temple. Vivekananda took stronger social and nationalistic stances by traveling the country on foot and then going to America.

Eugen Sandow was in Calcutta and Bengal during the time of Vivekananda, Rabindranath Tagore, whose niece was his admirer, and Mukunda Lal Ghosh, who later became Swami Yogananda Giri. In 1917, Yogananda founded his first "How to Live" school for boys in Dihika.[49] He taught there, nurturing his dream of setting up a residential school that taught moral and spiritual principles, as well as his unique form of tensing and release techniques and muscle-control exercises. The school was inaugurated on March 22, 1917, a date specifically chosen by his guru Sri Yukteswar according to the jyotish (astrological) value of Mahurta. It accorded with the Leo rising sign in Yogananda's astrological chart and the auspicious occasion of the spring equinox. This brought great success to his teachings on a global scale.

Yogananda's youngest brother Bishnu was a student at the school, eventually named Yogoda Satsanga Vidyalaya, in 1917-18, after it had been moved to

---

48 India's capital shifted from Calcutta (now Kolkata) to Delhi in 1911.

49 Dihika is a village in the Asansol subdivision of the Bardhaman district, West Bengal, India. It was made famous by Paramahansa Yogananda, who came to this small plot of land by the river Damodar with just seven students.

Ranchi, and was deeply influenced by these teachings. "I myself learned this system of yoga Exercises at the Ranchi School for Boys in India, founded by my Guru (Spiritual Preceptor) and brother, Paramahansa Yogananda." In 1916, Yogananda met Sri Manindra Chandra Nundy, the Maharaja of Kasimbazar, who was the principal patron for the boys' school, permitting free use of his premises. He also contributed about 4,000 rupees a month, a substantial sum of money then and approximately US$64 today, to meet salaries and other operating expenses.

The Maharaja had also separately appointed a hatha yogi named Alokananda Brahmachari to teach at the school, most probably after it moved to Ranchi. Brahmachari taught various asanas to many of the students. Bishnu Ghosh, then 14-15 years old, was one of them. Yogananda conducted spiritual classes, taught meditation, and was the school's supervisor. He also inspired students, particularly those spiritually inclined, to practice the set of Energization Exercises he had formulated in 1916. During this time, Yogananda certainly had influence over how asanas were being practiced. All this was later taught at his ashrams in the Americas.

Bishnu Ghosh's education professor, R.N. Guha Thakurta, was a huge inspiration to him. Then, after seeing a demonstration from Burmese body builder Chit Tun, he creatively combined physical culture with the muscle control techniques his brother Yogananda had taught him.

Yogananda himself was quite athletic and had a broad range of interests and skill in music, sculpting, and photography, not to mention esoteric practices. With no formal training, Yogananda would suggest powerful holds to skilled wrestlers, and prescribe curative postures and breathing exercises for chronic ailments. He also helped dance maestro Sri Uday Shankar, Ravi Shankar's elder brother, to incorporate certain pranayama and muscle control features in his dance forms.

Yogananda's creativity makes sense, given that his father, Bhagabati Charan Ghosh, was very knowledgeable in the therapeutic applications of asana, pranayama, and herbs. The elder Ghosh also influenced his youngest son, Bishnu, and Bishnu's friend Buddha Bose, encouraging the latter to start the Yoga Cure Institute.

Bishnu Ghosh and his friend Buddha Bose were even more inspired by an asana demonstration that took place in Calcutta in the early 1920s as part of the nationalistic movement meant to give young men the confidence to take on colonialism by increasing their physical strength. This seems to have been the birth of two major forms of physical exercise that have now aligned into a single comprehensive approach to mind-body medicine. The physical culture movement of muscle-building and control was combined with the wisdom of yogic breathing and concentration.

These physical pursuits, as well as others like wrestling and gymnastics, found a connection with the Hatha Yoga tradition in other parts of the country, such as the south Indian city of Mysore. This southern yoga tradition evolved from the large Wodeyar family dynasty,[50] which supported its development. This subsequently led to the popularity of some of today's asana forms, such as B.K.S. Iyengar's. The Mysore palace patronized Krishnamacharya, who was the teacher of many well-known asana instructors, including Iyengar, Pattabhi Jois, and Indra Devi.

In the north, Bishnu Ghosh's fame grew substantially with an endorsement from Jawaharlal Nehru, India's first prime minister. In the late 1930s, Bishnu Ghosh and his star pupil Buddha Bose began teaching asana yoga and muscle-control techniques in Europe and the USA, focusing on their therapeutic value. It was through these demonstrations, along with the popularity of Bishnu's brother Paramahansa Yogananda, who had already been living in America since 1920, that yoga gained momentum across the United States and Mexico. Some of the monks of the Vedanta Society established by Swami Vivekananda were also already doing asana demonstrations in America. However, the organization never emphasized asana yoga demonstrations or teachings.

Swami Kuvalayananda from the state of Gujarat was also greatly influenced by the Bengali yogis and the fervor for nationalism. The political leader and later guru Sri Aurobindo shaped Swami Kuvalayananda's views on nationalism while working as a young lecturer at the Baroda College, from which he graduated in 1910. Later, a yogi, Paramahamsa Madhavdasji, whom Swami Kuvalayananda had met in 1919 at Malsar, near Baroda, and who had settled

---

50   The Sritattvanidhi Manuscript of the Mysore Oriental Institute contains a section of about eighty asanas separated from others also listed. In total, 122 asanas are found in the yoga portion of this text. These illustrations seem to be consistent with some of those postures found in more ancient texts of the Hatha Yoga tradition, such as the *Hatha Yoga Pradipika, Goraksasataka, Gheranda Samhita*, and *Siva Samhita*. Many of the asana figures in this Mysore text are unfinished, and the date is unknown. Some of the asanas illustrated are part of an older tradition and similar to the 84 postures of the northern lineages of Yogananda and Sivananda. .The additional asanas listed in the Sritattvanidhi manuscript fall into several categories: "from the back," "from the stomach," and "standing asanas." There is some implication of repetitive movement in the asanas, as perhaps a type of callisthenic exercise. These might be linked to the Surya Namaskar sequence, as well as to the distinctive approach developed by Krishnamacharya.

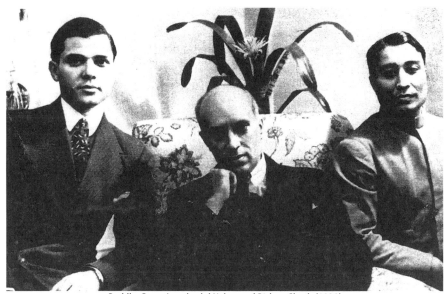

Buddha Bose, Jawaharlal Nehru and Bishnu Ghosh (1938)

on the banks of the Narmada River, gave him the deep insights into yoga that eventually developed into the scientific work that inspired the Yoga Therapy movement. Shri Yogendra was another of Paramahamsa Madhavdasji's disciples influential in promoting the therapeutic aspects of yoga.

It is clear that yoga asana and pranayama have gone through an evolutionary process since the time of the original yogic texts. What we see through the connection to Bengal in particular links yoga asana and pranayama to cultivation of both inner powers within the subtle body, and outer powers, such as muscular control and building the morale of the enormous lower and small middle classes in India during the nineteenth century. All this reflects the ultimate reunion of the mind-body dynamic that has influenced subsequent generations up to today. I have dedicated a later chapter in this book, entitled "Yoga Therapy," to presenting both the mystical and practical therapeutic benefits influenced by these groups of Bengali yogis, including Lahiri Mahasaya, Paramahamsa Madhavdasji, Swami Kuvalayananda, Paramahamsa Yogananda, his brother Bishnu, Buddha Bose, and later personalities like the infamous Bikram Choudhary, who came to the United States in the 1970s.

I practiced with Bikram for a number of years and was influenced by his emphasis on mind-body concentration as taught in the Ghosh-Bose line. However, I discovered the spiritual component of Yogananda's influence was completely omitted. I travelled to and sojourned in India, discovering much of what I am presenting here through years of my own yoga practice (sadhana) and clinical application. This mind-body emphasis reflects the very core of the yoga and Ayurvedic systems' approach of balancing therapeutic healing of body and spiritual transformation of the mind. This is not limited to recent and modern figures, but finds its roots in the Nath-Siddha lineages connected to Patanjali, Mahavatar Babaji, and Bhagavan Krishna.

We can only be grateful to the stalwarts of the Bengali and north Indian traditions, who have left us time-tested teachings to hasten our path to spiritual liberation. What was revived by them and has remained consistent is that Hatha Yoga is but one part of Raja

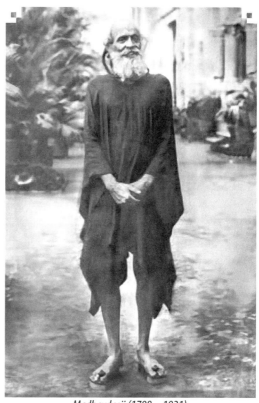

Madhavdasji (1798 – 1921)

Yoga, and yoga asana is but one component of the Hatha Yoga system. Not all meditative types do asana, but they might find it helpful to their meditation practice. Not all hatha yogis do asana, focusing more on pranayama, breath suspension, and other rituals. However, they might find some asana practice helpful in such pursuits.

Hatha Yoga should not be considered an end in itself if it focuses only on asana, although when combined with pranayama it can serve as a powerful vehicle in bridging the mind-body synergy and for spiritual transformation through meditation. I, like Bishnu and Bikram, used muscle-building exercises in my teenage years to build a scrawny physique and increase mental discipline over my body. I gradually started to shift my interest towards Raja-Hatha Yoga as I came across Yogananda's teachings, just after completing my B.A. at the University of Florida. I think you will find these methods for controlling both muscle and mind astonishing, especially today, when a great divide exists in the mind-body synergy.

As we can see, prior to the twentieth century, the health and wellness movement was divided into two halves. Some were attracted to the physical and others focused on the ancient spiritual and scientific principles taught in yoga. There now seems another, more recent divide in America between asana enthusiasts and yoga-meditation practitioners. The former use the body as the vehicle for transformation, the latter use the mind. I feel that unless the two are united, the movement will lead nowhere.

The Physical Body as a Mystical Form

In the yoga tradition, various techniques of carrying energy have been used for shifting both energy and consciousness. Mystical diagrams were commonly used along with ancient mantras, words of power that unlock knots or psychological energy blocks. Mantras are used to reprogram the brain and shift energy on a subtle level. Just as a noisy and disturbing city can displace our mental harmony, so songs of the soul can bring out the mind's naturally fine and peaceful qualities.

The mind produces its own obstacles because of the ego, conditions, patterns, and memories. In the Tantra tradition, yantras (geometric designs) were another unique device to focus and expand the mind and transcend body consciousness. The senses are not themselves bad, if they are used properly and with a higher purpose.

As we look deeper into the mystical side of Hatha Yoga, we find that the asanas are not merely physical stretches with certain purifying qualities, but each pose is likened to a yantra, which can transport the mind beyond the form itself. This is one reason that postures are named after and associated with animals, nature, and planets, symbolizing qualities and aspects of the Divine. Each asana represents a different archetype, a vehicle that can move our awareness beyond the limitations of the body. Nature is Divine and can be used as a doorway into higher consciousness. But we should not visualize the body itself doing the asana. Rather, the body identifies with and merges with the asana, becoming like a fish, tortoise, rabbit, and so on. Such an approach provides us with the power of yogic mythology for healing and self-realization.

This is one reason we do not find asana explained in much detail in the original texts. The emphasis on a single fixed form would deter from our finding our individual relationship with the asana, as it serves us according to our needs, capacities, and intentions. In yoga, the body has always been considered a temple. Different gods have been worshipped in the form of a statue (*murti*), which is the visual form of the Divine. This is similar to the *ishta devata* or "favored deity" concept, with each person finding his or her own personification of the Divine. Yoga strongly dissuades association with the physical body, unlike in modern asana yoga forms, which praise it, associating physical capacity and flexibility with progress.

Power of Surrender

I can't think of anything more powerful to do in life than to surrender to its fluctuating nature. What I mean by surrender is not to give up on life and become a drifting fool, but to give up on the idea that this material world will bring us everlasting happiness.

Learning to surrender can help us work with the forces of nature and our individual karma, rather than oppose them. The great saint Sri Ramana Maharshi made a bold statement in this regard: "The ordainer controls the fate of souls in accordance with their prarabdhakarma.[51] Whatever is destined not to happen will not happen, try as you may. Whatever is destined to happen will happen, do what you may to prevent it. This is certain. The best course, therefore, is to remain silent."

By remaining silent, we surrender to life's journey as the observer who partakes in the world but remains above its fluctuations—a monumental task. Alternatively, haven't we seen enough evidence that the "I," "Me," "Mine" mentality is destructive to our physical, mental, and emotional health, not to mention our ecology? Yogis, saints, and great teachers have proclaimed selfless surrender to be the solution to every problem and the secret to every mystery. The act of surrender strongly aligns with having faith and devotion, along with discipline or tapas,[52] as the cornerstones of spiritual development. Tapas strengthens the mind to overcome obstacles that can retard our progress. The obstacles in life are the tests that make us stronger and help us to understand ourselves better.

There is a story that the great young Swami Rama Tirtha tells about his daylong struggle to solve a mathematical equation. Finally, when he decided to give up—some accounts say he also was about to surrender his life—the answer

---

51   One of the three main types of karma, along with *sanchitta* (sum of our past karmas, good and bad, which are changeable) and *purushakara* (results of our current actions). *Prarabdhakarma* is charted in the birth natal chart or horoscope, the picture of the sky at the time of one's birth.

52   One of the fundamental components of the yoga system. It is considered the platform to spiritual living and a necessary aspect of attaining health and wellness in the mind-body. In yoga, it is also related to asceticism. The great sage Patanjali considers it one of the three main constituents of the Kriya Yoga system. It is said that when pure tapas is developed, it leads to perfection or enlightenment.

came to him. He says that when you chase after Vedanta, it keeps running from you; but when you surrender and stop seeking it, you discover the truth directly inside you. "The greatest sadhu, the greatest Indian monk, the greatest swami in this world is the Sun, the rising Sun."

> *The sun is the soul that gives us light, guides us, and teaches us that it is always there. Everywhere we are, all we need to do is surrender to its presence.*

One of the other important principles that is a great complement to the attitude of surrender is self-study or introspective analysis, known as svadhyaya. If we analyze ourselves, our own lives can become our scriptures. Through self-analysis, we can understand who we have become, discover where we are headed, and embrace where we have been. Many have reduced svadhyaya to intellectual study and memorization of words and phrases in scriptures. However, the practical way to apply this very valuable principle is to find the answers we seek in the experience of our own *sva* or life.

The highest principle of surrender is ishvara pranidhana ("commitment to the Lord"). It is the last of the introductory yoga-dharma principles, because it is the most powerful stance one can take to succeed on the spiritual path. On my first trip to India, I learned to surrender through the many circumstances that kept arising. Various occurrences tested my understanding, not to mention my patience, and prompted me to question "who" I was. Eventually, I learned it was more important to change my attitude than to try to change my outer circumstances, although it is sometimes necessary to remove ourselves from certain circumstances. It seems that India has the capacity to teach us many things about ourselves, especially Western spiritual aspirants traveling there for the first time. I highly encourage it. Many of the deepest yogic teachings can be discovered in the subtle nuances of the culture.

Many of the expectations I carried had to be destroyed or transformed: everything from the timing of the train to ideas I had about the way my yoga and meditation should be, just because I was in India. Everything I did or tried to do on my first sojourn practically forced me to surrender, "let go," adapt, and change to become someone new.

These lessons culminated when I was counseled by a monk named Swami Vishwananda. He suggested several things about my meditation practice that in a metaphorical sense said a lot about how I was living my life at the time. My practice was not in full accord with my actions. He said, "It's important not to get caught up in the mechanics of things or that everything should be in some perfect order, but more important is the end result. For example, if you are meditating regularly and then spending the rest of your day in meaningless activities, without right thought or presence of mind, then your whole day has been wasted and the meditation was rendered useless. Practice meditation and the techniques but then surrender them and hold on to the unchangeable, God."

The key is to hold on to the quality of consciousness cultivated in meditation as long as we can. In later years, I understood this as staying in present awareness, in the present moment, observant of all things. Many of the experiences of my inaugural trip to the motherland began to make more and more sense to me later. I learnt that meditation was not just a matter of sitting and practicing various techniques and rituals, but was about arriving at a new place of awareness and holding on to that insight and consciousness in everything I did.

Everything in the universe is trying to guide us back to the soul magnet, a special place that everyone is seeking, some consciously and others unconsciously. As mentioned earlier, fear is the most destructive of emotions, as it cripples the mind by creating limitations and obstacles. Also, fear attaches the mind to materialistic things and superstitious outcomes. Fears create illusion. On the other hand, ishvara pranidhana is a practice of real surrender to God, embracing the idea that we are not completely in control of our lives. Proper yoga sadhana teaches us how to work with unseen and mysterious forces, removing the veil of illusion that fear creates. What we do have control over is how we adjust and adapt to life's circumstances as our life slowly transforms itself. How we do things becomes much more powerful than what we do or try to do.

People try to control out of fear of a certain outcome and the emotional pain associated with it. The more suppressed or unresolved emotional experiences become, the greater the need to control our outer environment. The yogic concept of surrender is the most powerful technique one can practice to release the mind from fear. Yogis like Krishna and Rama were warriors or Kshatriyas, fearless and peaceful as they dealt with many challenging life circumstances. They had families, they were kings, and they overcame radical challenges during their lives. A great king or queen sits at the throne of omnipresence by learning to shut off the mind through pratyahara and experience the profound surrender that is Divine.

The value of these core yoga principles comes about holistically, when they are practiced integrally, beginning with a sound foundation in the yamas and niyamas. Over time, they help us develop the necessary state of mind and character required for using the body as an instrument in asana and pranayama.

If our social and personal life is not in accord with natural law, the use of the postures and breathing techniques can create physical and mental complications.

The core principles I have discussed are the foundation for lifestyle reformation and a prerequisite for health and wellness. Yoga stretches alone are not enough to bring us health, and fall short of yoga's grand goal. In other words, the way in which we live our life, the yamas and niyamas, significantly influence what we become, regardless of how much yoga we are practicing. These first two yoga limbs, which enumerate social and personal guidelines for balanced living, can be studied at traditional lineage-based yoga schools or most ashrams. I have found the writings of Paramahansa Yogananda, distributed by the organization he founded, the Self-Realization Fellowship, to be the most thorough and concise teachings on how to live a balanced and purposeful life.

Service in Yoga

Our ability to surrender is largely dependent on the discipline that we can create in service to others (*seva*). The yoga traditions have thrived longer than any other ancient tradition mainly on acts of selfless service to humanity. Service has always been a part of any culture that lives for a higher purpose. It is becoming more and more evident that the concept of service and barter will become the business model of the new age, with companies, families, and individuals exchanging services and commodities with one another, rather than commerce being based on monetary currency that actually has no "real value" or credibility.

There was a time in America when all currency was actually backed by gold or silver, but eventually this was no longer possible. It seems that stock markets and the value of the dollar depend greatly on the psychological mood of the country as interpreted by the media. Any type of economics, either personal or societal, based on spending or taxation will eventually fail, as it goes against the law of exchange or karma. The law of karma means that for every action or intention there is an equal reaction: cause and effect. If the majority of the world holds to a consciousness of buying, taking, spending, and acquiring, the universe will need to find some way to keep the earth in balance.

The concept of seva will eventually save the business world and our economies from complete destruction. Until then, global economies continue to teeter, along with idea that everything will continue to rise. It is said that what goes up must come down. Living and working on the basis of the idea that value of homes, real estate, and the cost of goods and services will just continue to rise is blind as the wind. These things may be difficult to understand at the present time, but Vedanta is not confined to India. It is the most practical and efficient way for us to evolve as a species.

Seva extends to anything we do to propagate the balance of life. When we serve the whole, we serve ourselves. I am not discrediting the value of being an individual or the importance of making choices in work or life that benefit us directly. The power of seva, however, comes in a more subtle form. As we serve others, we take attention off our own selves, the "I" self. The secret lies in the mind shifting its attention off the body, senses, and desires. Seva is the Karma Yoga way to purify our samskaras or habitual tendencies and buried selfish desires. When we find ways to serve each other, we help ourselves understand that we are all interconnected, to nature and all living things.

Seva can give people a sense of purpose and direction. It is the vehicle that carries the yoga practitioner, or anyone for that matter, to an integral approach to yoga. In Karma Yoga, all expectations of an outcome should be removed. Seva is a doorway into metaphysics, a type of informal training where not only discipline is developed, but many other powerful yogic practices such as renunciation (*sanyas*) and surrendering our attachment to the fruits of our actions (*tyaga*). Both are core teachings of the Bhagavad Gita.

Another powerful yoga practice that aligns well with the act of service is *japa yoga mantra*. This practice involves repeating powerful Sanskrit mantras while service or a chore is being performed. These are affirmations that help remove the mental clutter that veils our peace and enable us to have greater awareness. The old adage rings true: "What we think, we become."

True seva free of any personal gain or profit can teach us great patience and how to surrender to the next phase of life. Seva helps us embrace the spiritual path, which is slow, long, and requires walking the razor's edge. In Hindu mythology, Hanuman is the monkey God who personified service and loyalty, as poetically expressed in the epic story the Ramayana.

Seva has been the backbone of the yoga tradition for thousands of years. There many major dharmic organizations throughout India that operate solely on service and donations. Such organizations, founded by yogis figures like Mata Amritanandamayi, Satya Sai Baba, and Sri Sri Ravi Shankar, to name a few, have built schools and hospitals, and provided aid in natural disasters and food, clothes, and shelter for millions throughout India and the world.

In India, yoga has never been a business, as it has become in the West. Yoga will only endure through selfless service by those working for the higher good of mankind. Rather than spending so much time making ourselves happy, we can serve others. In return, a blessed gift is received: greater compassion for the world. Swami Vivekananda said, "The law of life is giving." When we practice seva, we not only benefit ourselves karmically, but we serve the great ones who have upheld these truths as living examples of the great scriptures.

Chapter FIVE

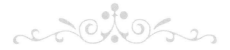

Purification and Restoration

Natural forces within us are the true healers of disease.
Hippocrates (Physician 460 BC - 370 BC)

What Is Detoxification and Why Is It So Important Today?

Detoxification is one of the most important themes in both yoga and Ayurveda. It is also a very popular topic for the modern urban dweller, who lives a life of excessive input and stimulation from the buzz of cities. Today, when most people speak of or hear the word "detox," they are referring to some kind of diet or juicing regimen that promotes weight loss.

The concept of detoxification is not new. Both the yoga and Ayurveda systems provide profound guidelines for it. Even the concept of rebirth or reincarnation, as it is commonly called, is based on the idea that we must remove desires, impurities, and karmas from our lives to attain ultimate enlightenment. The concept of detoxification is more like a process of "purification" that we go through in life as we become increasingly cleansed. Rather than removing something that is bad in us, we are actually focusing on increasing that which is good, pure, and positive in us. This is particularly important on the level of healing the mind.

Ayurveda provides two forms for healing the internal systems. These are known as *shodhana*, strong detoxification protocols, and *shamana*, gentler, lifestyle-based purification. For those who have a strong immune system and a sturdy constitution. Ayurveda uses a system called pancha karma (five actions), which integrates a multitude of treatments, diet, and other cleansing methods to remove toxicity from the body. Pancha karma is the go-to system of most Ayurvedic practitioners, and is usually offered in a clinical or retreat setting.

For those who may not require such a profound level of cleansing, a less aggressive form of purification is recommended. The seven shamana (palliation) lifestyle interventions are light diet, juice or water fasting, different types of exercises, sunbathing, fresh air, herbs that to increase metabolic strength, and herbs that remove bodily toxins or ama.

One of the ways I am able to express my creativity is in finding unique strategies for each client to integrate the appropriate healing procedures into their lifestyle. In some cases, where a person has no history of purification and some general toxic build-up from poor diet, air quality, and possibly prescription medications, I create a program that combines a bit of both shodhana and shamana therapies to ease them into cleansing over a longer period of time. Alternatively, when a person is highly toxic, overweight and mentally stressed-out, they benefit from starting off with a strong cleansing program and then continuing with gentler interventions integrated into their lifestyle over weeks and months.

In classical yoga, purification is mostly centered on removing disturbances from the mind. In contrast, Hatha Yoga considers physical detoxification a prerequisite to higher forms of practice like meditation. After we take in food and sensory impressions from our environment (*ahara*), they must also be released (*vihara*). This is one of nature's fundamental laws, the law of give and take. Mental and physical health and wellness require this exchange to maintain balance.

In Hatha Yoga, the postures, breathing techniques, and withdrawal of energy from the five senses form the three primary, vital aspects of purification. These three practical techniques form inseparable links that support purification and healing of the whole being, and serve as stepping stones to the higher inner practices of meditation. Yoga uses asana to purify the body by increasing metabolic strength, the jatharagni, and to remove dullness and tightness in the muscles, joints, and spine, while massaging the internal organs during various positions.

One thing that is unique about Hatha Yoga is its emphasis on creating flexibility and suppleness in the spine, which directly influences the functioning of the nervous system. Unlike modern fitness and sports, which can stress the muscles and internal organs with the impact of jarring activity, yoga gently massages the internal organs, improving their function and exposing areas that may be weak or dysfunctional. In other words, it's a powerful and direct way to impact the doshas that operate in the digestive organs, mainly the stomach, colon, and small intestine.

From a broader perspective, yoga aims at purification by establishing the mind in sattva guna, its natural state of stillness, calmness, and peace. Although yoga asana has the powerful effect of purifying the inner organs and nervous system, its higher intention is preparing the mind for meditation. Spinal preparation for meditation basically links the mind and the spine-body through the nervous system. The nervous system in turn affects the nadis[53] or energy channels that flow through the entire body and control physical health, quality of mind, and the balance of life.

The feeling that one gains from a good yoga asana practice is one of expansion and wholeness. As with most physical exercises, there is a feeling of contentment. In this regard, we can infer that the body also influences how the mind feels. While the mind is the master of the body, there seems to be an interesting energetic exchange between the two entities. When there has been an excess of ahara, as in too much intake of food or sensory impressions, the body begins to feel bogged down and the mind becomes agitated. Every "mind-body" relationship is unique and functions differently. So, depending on our lifestyle, environment, and karma, the harmony between the two can vary and the manner in which the mind and body fracture can also be very different. The transformative power of yoga asana depends on its being practiced along with pranayama or breathing techniques and pratyahara or restoration. These three techniques serve to relink the mind-body by detoxifying the body through the asanas and balancing the mind through breath control and nervous-system relaxation, which is an ancient form of what medicine now calls neuroplasticity.[54]

The simple practice of resting after postures has a profound effect on the purifying the central nervous system and the nadis, the more subtle pranic pathways. As the body's energy channels are expanded and cleared with fresh prana, they allow new, evolutionary adaptation, reprogramming how the cells and the hippocampus and cerebellum in the brain operate. The relaxation response given to the body through asana and pranayama practice is called pratyahara. This practice involves surrendering into stillness and shifting the mind into a witnessing state of awareness, which brings healing to the emotional body. Emotional as well as body and mind purification is a necessary part of a balanced yogic lifestyle. Asana, pranayama, and pratyahara provide physical,

---

53 Subtle energetic pathways that run through the body carrying life force energy. There are said to be 72,000 of these, of which three (ida, pingala, and sushumna) are the main channels, balancing the male and female qualities and serving as the major, central conduit that connects the chakras, the energy vortices along the spine.

54 It is now scientifically proven that the brain can change throughout life and is not a static organ.

mental, and emotional purification and furnish the well-being needed for spiritual evolution. Raja Yoga as an integral system is focused on purification or shodhana, but with psycho-spiritual intention. Hatha Yoga initially focuses on shodhana of the physical body as a preparation for higher and more subtle meditative practices.

Ayurveda purifies through diet, herbs, oil massage, sweating, and other body treatments such as in pancha karma or five actions. This removes accumulation of the doshas from their respective sites, the internal organs, and complements yoga asana and pranayama. The magic of the yoga and Ayurveda systems during purification is their capacity to rebuild the tissues or dhatus and restore energy equally. Both synergistically detoxify and restore mind and body.

Creating a Balanced Methodology for Detoxification

The process of detoxification can be challenging in many ways, physically, mentally, and emotionally, depending on the level of toxicity. An individual constitution and many other important factors should always be considered before beginning a program. Ayurveda has two main methods of bringing the doshas into balance. Removing excess toxins, fat, congestion, and anything that appears to be an obstacle to the balance of the doshas is called *langhana*. Ayurvedic therapies that have a cleansing or reducing affect are emetics or therapeutic vomiting (*vamana*), enemas (*basti*), nasal-cleansing procedures (*shiro-virechana*), and the other lifestyle protocols just mentioned. Balancing yoga postures,[55] such as one-legged poses and vinyasa-type sequences, produce body heat and have excellent reductive qualities. Strong pranayama like Kapalabhati and Bastrika also works well in this regard.

The other aspect of creating balance is directed towards those who lack strength or immunity, or have chronic fatigue. This can occur in all dosha types, although it is most commonly found in vata and pitta types. Tonification (*brimhana*) is about building strength in the body's tissues through diet and weight-bearing exercises like static weight-lifting or core-strengthening yoga postures, such as plank, chair, and bow.

With excess-vata conditions that create weakness, loss of weight, and lack of balance, a consistent regimen that strengthens the digestive capacity is critical. The ability to absorb nutrients more fully calls for a rich and nutritious warm-food diet and tonic herbs, including ashwagandha, bala, and shatavari. The depth and quality of rest should be increased.

---

55   See Chapter 7: Asana: The Vehicle of Yoga

Excess pitta conditions require rebuilding energy, after excessive wearing of the body and mental unrest, through a moderate approach to healing. This includes a diet of cooling and soothing foods, such as sweet fruits, grains, and bitter green vegetables. Gentle and relaxing exercise regimens are also called for.

Kapha types usually do not require much tonifying, owing to the greater density of their muscle, fat, and bone tissues. Whether the need is to reduce or strengthen the body, it is important to know which dosha is out of balance and the level of toxic build-up, so as to be able to create a balanced methodology for purifying the body.

Purification and Restoration in Yoga

In the Vedic teachings, two primary energetic principles come together: agni, the sacred fire of transformation, and soma, the soothing nectar of healing. Essentially, these are the subtle vibrations of the sun and moon, which influence the body and mind. Many of today's health issues are due to the strong emphasis on physical culture, including asana, along with over-stimulated lifestyles. It's not that asana is not a good way to combat the stress of the modern lifestyle. The issue is that asana can tax the body, deplete the tissues, and create adrenal fatigue or deficiency, especially with very intense power or hot-yoga styles. You may feel less stress, but at the cost of also feeling exhausted.

It has become all too common to see a "health" enthusiast or yogi begin their practice or day with a cup of coffee or energy drink. In order to purify the body properly, we must also consider the mind. Such stimulation can eventually lead to adrenal fatigue, and is associated with chronic fatigue syndrome. A balanced and purified body requires the same qualities in the mind.

On another level, the force of agni represents the transformative qualities produced by the energy of the sun. Heat transforms how we live and keeps all aspects of our life evolving. This sacred fire keeps us yearning for the answers to the mystery of creation. On the cooling side, soma reflects the qualities of the moon to sustain, support, and nourish us. For the purposes of increasing awareness, yoga aims at balancing the sun and moon energies. Yoga recognizes the capacity these forces have to purify the body through increased heat, sweat, and the secretion of other internal enzymes.

However, yoga considers the energy of the moon equally important for recharging and healing the body. Heat cleanses the body, but the cooling energy is what actually heals it. Medical practices focused on removing the symptoms of a disease through aggressive protocols, such as prescription medications and surgery, do so at an expense to the body, especially the nervous and immune systems. These interventions never really consider measures for restoring energy, and this often leads to other complications.

Medical doctors tell us to get plenty of rest and lie idle. However, doing nothing does not necessarily restore us. Although rest may provide us with a feeling of increased energy, this is often superficial and does not actually rejuvenate us deeply. Much of this is because the mind is not purified and rested along with the body, as it continues to be stimulated by media, caffeine, and exhausting verbal chatter. Yoga works with these energies on the level of mind, removing negative or disturbing currents by neutralizing (nirodha) them with positive ones.

Agni and soma later became known as the Gods Brahman and Vishnu in the teachings of *Sanatana Dharma*,[56] which is Sanskrit for *The Eternal Tradition*. There is no doubt that the moment we stand on our two feet, which are philosophically related to the element of fire, and place the body in a vertical position, we begin to feel the energies of the body change and become warmer. Thus, asana has a strong capacity to create warmth by raising the subtle heat present in each of the thirteen fires[57] that exist in the body.

The main difference between integral yoga, which connects asana with pranayama and relaxation exercises, and standard fitness-based exercise, is that comprehensive yoga should leave the practitioner energized. Standard physical exercise is usually exhausting and drains the life sap or *ojas*. The purpose of asana is not to exhaust the body and mind, but to awaken and distribute dormant energies. This brings enormous vitality to the body, rooted in balanced systemic function and reflected in a calm, present state of awareness. If asana is practiced independent of other tools, such as pranayama and relaxation response techniques, it is then not much different than physical exercise, and is reduced to a good sweat and stretch.

Hatha Yoga should have both detoxifying and restorative qualities, as was its original intention. You might wonder how the application of rigorous asanas can be restorative. In the first place, Hatha Yoga was not traditionally practiced as a variety of postures sequenced and piled one on top of the other, with little or no rest periods such as corpse pose or Savasana. This aerobic approach is a more recent methodology connected to the Mysore tradition of Krishnamach-

---

56   The original name of Hinduism.

57   In Ayurvedic physiology, there are agnis (fires) for each of the five elements and seven tissues (dhatus), as well as one for the digestive metabolic system. Each of these fires supports creation of the harmonious and balanced functioning of the entire physical body.

arya, which has created such spin-off styles as "flow," "power," and "vinyasa." In America, this non-stop, hyper-active approach to asana sequences has now replaced the aerobic movement of the 1970s and '80s, which has since practically disappeared, as most fitness crazes do.

My view is that we do not need to reinvent yoga, but rather we should practice yoga so it can change us.

The key to yoga's actually healing and energizing rather than depleting and reducing immunity requires embracing a sadhana or practice that combines activity and passivity. Rest in yoga is called Savasana or corpse pose. This could be considered the most important and mystical of the postures, because the name symbolizes precisely what yoga is trying to do for us: kill identification with the physical body. The posture itself induces the relaxation response, which can lead to the experience of peace. When the body is brought to a still position in Savasana, the body can recharge its energy.

The interchange between asana and Savasana is not about regaining energy that has been expended. It is actually a scientific system for gradually building and increasing energy levels as the practice progresses over time. The yogis were clever, and were not only aware of the effects of lactic acid build-up in the bloodstream, but understood how to reduce it by oxygenating the body through pranayama.

On the spiritual level, corpse pose is a practice of dissolving the mind-body identification, and this begins with the feeling of relaxation. We connect and then learn to disconnect from this feeling repeatedly, until the senses are finally so purified that we attain a feeling of contentment, peace, and equanimity. I will discuss Savasana further in the Yoga Therapy chapter, explaining its particulars and deeper healing attributes.

As we increase the capacity to internalize our awareness via the instruments of the mind and body, we increase our receptivity to prana, the life force. It is like closing one door of body consciousness to allow another to open. The second door, that of pure consciousness, is the one that sustains us as human beings and is the source of all health and happiness. It is not just the body that can become toxic. The mind can also become toxic through attachment to the body and senses, the fears of being alone and abandoned, and many other obstacles that force the mind into "I"dentification. Only from the domain of pure consciousness can any real healing occur. This is the source of power accessed by yogis in attaining magical powers called *siddhis*. Yoga teaches us how to access this saintly domain of consciousness, which exists within us like a portable paradise. Today's lifestyles keep us mentally exteriorized and superficially stimulated and entertained. We think and believe that we need to acquire something outside of ourselves to feel good, be happy, and so on.

The practice of Savasana is a powerful technique of sensory purification vital to restoring the soma energies in the body, which deal with the nervous and endocrine systems. If yoga practitioners over-stimulated with adrenaline continue to practice asana without rest, they will eventually do the opposite of promoting their health. The vital ojas energy that is our borrowed Divine nectar, and also sustains our heart and bodily tissues, can become depleted by a yoga practice that does not include restoration.

As a yoga teacher and director of my own center in Los Angeles for 15 years, I have seen much of what I have just described. Week after week, I continue to see students coming in for yoga class with all the indicators of adrenal fatigue and stress written across their faces. I know the last thing they need is to expend more energy outwardly through asana.

I recommend that most people practice yoga slowly and gradually build up to the amount of asana their body needs. Many factors should be considered, such as dosha type, background in other forms of physical culture, and general health history. I encourage everyone on two points. The first is to establish consistency of practice by attending class one to two times per week, with the intention of maintaining this schedule for at least one year. This also applies for those practicing at home. Secondly, I encourage everyone to implement daily and seasonal routines as taught in Ayurveda, so their lifestyle is conducive to purification and mental focus.

For the most part, the first few years of yoga practice and Ayurvedic lifestyle are a process of purification and detoxification. The mind gradually unwinds to a slower and more attuned level of awareness.

In many instances, I start yoga classes with the simple and gentle exercise of alternate-nostril breathing to balance and calm students' minds. This is done standing or sometimes seated. Then I ask the class to take Savasana and practice the tensing and releasing technique of energizing the vital energy points (*marma*) in the body. After this calming technique is completed, the entire room is still and quiet. I then have the students remain in Savasana for the entire duration of the sixty- to ninety-minute class. This is what most urbanites need, especially by the end of the day, after the body and mind have been over-stimulated. This type of mindfulness in yoga practice leads to a good night's sleep.

If, after sunset, yoga asana and pranayama are excessively stimulating or taxing, the mind-body relationship is disturbed. The mind and adrenals are reactivated. This not only makes it difficult to fall asleep at a reasonable time, but also, once the body is asleep, the mind remains awake in the dream state. It continues to send disturbing nerve impulses throughout the body, expending energy during a time of restoration. I will expand on this further in the chapter on lifestyle.

Restoration in Nature

Nature undergoes a process of restoration through internalization as she passes through the cycles of the seasons. In this process, the elements change, adapt, restore, and continue to perpetuate life. Nature has its own dharma or duty, and that is to support the balance of the planet earth regardless of what humans take from it. Whenever we take from Divine Mother Nature, we should give back in some way. It is not a one-way relationship, but involves give, take, and share. Yoga teaches us that everything is Brahman, of one creator, and each of us plays a role in the collective life of the planet.

Nature's seasonal cycles basically follow the sun, as the earth completes its rotation. The earth's seasons are the result of the tilt of the earth's axis. The intake of sunlight, rain, nutrients, and other subtle particles in summer allows nature to go through a period of absorption (*ahara*) of the sun's rays. These energies are gradually internalized through the autumn, and completely withdrawn in winter. In winter, nature is sustained through a direct link to the subtle magnetic fire (*vishnuabhi*). This core energy brings the pancha maha bhutas (five great elements) into manifestation, and is behind the life energies that control the creative, destructive, and sustaining forces on planet Earth.

Although the human body's anatomy is somewhat different from nature's, the physiological process for maintaining a balanced life is similar. My point is that the physical body and nature are intrinsically linked and function in a synchronized manner. The five great elements exist in nature and in our specialized human form. The only difference is the rate of vibration: the outer forms of the elements, visible in nature, are grosser.

The wisdom of Ayurveda is so effective because its teaching is based on scientific facts that serve to balance our body organically. The practice of asana can be compared to the growth and expansion of plants and trees in the spring and summer. Asanas expand the flexibility of our muscle tissue, increase mobility in our joints, and help circulate blood and oxygen. The postures give suppleness to the body.

Similarly, in spring and summer, plants grow and expand in shape and size. Nature performs her own dance of bliss (*ananda tandava*)[58] when she emerges from a period of hibernation and is in contact with the source of the inner sacred fire of knowledge, health, and higher consciousness. When we learn to turn our energies inward to the practice of meditation to resolve the obstacles and fluctuations life brings, we will experience joy and contentment, our own dance of Shiva.

It is the journey of turning our attention inward throughout the trials and tribulations of life that brings us growth. Success should not be measured by our material prosperity, but rather by our level of courage, endurance, and state of contentment. The greatest threat to maintaining our balance is the force of illusion or maya. Maya is quite mysterious. We must be clever so that we can use life's intriguing and thought-provoking experiences to look beyond the literal meaning of maya's illusionary effects and potentially to discover the Divine hand of nature guiding us towards resolution. All of life's experiences are linked. Resolutions bring restoration of our vital energies.

Many have misunderstood the use of the term "withdrawal" in yoga. Just to be clear, it by no means endorses escaping, running away, or acting irresponsibly. Withdrawal or ahara means to practice yoga in a mystical manner, so that it can bring solutions to all life's problems, while affording us many long-term benefits along the way. Yoga is not a quick-fix system. It is mainly concerned with the greater transformation of our life. When the scriptures and great gurus speak about the "inner journey" that all must eventually take for the attainment of bliss, they speak from an absolute state of awareness, which means they have reached the highest level of attunement. For us as aspirants (*sadhakas*), it is the practice of going inward that matters, because in time this brings us closer to the everlasting fountain of bliss.

Sexuality is the greatest externalization of our energy, and can be the most depleting physically and mentally if not used in accordance with nature's laws. Therefore, how we express and share it with another should always be with the right intention. An integral approach to yoga teaches us to become more observant of life, including our own thoughts, feelings, and actions. Certainly, the daily practice of integral yoga gradually brings us a calmer state of mind,

---

58   Lord Shiva as Nataraj is the cosmic dancer, and in this mythological dance he represents the rhythmic movements of the cycles of creation, preservation, and dissolution.

which improves our capacity to make decisions and attain greater intuition. Remember, the benefits come slowly, but are long-lasting. We can never blame outer circumstances, but must look at ourselves to question how certain circumstances were brought about.

Over billions of years nature has continued to endure countless changes in climate and oceanic fluctuations, while growing and sustaining different forms of life on the planet. Like pranayama, nature breathes through the process of photosynthesis,[59] a process of intake and output that sustains a rhythm of transformation and growth.

Pranayama techniques are specially-designed exercises that improve the quality of our blood. The various actions of these techniques help remove waste products dumped into the bloodstream by the cells, liver, and kidneys. When yoga asanas are combined with specialized breathing techniques and pratyahara, techniques of relaxation and sensory withdrawal, small valves in the blood vessels open and close, increasing the supply of oxygen in the blood. Red blood corpuscles carry not only oxygen but life force, prana, to the cells. Every corpuscle is a tiny battery of life energy.[60] Good blood is essentially good energy. One must wonder why we would ever need anything like caffeine, as everything needed for energy is in our blood. Poor diet, urban air quality, and a lack of proper exercise diminish the quality of our blood, as does lack of emotional balance.

In the winter, nature retreats, supported by stored solar energies and elements absorbed during summer and fall. Winter is dependent on the subtle lunar forces of nature, the cosmic intelligence (*mahat*) that sustains life. The practice of sensory internalization provides a resting place for us to witness the unfolding of who we are. It is the first step in the process of self-realization. Pratyahara is a natural process that supports the balance of nature and our own growth and development as spiritual beings.

On a smaller scale, a parallel can be observed in the twenty-four hour day. Each of the four seasons corresponds to different times of the day. In the morning, the spring season is reflected in cool temperatures, freshness in the air, and a call to begin the day with a clear conscience. The morning period is associated with kapha dosha, as water has spring-like qualities. Asana and bodily exercise

---

59   The process by which green plants and some other organisms use sunlight to synthesize food from carbon dioxide and water. Photosynthesis in plants generally involves the green pigment chlorophyll, and generates oxygen as a byproduct.

60   See: "The Divine Art of Erasing Age and Creating Vitality" by Paramahansa Yogananda, *Self-Realization Magazine*, Fall 2007 (Self-Realization Fellowship, Los Angeles.)

cultivate mind-body discipline optimally in the morning, strengthening the metabolic rate and keeping muscles and joints supple throughout the day.

As the clock arrives at noon, summer is represented, with the day's temperature reaching its highest point. During the middle of the day, blood flows fastest and our lungs operate more rapidly. This allows us to process ideas and perform and complete tasks briskly. Pranayama is likened to mid-day, as it exercises our lungs and increases our capacity to use the greatest amount of energy available to us. With every inspiring breath, there is an expiration of karma. The breath and karma are related: breath gives us life, and life is made up of series of actions that are inspired by our breath.

As the day transitions to evening, temperatures begin to lower, as in fall. Our energy also begins to retreat. Energy in the form of sunlight can be very healthy. Short intervals of sunbathing are an essential practice for physical and mental restoration. However, with over-exposure, sunlight can be depleting and drain our ojas.

This is why people sometimes feel the need to take a late afternoon nap, which Ayurveda recommends in the summer, because the powerful strength of the sun drains our energy, which, with a short rest, can be restored. It is a common practice today to counter the natural withdrawal that occurs in the afternoon by taking some stimulant like coffee that prolongs the momentum of midday energy. However, this superficial alternative takes energy from the adrenals, is short-lasting, and can eventually weaken the immune system.

The time from 2 – 6 PM is vata. To maintain balance, we need to redirect the mind-body energies inwards through various methods of energy withdrawal. Interestingly, some cultures like the European take a break from work every afternoon, and then work later in the night. The evening is a natural period to begin the process of unwinding the mind from external sensory stimulants and attachments, in order to keep the doshas in balance and maintain the body's energy.

At night, when the sun goes under the horizon, cooler or cold temperatures symbolize winter. The darkness of the night is the ultimate state of separation from the body and mind, which occurs during sleep. All identity with body, name, and association is lost. Meditation, the culmination of our yoga practice, is reflected in the darkness of night. Meditation guides us through the night to find the inner sunlight at the mystical point between the eyebrows. At night, the body and a balanced mind recharge their energies in the deep sleep state.

The modern urban dweller suffers from a very active mind, and while the body may be slowing down, mental movies continue playing, leaving the body far from restored. Meditation is the practice that allows us to access the positive energies of night. It not only improves the quality of but reduces the need for sleep. It is helpful to understand the energies of the daily cycle in order to adapt our practices and routines more efficiently. Ancient cultures, such as Vedic India, had a close understanding of the workings of these subtle energies and how they operate in time and space.

We should all have an appreciation of the benefits of physical exercise. But when practicing asana, we should never lose sight of its underlying intention and purpose: the inner journey. This inner process heals the physical body and has the potential for healing the soul and reducing karma. In life as physical beings, we are either reducing or acquiring new karma. There is no in-between. Asana can be combined with pranayama in many different ways to induce restoration.

Postures and breathing techniques work together as both gross and subtle forms of healing and restoration. These practices are extremely purifying and restorative when practiced in nature. While postures treat the body broadly, as a whole, pranayama is a more specific way to work with energies in the body through the breath. Asana takes care of the body and moves the water and earth elements, while pranayama works with the fire element to ignite the kundalini shakti in the astral body. Nature brings balance to ether and air by providing a deep grounding space to absorb restless thoughts in the mind. Posture, breath, and exposure to the elements in nature combine in an integral way to balance the three doshas. Yoga works with nature to purify and restore us.

The Sacred Link to the Doshas

Both yoga and Ayurveda emphasize balance as a requisite to self-realization. On the physical level, Ayurveda aims to balance the energies of the doshas—vata, pitta and kapha—as they function in their various capacities. The Hatha Yoga system aims to bring balance to the subtle or astral body's sun and moon energies, which flow through the two main channels known as pingala nadi, the sun channel, and ida nadi, the moon channel. This harmonious relationship depends on a balance of the male energies of reason and the female energies of feeling. Astronomically speaking, these are also the two forces that influence the ebb and flow of the tides and govern the cycle of the seasons.

Hatha Yoga implies a sun-moon balance. This result is not arrived at through asana alone. Hatha Yoga combines the practice of asana and pranayama in an integrative manner, including the use of bhandas or locks and mudras or gestures to sustain and direct prana properly. Hatha Yoga is a preparation for meditation and a valuable way to improve the mind-body relationship.

The core therapeutic benefit of asana comes from holding the postures. This requires being still and concentrating, a practice not commonly implemented in modern health and fitness. I believe this is one reason for the overwhelming popularity of the vinyasa or "flow" approach to yoga, which revolves around sequencing postures without holding poses very long or giving much time to rest in between in order to restore vital energies.

The point here is not to blame the practitioners, but the lack of training teachers receive in the other limbs of yoga and in Ayurveda. Yoga follows Ayurvedic anatomy, which considers healing on the level of body, mind, and soul. It is helpful to learn modern western anatomy, but we should not depend entirely on this model in understanding how yoga benefits the body.

The Ayurvedic anatomy of the seven tissues can be connected to the doshas, chakras, emotions, and mind. This is particularly useful for any practitioner who is working with a client to assess the root causes of a health imbalance. I have had a number of clients over the years who came in for skin issues such as eczema and psoriasis, which are typically connected to high pitta and toxicity in the blood tissue (*rakta*). Pitta, the fire element, usually goes out of balance because of anger and resentment connected to the second and third chakras in the subtle body.

All disorders are born in the mind and move through the emotional body to impact the doshas, anatomy, and physiology, eventually causing the appearance of symptoms. This is an example of how a physical issue can be linked back to various causative factors. The power of this medicine is that it teaches us that healing is not simply a physical matter. Healing our physical body is a window that allows us to see how we can cultivate a greater understanding of who we are, how we are living, and what we need to do to change our relationship with ourselves, our community, and our living planet.

This is why we must always maintain the attitude that we are not these physical bodies. They have been given to us as vehicles for the transformation of our consciousness. Everyone should become aware of their elemental energies, and understand how they become doshas and impinge on bodily health. There is a two-fold basis for the practice of Ayurvedic medicine. There is a unique mind-body type, prakriti, which, when the elements become imbalanced due to lifestyle factors giving rise to various symptoms, is called vikriti. This wisdom is the birthright of all humanity and the one way we can return humanity to dharma.

The sacred link to our doshas demands we understand the qualities of nature's elements and draw nearer to the science of energy. Traditional yoga and Indian classical music and *vastu*[61] were aligned to the elements of the day and seasons. This scientific alignment to nature's elements brings about a gradual and subtle purification that keeps our miniature bodily universe synchronized to the grander universe, as taught in Samkhya philosophy.

The Power of Sweat

The fascination with sweating is nothing new. It has been a healing practice in many ancient cultures and traditions for centuries. The hammam or Turkish bath, the Mexican temescal, and the Native American sweat lodge were all used to purify the body and as spiritual rituals for releasing negative energies. The Finnish sauna was a popular social practice and a place to relax and share time with family and friends. There is obviously a psychological aspect to perspiring, because sweat is regulated by the sympathetic nervous system and adrenal glands. The modern lifestyle's tendency to stress the adrenal glands can cause excessive sweating in some individuals, and over time this leaves a person feeling depleted, and can eventually lead to chronic fatigue issues.

The adrenal cortex produces cortisol, a hormone that functions to produce and store energy. When sweat therapies are used for detoxification purposes, they must always be combined with some form of restoration and cooling. This is what distinguishes Ayurvedic sweating or fomentation therapies from the practices of other cultures. Three main factors govern Ayurvedic use of sweat therapy for detoxification and maintaining health. The primary factor is regarding the head, which, as it contains sensitive organs like the eyes and brain, should not be heated. The second consideration is the season. Depending on the climate, excessive heat or sweat therapies should be minimized in the summer, as the season naturally induces sweat in daily living.

The third and most specific factor is the individual prakriti or constitution and vikriti or imbalance. This is also considered when determining the duration of

---

61   The Vedic science of construction or architecture. The Sanskrit word vastu means a substance or article. It considers the pancha maha bhutas (five great elements), astrology, geography, and even the individual's dosha type as part of its methods.

the treatment and also the type of sweating device to be used. Ayurveda has a full-body steam bath called *svedhana* implemented as part of the pancha karma system. Other types of fomentation are used in a more localized fashion to address specific areas like major arm and leg joints or the lower back muscles. This type of steam therapy is called nadi svedhana.

While all dosha types can benefit from sweating, length and frequency should be adjusted according to type. Kapha types take the greatest time to perspire and can enjoy steam baths at high temperatures without any concern of provoking an imbalance. Vata types also benefit from sweat therapies, but should take heat in lesser amounts and for shorter durations to avoid drying out. Pitta types should enjoy a small amount of sweating therapy administered infrequently, especially for those living in tropical climates.

The skin is often considered to be the largest organ in the body. The porous qualities in the epidermis allow it to take in oxygen and almost anything it is exposed to. The epidermis is composed of the outermost layers of the skin. It forms a protective barrier over the body's surface and is responsible for keeping water in the body and preventing pathogens from entering. The epidermis also helps the skin regulate body temperature. The dermis is the layer of skin beneath the epidermis and consists of connective tissues that cushion the body from stress and strain.

The endocrine system is directly linked to dhatu or tissue strength and density. In Ayurveda, the quality of these tissues is measured by the strength of the agni or fire that supports each of them. Although a good capacity to sweat and heat the body is necessary for maintaining the tissues and balanced endocrine function, pitta types who are not cautious when using sweat therapies or yoga practices can develop estrogen deficiencies. The role of estrogen deficiency in skin-aging and wound-healing can serve as an initial marker for the onset of greater complications with menstruation, fertility, and, potentially, immune disorders.

In Ayurveda, the skin is considered to provide a major entryway for the delivery of vital herbal medicines carried through oils. The importance of the skin must not be overlooked, as oils, herbs, and foods can be absorbed through the skin to nourish the entire body and its systems. This is called oleation (*snehana*) and sweating (svedhana). These are preliminary practices (**purvakarma**) for preparing the body for detoxification in the pancha karma system.

The practice of self-massage is called *abhyanga* and is endorsed as a powerful practice in a daily preventative-medicine routine. The external oleation of the body serves two primary purposes. Oils infused with herbal medicines begin to penetrate the epidermis, into the dermis and beyond, to loosen subtle toxins known as *ama* that get clogged in the bodily tissues. Consistent and repetitious strokes aid in loosening these toxins. When this is followed by svedhana or steam therapy, the heat opens the pores, pushing sweat through to cleanse bodily channels and pathways.

Oiling the body also has a powerful nourishing effect, bringing nutrition (*rasa*) to the tissues. This is like feeding the body through the skin to nourish the plasma, purify and strengthen the blood, improve muscular flexibility and joint mobility, balance nervous system function, increase immunity, and calm the mind. Steam or any heat therapy, including yoga asana practice, aims at detoxification. While oiling the body promotes energy intake, the process is complete only when sweat, moved by subtle pranic currents, releases toxins.

In the broadest sense, the main function of this staple Ayurvedic practice is intake and output, which also impact the direction and flow of prana. Snehana and svedhana both improve digestion by strengthening the jatharagni or digestive fire, and increase the main respiratory function in the heart and lungs (*pranvaha srota*). This is especially the case when oils containing stimulants like camphor, eucalyptus, tulsi, mint, and thyme are used. Oleation and yogic practices combine powerfully to increase the function of the pranvaha srota.

Abhyanga or self-massage is an important prerequisite to asana and pranayama, as the oils increase the body's agility and help stimulate lymphatic function, which helps release toxins from the body. Fomentation can also be done with a warm to hot bath to which oils and vata-alleviating herbal decoctions have been added. The use of any heating therapy or yoga practice has its precautions and should be adjusted with the factors just mentioned: head, season, and dosha type. Other specific precautions on the use of heating therapies include: high pitta vikriti, physical weakness, excessive thirst, use of strong drugs or alcohol, pregnancy, diarrhea, jaundice, skin rash, and low ojas or diminished immunity.

There are many practical ways to integrate body-oil massage and sweat therapies into a lifestyle routine. I often tell my clients that there is no better way to begin the morning than with detoxifying practices such as these, which enhance the sadhana and set the course for the entire day. The easiest type of sweat therapy is a hot shower taken after performing oil massage in the morning. The frequency of the therapy depends on the dosha and also the climate you live in.

Community Cleansing

For the most part, people like to spend time with other people. As the ego enjoys stimulation by the five senses, so it thrives among others like itself. The law of attraction is based on the scientific principle that like attracts like. The soul is a magnet that, through the choices we make over many lifetimes, creates a vibrational quality or frequency, somewhat like the distinct sound of a motor. Each soul has its own distinct vibratory sound. In yoga, community is referred to as *sangha*, a term that reflects a much higher spiritual principle than simple association. It means rather the company of wise or advanced yogis.

Because the experience of awakening ourselves to a higher purpose is somewhat rare, especially during the materialistic era of the current Dwapara Yuga[62] or bronze age, arriving at the sacred juncture of becoming more conscious also comes with initial periods of feeling alone and removed from society. For this reason, the awakened soul is then spurred to mingle with vibrations akin to his or her own, converse on a higher level, and exchange and reflect on thoughts, visions, and feelings that may not be understood except in spiritual circles.

There is no doubt that environment is our biggest influence. When we surround ourselves with souls on the spiritual path, we are uplifted and purified. In the Srimad Bhagavata, Bhagavan Krishna says to Uddhava, "I am not so easily attainable by Yoga, Samkhya or discrimination, Dharma, study of the Vedas, Tapas (austerities), renunciation, liberal gifts, charity, rituals, vows, mantras, pilgrimages, as by Satsanga." Around each soul, there exists a pranic aura that influences the environment. Saintly beings can permeate an area for hundreds of years after their presence. Bedrooms, furniture, land, elements, and even empty caves can hold a strong vibration. This is the reason certain areas have become sacred pilgrimage sites. The collective positive energy of visiting aspirants also sustains the pure energy of a place.

In my counseling work, if I recognize that a person does not have a good track record in health and wellness disciplines, although they have the desire to attain greater spiritual purpose in their lives, the first thing I say quite candidly is: "You can't do it alone." I encourage them to be part of a community that endorses the changes they want to attain. Collective energy works in mystical ways, uplifting the mind into its naturally calm and reflective state. Sangha stirs the soul, expands our awareness, and nurtures compassion and love. All the great ones have endorsed the value of sangha as well as *satsanga* or spiritual discourse.

---

62   The ascending Dwapara Yuga or cycle began in 1700 AD.

The majority of people today are buried deep in the gadgets of the sensory world. Most work and conform to today's trends like programmed robots, filling themselves with headlines and life dramas, while rarely pondering, even for a moment, the nature of their existence. In spiritual communities, the mood is high and people are optimistic. They discuss the beauty of nature, and enjoy simple and sweet humor without criticism of others, as well as the promise each day can bring of attaining higher consciousness. Solitude also has a place in spiritual development. However, this comes after the aspirant has attained a stable level of discipline that includes a daily yoga asana practice, Ayurvedic wellness therapies, study, and meditation, all of which require the support of good sangha and a counselor or the guidance of a guru. Spiritual communities are springing up throughout the world along with the globalization of yoga centers, vegetarian restaurants, and special festivals and conferences.

Chapter SIX

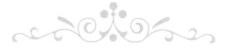

Yoga Therapy

An imperative duty of man is to keep his body in good condition; otherwise his mind is unable to remain fixed in devotional concentration.
Paramahansa Yogananda (1893- 1952)

The Physical Body in Hatha Yoga

Yoga is an enormous science that spans over thousands of years. It is one of the wisdom sciences born of the ancient Vedic culture of India. The purest form of Yogic thought is known as Advaita Vedanta, which essentially expounds the unity of existence and that no division or differentiation exists between life on the planet earth and the grander universe. The world originally discovered yoga through the wisdom tradition of the Vedas. These holy scriptures sprouted the seeds of what would become the trunk and branches of the now very expansive yoga tradition.

Due to the fluctuating cycles of consciousness, described in the teachings on yugas, the understanding and practice of nature's perennial wisdom in consonance with universal law has evolved according to the capacity of mankind. Regardless of how these laws expanded into societies and different cultures across the globe, the physical body has always been the vehicle for human evolution, and the mind is the wheel that steers it. The body transports the wisdom of world cultures from one country to the other and, through various ambassadors, brought yoga to the West. The body has also been the vehicle for creative expression in the martial arts, dance, theater, and the building of great monuments throughout the world like the Egyptian and Mayan pyramids. The body is used to procreate and perpetuate the human species, build community, create the family bond, and grow beyond it.

Yoga these days is mostly associated with the body, but if we look to the scriptures that have carried these teachings, very little is mentioned or described with regards to the body. In fact, the greater tradition of yoga is much more about the mind, its operations, fluctuations, powers, and the realms of consciousness it can access. The Bhagavad Gita describes asana very clearly as a seat: "In a pure secret place by himself established in a fixed seat of his own, neither too high nor too low, with cloth, black antelope-skin and kusa grass one over the other, there, making the mind one-pointed, with thought and the functions of the senses controlled, steady on his seat, he should practice Yoga for the purification of the Self, holding the body, head and neck erect, firm, gazing steadily at the origin of the nose without looking around."[63]

The law of karma culminates in the physical form. We can learn from the body, which reflects our past thoughts, habits, patterns, and lifestyle. In the purest sense, the wisdom tradition emphasizes cultivation of knowledge or Jnana Yoga. In the practical sense, it considers the value of our actions, or Karma Yoga, in the operation of the senses, ego, and living material world.

The form of yoga centered on use of the body is Hatha Yoga, and was an alternative approach to the Raja Yoga system popularized by Patanjali. After many centuries of Buddhism and its meditation practices as the predominant form of spirituality, by the 4th, 5th, and 6th centuries AD Raja Yoga began to decline, as consciousness dropped to its lowest point as determined by the cycles of the yugas. It was at this point that Hatha Yoga separated from the broader Tantric tradition, and Matsyendranath and Gorakhnath founded the Nath cult. Hatha Yoga became a system about purifying the body as an alternative path from that of Raja Yoga.

Hatha Yoga simplified its approach, removing esoteric rituals and emphasis on yama and niyama codes of ethics. It emphasized the importance of physical and mental purification through asana and pranayama and six cleansing rites called shat karmas. Through this inspired modification, Swatmarama, author of the **Hatha Yoga Pradipika,** made Hatha Yoga more fashionable and adapted to an age of consciousness immersed in "body" and "I" awareness.

Rather than trying to teach a culture to work through the difficulties of mastering the mind and develop discipline and the noble virtues of the yamas and niyamas, this approach was about simply connecting the mind to the body. Through purifying actions on the body, the mind can become fixed and connected to

---

63   Bhagavad Gita Ch. VI, Verse 10: *yogi yunjita satatam atmanam rahasi sthitah ekaki yatacittatma nirasir aparigrahah,* Verse 11: *sucau dese pratisthapya sthiram asanam atmanah natyucchritam natinicam cailajinakusottaram,* Verse 12: *tatraikagram manah krtva yatacittendriyakriyah upavisyasane yunjyad yogam atmavisuddhaye*

it, and develop the initial requirements for mind mastery endorsed in the Raja Yoga system. This seems possibly to be the original rebirth of the mind-body trend we are still experiencing today. This trend was reignited again during the physical culture era of the 19th and 20th centuries, which coincided and was fueled by British colonialism and the nationalistic fervor that culminated with Indian independence in 1947.

Yoga can be focused on the body as a vehicle for transformation, but we must be careful not to misinterpret Hatha Yoga as the body-body system it has in many cases become as it has globalized. The aim of Hatha Yoga is bridge the mind-body gap by using the body and breath as a vehicle for creating synergy.

Again, it is through the purification process and techniques described in Hatha Yoga that the mind-body relationship can be nurtured and bonded in preparation for transcendence from the body. The Hatha Yoga movement has brought an enormous tradition to a very fundamental place, establishing the importance of physical purification and detoxification of waste products, namely gas, acidity and mucous, the by-products of the wind, fire, and water doshas. Hatha Yoga considers asana and pranayama as practices to purify the body and mind.

The Hatha tradition, as a sub-form of the broader Tantra system, accentuates outer expression and external practices that are gross, robust, esoteric, and at times intimate. While Raja Yoga also considers asana and pranayama important, it considers the yamas and niyamas prerequisites, and spotlights the auspicious internalization of prana and transcendence beyond the senses as entry into deeper inner forms of meditation and exalted blissful states of consciousness.

These are two different paths with varying intentions, focused on the same goal, the realization of spirit. Hatha Yoga serves to purify the body of impurities, as does Ayurveda, although in a more comprehensive and integral manner centered on lifestyle, routines, and seasonal adaptations. Physical purification through asana and pranayama is a vital step on the spiritual path, which can eventually lead a person to embrace the principles of Raja Yoga.

It seems more apparent now in this era that Lord Shiva set the intention for bridging Hatha and Raja Yogas through his maha siddha ambassador Babaji, who continues to initiate yogis on the path towards higher knowledge. The first verse of Swatmarama's *Hatha Yoga Pradipika* states: "Salutations to the glorious guru, Sri Adinath,[64] who instructed the knowledge of hatha yoga,

---

64   One of the names of Lord Shiva, who is the eternal and supreme consciousness. Shakti is the creative power and the feminine side of Tantra.

which shines forth as a stairway for those who wish to ascend to the highest stage of yoga, raja yoga."

The practice of yoga asana should strengthen the realization that the mind is the ruler of the body. For the majority of the human population, the body dictates to the mind what it should do and feel. Our culture has created a state of mind dependent on physical sensation and appearance. If the body is in pain, the mind becomes weak. If we believe the body looks undesirable, the mind becomes depressed. If the body is sick, the mind also becomes infected. When the body is tired, the mind also becomes lazy and lacks enthusiasm.

The original culprit is actually the mind, which brings the body into such states of poor health and disease. The mind essentially locks itself in the prison cell of the body, struggles to get out, and is always blaming the body. These never-ending excuses lead us into circular patterns of affliction known in yoga as *kleshas*. In yoga the kleshas are considered as five types of mental disorders that create suffering mentally and physically.

1. **Ignorance** (*avidya*): Pondering the idea of human life can begin to create an affliction with in us because of its temporal nature. Human life lacks a definitive term, leaving us to think we live for an indefinite period of time. Avidya refers to a general type of spiritual blindness that leads us into unconscious living. This type of thinking segregates us from nature and universal laws.

2. **Egoism** (*asmita*): This is an overwhelming identification with a name, title, or any particular role in life as part of a tribe or group. Egoism breeds particularity and superiority, and causes us to struggle to enjoy silence and solitude.

3. **Attraction** (*raga*): This is a form of attachment that relates to the temporary pleasures of the sensory world and reflects conditional, patterned existence (samsara).

4. **Aversion** (*dvesha*): This is the feeling of reluctance or repulsion from painful memories and bad experiences, which can make one want to escape or run away.

5. **Attachment** (*abhinivesha*): Through the repeated cycles of attraction and repulsion, we become attached to a specific outcome and life itself. Such repeated patterns breed pride, which even the wise can find hard to escape.

The kleshas determine the quality of our current lives and also reflect hidden factors buried in the karmic bank, based on actions from previous lifetimes. We must always remember the body and the mind are connected and share an integral relationship necessary for healing. Yoga is a system designed to unify the mind and body and transcend them in order to destroy the effects of the kleshas.

What I often see in yoga classes, particularly with new practitioners, are bodies imprisoned by and limited to the current capacity and power of the mind. This can be largely attributed to the kleshas creating a false sense of being or awareness. Initially on the yogic path, there is a lack of expanding awareness beyond the body or even being able to connect to the energies in the body. The repeated use of asana can perpetuate this limited body ideology, which is in complete contrast to principles of traditional yogic teachings.

> *The essence of Vedantic teaching is that we are not the body or mind. We are the Soul or transcendental Self.*

The Therapeutic Side of Yoga

Although Hatha Yoga aims at physical purification as a preparation for attaining high levels of spiritual energy, it also provides many benefits to our health and the quality of lifestyle. While the practices of asana and pranayama are external ones, they most benefit our inner anatomy and systemic functions. Each position has the power to press and massage the internal organs and affect how blood flows, aiding its impact on overall bodily health. From the scientific perspective of matter and energy, we know that like attracts like. Similarly, if one organ begins to fail, then other organs begin to malfunction in a domino effect. This is typical of what we see today in medicine. When a patient complains of pain in one area that has gone on for some time, eventually issues arise in other parts of the body. This is particularly difficult to change when only symptoms are being treated and root causes are not. The dominos continue to fall.

In order to reverse the "like attracts like," we need to follow the opposite approach of *"what we resist the most, we need the most,"* also known as *yukti vyapashraya*. This is precisely why Ayurveda considers the digestive system and its organs—the colon, small intestine, and stomach—the "mother of the body." According to Ayurveda, disease begins and ends in the digestive system. If one of the doshas becomes imbalanced, this increases its elemental qualities, producing ama or undigested food waste. The general sense is that when the doshas go out of balance there is some disturbance to the jatharagni or digestive fire that governs metabolism.

There is no exercise or system more powerful for enhancing the digestive function than yoga asana. As a whole, asana is a bull's-eye therapy for repairing and maintaining metabolism. This is the key to the kingdom of health. As organs synchronize, following in rhythm with each other, their leader is their mother, the digestive system. In this regard we should always look to these three organs and the digestive system as a whole for improving health. This is usually the first place I look when doing a comprehensive Ayurvedic assessment. In most cases, the symptoms of health disorders can be traced to the digestive tract. Unlike vata and kapha, which can benefit from regular and strong yoga asana practice, pitta types generally require reducing asana because of its capacity to increase heat in the body, unless very specific poses have been prescribed by a practitioner specifically to correct such imbalances.

On the more subtle level, therapeutic yoga aims to balance the positive and negative energy channels known as pingala and ida. Working with prana and apana can address the causative factors of diseases, because these are the master forces ruled by the mind, which influence physiological processes. Asana, especially when combined with pranayama, can increase and improve the balance of prana. When prana is spoken of as "balanced," it indicates the unification of both currents, which has both physical and spiritual implications. When addressing therapeutic healing through asana, it is a good idea to consider the body's two main energy gateways. The hips and shoulders are two areas where prana becomes blocked, which can lead to a variety of complications.

The hips are a structural area where prana is commonly trapped or obstructed. This is also often indicated with knee issues, tension and hypersensitivity in the buttocks, weakness in the legs, and lack of balance. Many of these hip-related problems are connected to vata dosha, and reveal themselves in the yoga room. I have seen many situations with students in my yoga classes struggling from hip issues. When I do a complete Ayurvedic assessment, vata is usually the culprit. In many cases, they have a vata constitution (prakriti). More asana hip openers are not always the best solution for addressing such issues. Rather a more specific prescription of postures practiced slowly, with the right attention, is indicated, combined with application of therapeutic oil to the affected areas. Lifestyle routines, diet, and herbs are also brought in to enhance the mind-body synergy.

The shoulders are the other gateway of prana and, when blocked, can affect the heart, devotional capacity, the throat and use of speech and mantra, and thyroid function. In the shoulders and upper back, we often see that kapha dosha increases both muscle and fat density, creating inflexibility. Such structural impairments also reflect a host of psychological patterns or samskaras. Always keep in mind that in the Ayurvedic view, the mind shapes the quality of the spine. Inversions (headstand, shoulder stand, plow) and arm balances (crow, side plank, bridge) are excellent for opening these areas, reducing excess fat, and creating leaner muscle mass.

Another important factor with respect to these two areas is integrating pranayama with prescribed poses. It is often good to work on both of these areas with different postural combinations, with the intention of centering energy so that prana is neither too high nor too low, but balanced in the center. In this section, we will discuss further details of the implementation of pranayama with asana for therapeutic healing. Use of asana and pranayama for therapeutic purposes can lead a practitioner to the deeper, mystical side of yoga. This seems to have been a clever correlation on the part of the great sages and yogis who have helped reintroduce yoga into the modern era.

Treating the Individual, Not the Disease

I think one of the most beautiful things we can all appreciate in this world is that it is filled with diversity. When we look around at our circle of friends, family, and community, we realize that every person is unique. Everyone has a distinct quality of mind, body, and the specific events that have shaped their lives. Many of us share striking similarities with certain people or family members, but no two people are exactly the same. It is through this understanding that the teachings of Ayurveda and yoga operate, linking teacher and student or guru and disciple for millennia

After the long Vedic golden age, there came about a number of philosophical perspectives that expressed this traditional understanding of creation and existence. One in particular that has had a long standing impact on the expansion and practice of yoga and Ayurveda is Samkhya philosophy. It clearly enumerates twenty-four principles that explain the basic relationship between human existence and nature. It recognizes a supreme consciousness known as purusha and creative power known as prakriti.

Samkhya incorporates the Shiva and Shakti principles, although its explanations are more scientific in value and jibe with our common sense. Essentially, Samkhya states that we are all miniature living replicas of the universe. Based on this, yoga practices and Ayurvedic routines and rituals can be integrated into our lives in a most specific and effective manner, according to what our body and mind need. The Samkhya philosophy gave birth to the prakriti-vikriti principles and brought the importance of treating the individual person, not the disease or disorder, to Ayurveda. The person must be recognized and acknowledged.

Medical prescriptions and recommendations that endorse a general concept or program for everyone are short-cuts born of branding, capitalism, and greed. It's a fast way to sell a concept that may work to a certain degree, but disregards understanding a person from the inside out. Such generic forms of health and wellness are like maintenance for robots. All therapeutic practices need to be founded on the idea of individualism in order to be truly effective.

In counseling, when each person's distinct and individual qualities are recognized, advice and information become specific and unique. From this perspective, people can become inspired to live responsibly. What I am saying is, when healing is based on teaching people to recognize the impact their mind has on the body, they are empowered. When we teach others of the power of making healthy choices, they will begin to give their choices greater consideration and their health will change. Then societies and eventually the world can begin to change.

Recognizing the unique qualities of each human being allows us to respect each other in the manner of the eternal tradition, spirit to spirit. Nobody likes to be known by a number, code, or condition, as is the case when health care companies place clients in the "elderly group," with the "diabetics," and so on. How these companies disperse funds depends on business codes and costs, and ignores the original intention of health care, to provide an opportunity for healing. Why don't we help people heal themselves and end the dependency we have created on programs, diets, surgeries, and drugs? Because it's a lot more work and requires more time than most people have reserved for healing themselves.

In the guru-shishya[65] tradition of yoga, a sacred link is created for the transmission of knowledge through the sage, rishi, or guru to the disciple or student. This tradition defines a succession of energy transmitted from soul to soul. This relationship involves direct and personal contact with the teacher or guru, and knowledge is imparted according to the student's disposition

---

65   Also known as *sampraday* or *parampara* in traditional Indian culture, as expressed in Vedic-Hindu, Buddhist, Jain, and other traditions.

and karma. This transmission of knowledge is specifically made to heal and promote self-realization, with no other expectation. The requirements for this sacred relationship are loyalty, respect, and love. This teacher-student link in yoga is another expression of the prakriti concept Ayurveda uses for healing.

While in ancient times, teaching and training were always imparted through this sincere relationship, in much of today's yoga we are far removed from such a link. These days we superficially honor schools, programs, degrees, and institutions, and have disregarded the bonds we share with an actual living teacher. Both the prakriti concept in Ayurveda and yoga's guru-shishya tradition are based on the eternal and perennial relationship of the sun and moon, moon and earth, mother and child, and spirit and nature. This sacred link is something we must all aim to preserve in our lives, especially while embarking on a journey into yoga and Ayurvedic healing. In this way, we can deepen our connection to the wisdom of the ancient traditions, which can uplift humanity from its current health dilemma.

Effects of Yoga Asana on Anatomy

According to Ayurvedic anatomy, there are seven bodily tissues called dhatus that comprise layers in the body. Each of the dhatus plays a vital role in maintaining the balanced state of tri-dosha. The strength of the tissues is a reflection of the state of our health, which can be substantially influenced through the practice of yoga and pranayama. The dhatus are made up of the five elements and are connected to the doshas. Externally, asana benefits the muscles through flexing the spine to increase physical flexibility. On a structural level, asana's therapeutic focus begins with the spine, where the entire nervous system is soothed and steadied. The spine is symbolic of the tree of life and, on a more subtle level, is seen as a pathway for prana, healing, wisdom, and enlightenment.

Our spine is also a reflection of our attitude towards life. It is a type of body language that demonstrates our capacity as spirit beings to stand strong to life's tests and trials. In essence, our spine is a reflection of our karma, attitude, and outlook on life. It reflects the manner in which we breathe and absorb experiences. Vata-related issues typically originate in the lower lumbar spine and have the potential to move through the nervous system, shaping the alignment and influencing digestion and our overall disposition.

The muscle tissue or *mamsa* dhatu is the one most affected by asana yoga. It is brought into balance through the stretching and strengthening action of the vigorous physical postures. Asanas are very preventative for arthritis and osteoporosis, which are common vata disorders and involve *ashti* dhatu or bone and cartilage tissue. Asana can help to reduce inflammation and improve the lack of mobility associated with these diseases. The static action of asana is grounding to the *majja* dhatu or bone marrow and nerves, allowing for a steadier flow of energy through the nervous system. A steady practice of asana brings consistent and dependable function on a systemic level. A balanced majja dhatu creates a more stable mind, as asana improves the mind-body connection. Asana that is grounding, calm, slow, and targets the spine and hips, is of great value for an age of media and electronic over-stimulation.

The practice of asana produces enhanced functionality in the heart and lungs. Asana naturally increases blood pressure, and this increases the blood flowing to and from the heart and the flow of oxygen-poor blood from the body into the right atrium of the heart. It also enables the pulmonary vein to empty oxygen-rich blood from the lungs into the heart's left atrium. The right combination of postures, along with a strong emphasis on proper breathing, allows the *rakta* dhatu or blood tissue to be strengthened and purified with increased levels of hemoglobin.[66] Kapalabhati pranayama is also a very important breathing technique for purifying the blood, and can be integrated into asana sets.

Through a vinyasa approach of sequences linking movement with breath, a more cardiovascular effect is created as the heart rate naturally increases when rests, such as Savasana, a form of pratyahara, are reduced or even eliminated from practice until the very end of a session. With higher cardiovascular function, the body's agni levels increase, creating more heat. Heat and sweat, its by-product, balances the *medas* dhatu or fat and is a key factor in kapha management. Through improved digestive power the body is able maintain *rasa* dhatu or plasma to nourish all the dhatus.

Asana could be considered the single most effective means for increasing the jatharagni or metabolic function. Proper asana aims to center the energy in the body, bringing more blood flow, heat, and circulation to the central or digestive organs. The *shukra* dhatu or reproductive fluid is the essence of all the tissues and gives us the inspiration and motivation to improve ourselves. All energy that the body expends is derived from ojas and expressed through the shukra dhatu. Shukra ignites the agni and provides a way of eliminating all impurities and diseases from the body.

Asana can enhance the ojas-shukra relationship, but it must be done carefully and according the prakriti-vikriti of the practitioner. For example, if asana

---

66   A protein responsible for transporting oxygen in the blood of vertebrates.

is done excessively by someone with a vata constitution, this may over time deplete the ojas and weaken the shukra dhatu. Excessive asana should also be cautioned for pitta types, who are susceptible to raising their agni too quickly. Asana with respect to pitta-type conditions requires rest between each posture so as to keep the agni force from burning up soma energy.

Shukra depends on soma for its support, strength, and function. If an asana practice is too agni-focused, it will leave the body wasted and exhausted. Excessively heated yoga rooms and lengthy practice that includes many spinal compressions or backbends and inversions can cause shukra depletion. One of the main practices for enhancing the shukra dhatu is Savasana and a proper cooling period, which enhances soma energies to balance agni in the body. A proper cooling period should also include spinal twists and lunar pranayama practices. Sheetali and Sikari pranayama are very good in this regard. Keep in mind that heat rises and, as it does, it must be met with soma forces descending from above to enter the heart and balance the body, mind, and consciousness.

In esoteric thought, the lower half of the body represents the solar or heating energies, while the region above the heart represents the lunar or cooling energies. Balancing the energies requires centering them in the heart. We create heat and circulation through the activity of the heart, but we must also cool the body and mind by releasing pressure and relaxing the mind into the heart. The merging of the mind into the spiritual heart is a key theme of Vedantic teaching.

Asana and pranayama are natural tools for healing the dhatus. Any program aimed at improving the health of the dhatus must include some aspect of placing the body in dynamic positions, combined with an awareness of breath to develop synchronicity between mind and body. In yoga, being able to sit or come into stillness is actually a transformational use of the body and mind for evolution. As the body and mind arrive at a state of perfect stillness, quite the antithesis is occurring on the molecular level within the subtle mental body. The molecules dance in a very high state of vibration. The mystery of the light of the soul lies in this contrast. On one side, we can experience tremendous therapeutic healing, and on the other a transcendence of consciousness. This dazzling light begins to appear as the guiding force of inspiration, which leads us to a life of truth or *sat*. It is from this that all myths are born.

Asana and the Spine

Yoga asana is all about the spine, which is symbolic of the perennial tree of life. There are several aspects of asana that should be considered relative to healing.

One is its healing capacity on a structural and anatomical level, and the other regards the energetics of the subtle body. While yoga is mainly concerned with the balance of prana and expansion of awareness, consideration of the physical body, its tissues, the spine, and general physical health history is important and should not be overlooked when beginning a practice. If the body is malnourished, injured, or debilitated in some way, focus should be placed primarily on establishing a stable physical foundation for energy to be contained, as yogic practices like asana and pranayama enhance the body's energy.

The physical body, its anatomy, the dhatus or tissues, and spine are measures of the consciousness an individual carries. All aspects of the physical body are components that work synergistically to support the harmonious flow of prana shakti within us. Our human potential and prana shakti are dependent on healing the physical body and improving the mind-body relationship, balancing the cosmic forces of the sun and moon. Whether you work on the inner body or the outer aspects, each will benefit the other. This may be true, but more importantly, we should always consider both aspects as they are intrinsically linked.

The other factor when using asana for healing the mind-body relationship is the level of attention one maintains while holding the poses. In essence, all yoga is spinal yoga, in that developing awareness of the spine brings balance to the pingala or solar and ida or lunar channels. The primary purpose of hatha yoga is to prepare the royal pathway within the spine. If the sun and moon channels are balanced, then prana is centralized in the most sacred of yogic channels, known as the sushumna, the river that flows to Brahman.

In asana, as postures are practiced, a general awareness and feeling of the spine is key to attaining the inner benefit of balanced prana. This is not only important for developing stability in certain poses, but also to becoming aware of specific areas in the spine that may indicate weakness or accumulation of a dosha. The asanas affect each person differently, depending on prakriti and vikriti. The overall practice of yoga asana is extremely helpful in bringing balance to the body in terms of strength, flexibility, physiological function, and balance between mind and body. The Kriya Yoga referred to in the Bhagavad Gita and by the sage Patanjali in his Yoga Sutras was popularized in this age by Paramahansa Yogananda as a form of Raja Yoga that strongly emphasizes concentration on the spine, which directs prana into the sushumna nadi, reducing the karmic burdens that keep us limited to body consciousness. It was in fact Yogananda who pointed out the relationship between the following passages from these two essential teachings:

A muni—he who holds liberation as the sole object of life and therefore frees himself from longings, fears, and wrath—controls his senses, mind, and intelligence and removes their external contacts by (a technique of) making even, or neutralizing, the currents of prana and apana that manifest as inhalation and exhalation in the nostrils. He fixes his gaze at the middle of the two eyebrows (thus converting the dual current of the physical vision into the single current of the omniscient astral eye). Such a muni wins complete emancipation.

Bhagavad Gita Chap. V verses 27-28[67]

Liberation can be attained by that pranayama which is accomplished by disjoining the course of inspiration and expiration.

Patanjali, *Ashtanga Yoga Sutras* II:49

Ayurveda and the Spine

Similar themes appear in other lineages and classical teachings. When asanas are combined with an Ayurvedic approach, they can be used to treat the doshas more specifically, since they affect the three main spinal regions, the lumbar, thoracic, and cervical. Ayurveda determines this based on the physiological locations, both primary and secondary, in which each dosha accumulates. Without going into a complete explanation of Ayurvedic anatomy, I will list only the primary sites where the doshas accumulate, as this is all that is necessary to explain how the doshas affect the spine.

Vata dosha's primary site of accumulation is in the colon. Pitta's primary site of accumulation is the small intestine, and kapha's primary site is the stomach. Given the primary site of vata (air) dosha, we know, based on colonic function, that its accumulation can have an indirect influence on structures such as the sacrum and coccyx, as well as the central nervous system and sciatic nerve in the lower spine. Because this system is energetic, it is not possible to confirm that this will always be the case with regards to vata. This erratic quality is particularly the case with vata, as the air element is the most inconsistent of the three doshas.

The Ayurvedic view of asana is based on each posture's effect of either increasing or decreasing dosha. The common-sense energetic principles that underlie the entire science are the basis of this analysis. Ayurvedic teaching is applied in a practical sense, and not to specific asanas. The basic understanding is whether

---

67   From God Talks With Arjuna: The Bhagavad Gita, by Paramahansa Yogananda (Self-Realization Fellowship, Los Angeles, Calif.)

sequences or postures are heating, cooling, or balancing in their effect on the spine and body.

The Birth of Yoga Therapy

Asana can be considered one of the most effective forms for healing the body inside and out. I will later discuss the specific benefits of selected asanas on anatomy, physiology, and the Ayurvedic doshas. I have selected many of the most practical and widely known postures listed in the original texts of the Hatha Yoga tradition, such as the *Hatharatnavali, Hatha Yoga Pradipika, Gheranda Samhita*, and *Shiva Samhita*. I will also discuss the spiritual implications of each posture and their capacity for preparing the body and mind for meditation.

The cause of the rise of yoga as therapy is two-fold. First, it is related to the shift in consciousness that as mentioned occurred in 1700, according to the Vedic yuga system, as the planet earth entered a second age of spiritual development, reflecting the need for humanity to reinvestigate the mind-body relationship. Second are historical reasons related to the Indian society's struggle during centuries of Islamic oppression and British colonialism, which undermined the nation's spiritual dharma.

Also significant was the insight of yogis like Lahiri Mahasaya, the direct disciple of Mahavatar Babaji, who was able to expound Kriya yoga in light of Charaka's[68] Ayurveda teachings as well as other philosophies. Swami Sivananda, a trained medical doctor and founder of the Divine Life Society, had an Ayurvedic health facility at his ashram in Rishikesh and wrote one of the earliest books on the relationship between yoga and Ayurveda. Another great figure, Paramahamsa Madhavdasji, influenced his young disciples Swami Kuvalayananda and Shri Yogendra to research and develop yoga's healing properties. Shri Yogendra actually founded the earliest known "Yoga Institute" focused on therapeutic principles, in 1918 near Mumbai. A year later, he opened another institute in New York, which did not endure.

Bishnu Ghosh and Buddha Bose in Calcutta and Kuvalayananda and Shri Yogendra in the southern state of Maharastra all opened the first yoga therapy centers between 1918 and the 1930s. The yogi Krishnamacharya, appointed to teach yoga at the Mysore palace, integrated the influence of gymnastics and wrestling into his signature "vinyasa" approach and embraced the importance of teaching based on the individual qualities of students. After his center closed,

---

68   Ayurvedic medicine's preeminent physician. The *Charaka Samhita* is one of the primary texts of Ayurvedic medicine.

his disciples, such as B.K.S. Iyengar, Pattabhi Jois, Indra Devi, and others, carried on, creating distinct approaches to sadhana based on their perspectives on what their teacher taught.

It seems that of the commercial asana forms that exist today, particularly in the West, the vinyasa approach has won out in popularity. In my view, this has much to do with the vata mind-set of our modern societies, which lack attention and resist learning how to be still. According to Ayurvedic understanding, this is due a number of factors, such as improper diet, lack of yogic lifestyle, and disregard for nature, missing from today's fragmented yoga teaching. This can lead to sustained restlessness, anxiety, and fear, which deplete the body of its vital energy.

Yogananda's father, also a direct disciple of Lahiri Mahasya, carried on his Guru's influence by recommending practical healing formulas and simple uses of asana and pranayama for various health issues, providing natural and practical caring guidance to many. Undoubtedly, his son Makunda Lal Ghosh, prior to taking *sannyasi* (monastic) vows and becoming the monastic Yogananda, was exposed to this wisdom and approach. In fact, this is evidenced in Yogananda's "How to Live" lessons, where he gives remedies for various ailments and different diets for everything from weight loss to building immunity and fighting off colds.

The Kriya Yoga lineage of Babaji, as disseminated by Paramahamsa Yogananda to the West, was an integral and comprehensive approach to spiritual development through yoga. It taught balance through a harmonious mind-body relationship that depends on proper lifestyle according to nature's laws. Yoga as a therapeutic tool must embrace Ayurveda, as initiated through the channel of these great gurus and energetically transmitted by their lineages, in order for their teachings to endure and provide us true emancipation, as originally intended. It is important for us not to get tangled up in historical data as Hatha Yoga evolves. However, there is value in understanding the importance of uniting the yoga and Ayurveda systems to produce harmonious mind-body relationships in practitioners, and for the facilitation of higher consciousness on the planet.

> *Curative remedies and practices for spiritual evolution of mind and body should not be done independently of nature, but must be done with full consideration of the Divine's presence in all aspects of creation.*

According to the Sanskrit yoga scripture *Hatharatnavali*,[69] "The Almighty

---

69 By Srinivasa from Andhra, South India, written approximately between 1625 and 1695 CE. The Kularnava Tantra also makes reference to the 8,400,000 forms of life.

Shambhu (Shiva) has described eighty-four asanas, taking examples from each of the 8,400,000 kinds of creatures." The *Gheranda Samhita* states: "There are eighty-four hundreds of thousands of Asanas described by Shiva. The postures are as many in number as there are numbers of species of living creatures in this universe."[70] "Among them eighty-four are the best; and among these eighty-four, thirty-two have been found useful for mankind in this world."[71]

Interestingly, the *Hatha Yoga Pradipika* of Svatmarama Yogindra lists only fifteen postures. Gheranda lists thirty-two postures as the "best" of the eighty-four referred to in the above sutra, being practical for mankind. Of the thirty-poses he describes, the fifteen poses described in the *Pradipika* of Svatmarama are included. Some yoga scholars believe the number 84 is purely symbolic and stands for completeness.[72] Another viewpoint of yoga scholars is that the therapeutic approach to posture may have emerged as part of the Tantra tradition, which considers the mind-body relationship as one of its central tenets, with the body as the temple for experiencing the Divine.

The tradition of the eighty-four asanas can be traced to a number of texts from different regions throughout India and Nepal. From the Jodhpur tradition, the connection of the eighty-four asana is drawn to the eighty-four adepts (*siddhas*). The number 84 is evidently connected to many aspects of Eastern spiritual culture. It is mentioned in various yoga texts and the *Kamasastra*, and can also be associated with the 84,000 stupas built by Asoka. In my view, 84 seems to stand for completeness, even though many of the texts differ in the names and types of postures. An interesting point that can be drawn from the 84 postures is their relationship to living creatures and nature, which links yoga to nature and life.

Asana was only one of many techniques, and not the most important, considered in the Tantra tradition for expanding prana, both for healing and realization of the feminine Divine. In some respects, the asanas were gestures for cultivating energy or Shakti to be offered to Lord Shiva. Many of the Bengali Yoga masters worshipped the Divine Goddess in her various aspects as Kali, Saraswati, or Durga, as Bengal has thrived as a region of bhakti or devotion. Many asanas are described in the ancient texts, with some differences in nomenclature and technical description. However, all seem to agree on the importance of 84 for whatever reason, with the best postures being seated asanas like Siddhasana

---

70   *Gheranda Samhita* Ch 2, verse 1
71   *Gheranda Samhita* Ch 2, verses 1-2
72   The late George Feuerstein (1947 – 2012), in an essay titled "Eighty-Four Asanas," also mentions there were 84 great adepts or maha-siddhas, who lived in the period from 500-1200 A.D.

(posture of attainment) and Padmasana (lotus posture). Simple descriptions of the asanas are given in these ancient texts in a sort of epigrammatic style. There is a subtle implication that details of alignment and precisely fixed arrangement are inconsequential. What is intended is the use of the postures as vehicles for transcending consciousness.

Anandamayi Ma and Yoga

Before the Hatha Yoga tradition began its modern adaption in the nineteenth century, asana was considered mainly a system for purifying the body with systems such as the shat karmas or six detoxifying actions. There was also a focus on the more subtle level of prana and how its variegated effects can be modified to create a unified stream of consciousness. Cultural and exercise-based practices were not preserved in writing as much as they were disseminated through extensive family systems and through the teacher-student or *gurukul* tradition. Less significance was given to reading and writing than to listening and watching.

One of the greatest female illumined masters of yoga, also from Bengal, Sri Anandamayi Ma, once said: "When an asana forms spontaneously, that is to say as an expression of a particular state of mind, it will be perfect. In other words, the position of the legs, feet, hands, the head and the gaze…every single detail will be precisely as it ought to be. Whereas the asana performed by an effort of will can never have the same perfection. Asanas are closely connected with one's breathing, and the breath with one's state of mind, at any particular time. If asanas are engaged in as a yogic practice, that is to say in order to attain the revelation of the union with the ONE which universally exists, then only will they yield the desired result. If, on the other hand, asanas are done merely as physical exercises, they may bring about greater health and fitness, but not union (yoga)."

As mentioned previously in the Physical Culture section, this approximately century-old body-building culture, which includes the muscle-control taught by Maxick and Sandow, began to draw on the connection the mind and concentration played on developing the muscles. These masterful techniques were tools for personal transformation professed to build strength, confidence, and other self-help virtues that eventually would find a connection with yogic practices.

Bishnu Ghosh, his father Bhagabati, the younger Buddha Bose, Swami Kuvalayananda and Shri Yogendra became envoys for the yoga "therapy" concept taught and described from a more scientific perspective. The spiritual viewpoint always remained intact with illumined souls like Anandamayi Ma and Yogananda, who shared similar perspectives on asana. Asana's spiritual intention was captured during a conversation between Sri Anandamayi Ma and Sri Daya Mata[73] in Calcutta in 1961.[74] During an informal gathering between these venerated sisters and a few close devotees, Anandamayi Ma asked Daya Mata how many asanas she used to practice. Daya Mataji replied, "Only a few." As a young girl, she used to try to do some asana, but Yogananda had expressly told her that it was not necessary to do them all, as "Energization"[75] exercises would suffice for her spiritual advancement.

Daya Mata went on to say that Yogananda advised only a moderate use of asana exercises to remove the body from being an obstacle in the practice of meditation, so that other, more subtle inner techniques, such as pranayama, mantra, and concentration, could be integrated, and the evolution of body, mind, and soul could be further refined. In noting Anandamayi Ma's interest in knowing more about Energization exercises, Daya Mata elucidated that it was not a matter of which body part was being tensed or energized or what was being gained on the physical level. It was more a matter of exercising the mind in such a manner that, through concentration, one could actually feel the prana that is linked to Will power.

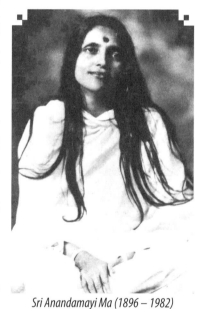

Suddenly, upon hearing this, Anandamayi Ma responded by saying that indeed, through such "*antar-dhyana,*"[76] yogis could live very long in the body. Similarly, Anandamayi Ma greatly appreciated that, in response to somebody seeking Yoganandaji's blessing for sitting long in Padmasana, he said that it would be better to ask for the blessing to have love for God. Anandamayi Ma went on to point out, "This was a very important message; asanas then happen all by

Sri Anandamayi Ma (1896 – 1982)

---

73 Sri Daya Mata was the third president of the Self-Realization Fellowship/Yogoda Satsanga Society in India, organizations founded by Paramahansa Yogananda.

74 I have paraphrased this story as it was imparted to me by a monk in India who heard an original audio recording of this discussion.

75 A unique system of muscle tensing and releasing exercises devised by Yogananda in 1916 for developing the mind-body relationship, increasing will power, and inducing sublime pratyahara (sensory purification and withdrawal). This topic is described further in Chapter 10.

76 Inner meditative state that links the meditator to the maha prana or essence of immortality.

themselves." In other words, through surrender, love, and devotion to God, the sadhaka finds the right asana or attitude for experiencing the Divine.

The conversation continued to deepen when a devotee in the group asked whether it could be said that if one can sit in meditation, they naturally have the requisite love (*prema*) in their heart, Anandamayi Ma responded by saying, "No, it may not always be the case. One will not necessarily have steadiness of prana by performing padmasana (lotus posture) or other asanas, whereas, one who is able to steady their prana, for them padmasana can naturally take place, leading to deeper meditation." She asserted that 'if the yoga practice does not lead towards meditation and enlightenment, then the asanas will not perfect. The intention of sadhana is on steadying the prana—and not on balancing the asana—in this manner, the **atma-swarup** (soul) is revealed."

This brings to light an essential premise of the yoga teachings, that the body follows the mind, therefore the mind is master of the body, and in order to balance it energetically, we must look to the subtler life force contained in it. By balancing prana, bringing it into a stillness whereby mind and breath are merged into the heart, the soul is discovered. Anandamayi Ma elaborated on the importance of having the right mood or attitude (*bhava*) and said, "One may perform a lot of different postures and mudras, but they may not have formed a connection in the first place. The real objective is not asana but to connect to the Supreme." Another great Bengali female saint who is a kriya yogi, Sarbani Ma,[77] does not consider Hatha Yoga necessary for spiritual evolution, although she does recommend it to certain individuals needing therapeutic aid.

The Rise of Bengali Yoga

To set the stage for a moment, the state of Bengal is an eastern state of India and is one of the most densely populated regions on the planet. It is home to the Ganges river delta at the confluence of the Brahmaputra and Meghna rivers. Rivers have always been a sacred part of yoga and the Indian lifestyle. The capital of Bengal is Kolkata, which was the center of the Indian independence movement. As yoga began to expand at the turn of the century through the 1950s, as a counter-cultural force opposed to British occupation, the region also struggled against a tremendous set-back, the Great Bengal Famine of 1943-44, which took an estimated two to three million lives. India battled through this and eventually gained independence in 1947. Bengal managed to become a womb for bhakti yogis and the nectar that would sustain the renaissance of yoga in India and across the globe.

---

77   Took initiation in Kriya Yoga in the lineage of Swami Pranavananda, as mentioned in the chapter "The Saint with Two Bodies" in *Autobiography of a Yogi*.

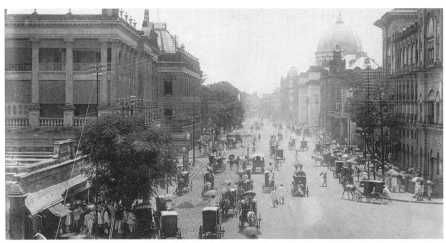

Calcutta, India in 1920's

Bengali seers like Sri Aurobindo promoted yoga as an integral system, a way of life that cultivated a dynamic relationship between mind, body, and soul. Some of the many styles of yoga that provide this pure synthesis remain extant in India, but only through a few living yoga teachers and lineages. This synthesis may even still exist sporadically in commercial yoga.

One of the most influential figures of yoga in the West was Paramahansa Yogananda, who formulated a practical means of integrating ancient themes and techniques for the spiritual growth of people in Western societies, and for Eastern cultures to reestablish their balance between spirituality and the material. In my view, Yogananda somewhat influenced the application of the 84 postures as a precursor to Kriya Yoga, and at the very least gave some simple suggestions on how theses postures affect the spine and prana. However, it does not seem likely that Yogananda, who was sent on a specific mission to spread Kriya Yoga, would have meddled much in such gross matters, considering his discretion about over-emphasizing the physical body.

Rather, what is consistently evident in Yogananda's teachings, as well as those of other great Indian saints like Anandamayi Ma and Sivananda, is asana as a worthy tool for disciplining the mind, transcending the senses, and preparing the spine for meditation. Asana is an instrument for purification of the body and a means of separating our attention from it. We also see no concise, factual description of asana in any of the Indian classics like the Ramayana, Bhagavad Gita and Mahabaharata, or even the Yoga Sutras of Patanjali.

It is important to note that sages like Yogananda often devise new paths and techniques of yoga practice that have no direct reference to any previous teaching or scripture, as was the case with the "Yogoda" system he adapted into the Kriya Yoga taught by his gurus. The "Yogoda" approach was a pilot representation of what Yogananda later disseminated to the West. It represented an integral approach to cultivating a strong body and the power of concentration to transcend sensory perception, as a foundation for the mystical teachings of Kriya Yoga.[78] The ancient science of Kriya Yoga was re-adapted by Yogananda for the modern era, while still maintaining the vital logic presented by sage Patanjali in his Yoga Sutras in approximately the second century B.C.

Subsequently, traces of Yogoda wisdom spread through Yogananda's brother Bishnu Charan Ghosh,[79] who opened a school called Bishnu Ghosh's College of Yoga and Physical Culture in 1923, which continues to operate today. Although the school was focused on the fitness aspect of the physical culture movement, Bishnu did teach an eclectic combination of asana and muscle control for greater mind-body synergy. Bishnu obtained the title Yoginder Bishnu Charan Ghosh (Rishikesh) from Sri Swami Sivananda, who was not from Bengal but Pattamadai, Tamil Nadu, and later, in 1938, founded the Divine Life Society ashram in the northern city of Rishikesh along the banks of the sacred Ganges River in the state of Uttrakand. Sivananda also played a major role in the development of the mind-body movement through an integral approach to yoga that launched the famous slogan "Serve, Love, Meditate, Realize." Sivananda called his yoga teachings the "Yoga of Synthesis." During these years, Sivananda began his first yoga teacher trainings, which Bishnu seems to have participated in. I currently study with Swami Jyotirmayananda, one of Sivananda's last living direct disciples, and have worked closely with him to interpret Sivananda's writings.

---

78 Swami Yogananda, who received the title "Paramahansa" in 1935, was chosen by Mahavatar Babaji to spread the teachings of Kriya Yoga. "East and West must establish a golden middle path of activity and spirituality combined." Chapter 36, *Autobiography of a Yogi* by Paramahansa Yogananda (Self-Realization Fellowship, Los Angeles, Calif.)

79 Yogananda wrote, "The students were also taught yoga concentration and meditation, and a unique system of physical development, 'Yogoda,' whose principles I had discovered in 1916. Realizing that man's body is like an electric battery, I reasoned that it could be recharged with energy through the direct agency of the human will. As no action, slight or large, is possible without willing, man can avail himself of his prime mover, will, to renew his bodily tissues without burdensome apparatus or mechanical exercises. I therefore taught the Ranchi students my simple 'Yogoda' techniques by which the life force, centered in man's medulla oblongata, can be consciously and instantly recharged from the unlimited supply of cosmic energy. The boys responded wonderfully to this training, developing extraordinary ability to shift the life energy from one part of the body to another part, and to sit in perfect poise in difficult body postures. They performed feats of strength and endurance, which many powerful adults could not equal. My youngest brother, Bishnu Charan Ghosh, joined the Ranchi school; he later became a leading physical culturist in Bengal." Autobiography of a Yogi by Paramahansa Yogananda (Self-Realization Fellowship, Los Angeles, Calif.)

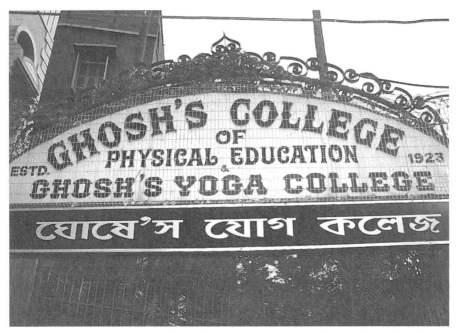

Bishnu's primary pupil, Buddha Bose, also eventually opened his own school, called the Yoga Cure Institute, in 1937, in the same location as Ghosh's College of Physical Education. The two continued to share the same location until the 1970s. Buddha Bose's Yoga Cure Institute was more focused on the curative aspects of yoga asana and its integration with pranayama and relaxation techniques. As a former body builder and physical culturist myself; I was enthralled to know more about the deeper spiritual side this yoga system was aligned with. What captivated me was that asana had a much deeper purpose internally and externally, and these "positions" could have much more profound implications on the mind if practiced properly.

Yogananda's very partial interest in the use of these asanas came from exposure to the nationalism that was afire during his youth. Bhagabati Charan Ghosh, Yogananda's father, was also influential. An advanced yogi himself, he mentored

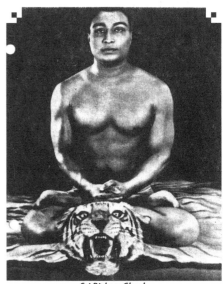

Sri Bishnu Ghosh

Buddha Bose and his interest in the curative aspects of yoga asana. Another mentor was Maharshi Nagendra Nath Bhaduri (1846-1926), to whom Yogananda dedicated a chapter in his autobiography.[80] Nagendra Nath was an educator who established a free primary school in Calcutta and encouraged students to build strong physiques. He advocated the physical culture movement as part of the nationalism developing at the turn of the 20th century. Nagendra Natha at heart was a bhakta or devotional yogi, who shared his wisdom in a humble and obscure manner to those close to him.[81] It seems that Nagendra Nath was another of the formidable influences to Yogananda, a hidden gem who propagated the rebirth of the mind-body synergy that later spread to the West.

I give credit to all the yogis who had full mastery of the mind, and not as much to those bent on the muscular body's external mechanics. My teacher Vamadeva and I often say that many of the greatest yogis are the least known. However, in some mysterious and Divine way, they influence the world and those like Yogananda, who could spread the teachings.

Many others, like Sri Aurobindo,[82] who was very distantly related to Yogananda, imbued bustling Calcutta with important themes that promoted spreading the value of mind-body synergy. The famous poet Rabindranath Tagore, whom Yogananda met with personally and wrote about in his autobiography, promoted some interesting views on education that Yogananda carried close to his heart. Tagore was an international figure closely connected with towering personages like Gandhi and Sri Aurobindo. He delivered talks in America[83] and always recognized the importance of the mind-body relationship in his educational system. He was widely admired by many contemporaries.

Tagore's educational concepts at Santiniketan were comprised of a well-rounded approach to learning, including physical training, judo, dance, gardening, and other arts. Interestingly, he did not believe in examinations, as these place pressure on learning or cramming as we know it in the West, and stifle individual expression and development. Tagore was also interested in the moral and ethical principles of yoga, the yamas and niyamas, for development. He was influenced by Neo-Vedanta, the interpretations of Hinduism that developed

---

80 "The Levitating Saint," Chapter 7, *Autobiography of a Yogi*.

81 Maharshi Nagendranath [His Life & Advice], Prof. Tripurasankar Sen Shastri, Nagendra Mission.

82 Born Aurobindo Ghose in Calcutta, Bengal. He lived from August 15th 1872 to December 5th 1950. He was an Indian nationalist, philosopher, yogi, guru, and poet. Developed a spiritual system he called Integral Yoga that is focused on the transformation of the entire being. This differs from the Integral Yoga taught in the United States during the 1960s and '70s by Swami Satchitananda of the Sivananda Saraswati lineage of Rishekesh.

83 Tagore was hosted by Sister Gyana Mata in Seattle, who was one of Yogananda's very advanced and early disciples.

in the 19th century, and by his own father, Debendranath Tagore, the founder of Brahmo Samaj movement.

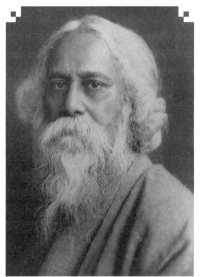

Rabindranath Tagore (1861 – 1941)

During the late 1800s and early 1900s, yoga asana was becoming more recognized in Bengal, and was being reborn alongside the physical culture movement. However, it seems that the practice of asana also grew through the devotional practices that began with Ramakrishna and his disciples, Nagendranath, Srila Bhaktisiddhanta Sarasvati, A.C. Bhaktivedanta Swami Prabhupada the Guru of ISKCON, and Swami Ram Tirtha.

The idea of the body as temple, with the mind and spine intricately connected, began to gain currency and is evident in what Yogananda brought to the West. However, the physical factor of using the body to develop morality and courage, improve health, and for a host of other common-sense reasons, was never considered primary to the core Vedantic themes that were disseminated by these great progenitors of modern yoga. The physical body was considered a part of an integral development that included the mind and spiritual wisdom. These integral themes of mind-body relationship, nature, devotion, and wisdom were the cornerstones of the greater yoga tradition that has been propagated into global awareness.

Sri Aurobindo once said, "The process...accepts our nature...and compels all to undergo a divine change... In that ever progressive experience, we begin to perceive how this lower manifestation is constituted and that everything in it, however seemingly deformed or petty or vile, is the imperfect figure of some element in the divine nature." It seems that while Indians were emphasizing these strong body practices to raise the morale of the people to fight against the proselytizing activities of the Christian missionaries and the oppression of British Raj, the Western world was fascinated with the observation of the body merely for entertainment purposes.

Ghosh's College of Physical Culture and the Yoga Cure Institute were literally around the corner from the family home. Both Bishnu and Buddha were also initiated into advanced forms of Kriya Yoga by Yogananda, and implemented its various themes in their teaching at their schools. These approaches represent specific prescriptions according to the principle of prakriti or individual constitution, which gives special emphasis to healing unique to an individual's needs. In yoga, asana, pranayama, relaxation techniques, and meditation are used as tools for establishing balance. Although the pioneers of yoga therapy did not specifically acknowledge the practice of Ayurveda and yoga, they obviously understood the philosophical[84] importance of such an approach and unknowingly formulated the concepts behind the practice of yoga as "therapy."

This interesting point is connected to the fact that the great yogi Lahiri Mahasaya, guru of Yogananda's parents, and Swami Sri Yukteswar, Yogananda's guru, were well-versed in Samkyha philosophy and the *Charaka Samhita* or Ayurvedic book of medicine. Lahiri Mahasaya expounded fascinating and esoteric commentaries on both subjects from the perspective of prana as related to the scientific practice of Kriya Yoga.[85] The power of asana to affect our inner anatomy is unlike any other ancient system in world history. Yogis like Lahiri Mahasaya extolled the development of prana through the practice of Kriya Yoga as the greatest medicine for bodily health and realization of the Self.

Although it may seem that muscle-control practices were invented in the 19th century, similar techniques appear in an ancient yoga text called the *Vasishta Samhita*, which indicates the system's antiquity. This text itemizes 18 vital energy centers evenly distributed throughout the body. Each center is part of a pranic network that influences the flow of energy through the entire body and withdrawal of energy from the senses. In a text entitled "Key to the Kingdom of Health," Buddha Bose outlines twenty similar points taught in Yogananda's energization system, which are also similar to those found in Sivananda's and Kuvalayananda's teachings. The centers are stimulated in a variety of positions, from standing to lying on the back in Savasana, for the enhancement of sensory withdrawal. The unique point relative to Yogananda's teachings was to draw the power of attention to the maha or grander form of prana entering the body to expand strength, vitality, awareness, and the energy centers or chakras along the spine.

On a different level, asanas can be used selectively according to our preference, and also for specific remedial measures. Asanas can be practiced individually or, for greater benefit, they can be combined into a series or set of postures. For every pose, there exists a counter-pose, depending on the effect on the spine. When we practice a spinal compression posture like Bhujangasana (cobra),

---

84   Samkhya philosophy.
85   *Complete Works* of Lahiri Mahasaya, Swami Satyeswarananda.

it should be combined with a spinal extension posture like Pachimotthana-sana (seated forward bend) to release pressure from the vertebrae and create flexibility in the joints and muscles. Twists can also be used as counter-poses.

The other important factor in enhancing the effects of asana is the symbolism or meaning behind each posture. I have chosen to include limited details of specific instructions on performing the asanas, because it is much more effective to learn them directly from a yoga asana teacher. Also, the basic points of positioning the body can be gathered through study of the images provided in this book.

Yogananda taught some of the 84 scriptural asanas, along with penetrating insights on their therapeutic value, in America[86]. This was a supplementary (not complementary) part of the disciplinary practices undertaken by monks entering his ashram for training. There were also regular public asana demonstrations at the Hollywood, California temple and perhaps elsewhere. The Self-Realization Fellowship published this content regularly in its magazine. Other demonstrations were given in America by Bishnu Ghosh and Buddha Bose in 1939. After having taught in England and Germany, they taught in Washington D.C. and at Columbia University in New York City. In the USA, Yogananda sometimes brought SRF monks with him to perform various asanas when he was invited to lecture in different cities. Indra Devi, the only female yoga teacher accepted into training in India with Sri Tirumalai Krishnamacharya in 1938, eventually moved to America. She opened an asana school in Hollywood in 1948 and taught there until at least 1960, before moving to Mexico. This book includes many years of my own research and personal sadhana with these postures as well as integration of work done at my Dancing Shiva yoga studio and Ayurveda clinic.

The Mysticism of Asana

The mysticism of asana is derived from its capacity to develop will power, which also strengthens the body. Saints like Jesus and sages like Yogananda have stated that the physical body is not sustained by food and exercise, but depends more on the subtle life-force energy within, which is a loan given to us by the Divine. What is unique about the system Yogananda taught was, as he said, "It teaches one how to concentrate his or her attention, not on instruments, muscles nor body movements, but on the awakened energy which is the direct giver of power, strength and vitality to all bodily tissues, including

---

86 As seen in the documentary film *Awake: The Life of Yogananda*, by CounterPoint Films.

the muscular."[87] What is being referred to is the flow of energy within the body rather than positioning the outer body. Good mobility in yoga asana is more important than extreme flexibility. The greatest importance lies in focusing the mind's attention on the source of the energy that comes into the body. An effective use of asana relies not on physical transformation but mainly on the energy behind each posture.

Asana, as practiced by yogis, and mentioned in the scriptures, did not emphasize physical alignment in the sense that everyone must conform to particular physical positioning. It was based on the higher awareness of experiencing the transformation of energy through exercise of the will, which ultimately creates the posture. Will creates energy and energy manifests the postures. It is these movements that give rise to a new direction and placement for the prana, in which the energy becomes seated or focused. When prana flows into various nadis or marmas, that is, prana power points, the practitioner gains mastery over the body and accesses asana's healing benefits.

The breath during asana should remain as normal as possible. Obviously, this will vary depending on the nature of pose. One slight difference does exist between breathing "normally," as we do while walking, sitting, or performing a random activity, and breathing in the practice of asana. Breathing in asana should be done in a proactive manner. This is particularly important during the beginning of any asana practice, because it is necessary to circulate the blood and oxygen to warm up the muscles and prepare the joints to enhance the practice and reduce the risk of injury. It is easy to forget to breathe, and so, with a proactive breathing approach, we must remind ourselves to keep breathing deeply all the time.

Normal breathing from the yogic perspective is defined as deep and expansive, so as to fill and expand the lungs and diaphragm. Such breathing is of key importance for scattered and restless people, naturally quick breathers with a predominance of air or vata. Although certain branded styles of yoga endorse the practice of certain breathing techniques like Ujjai during the performance of asana, this is only one approach and can be somewhat challenging, especially for people trying to learn a posture for the first time. Repeated practice of a technique such as Ujjai during asana practice can also be very heating and should be cautioned for types that may have a predominance of fire, naturally occurring internal heat, or pitta.

---

87 Paramahansa Yogananda, "Descriptive Outline of Yogoda," published by Self-Realization Fellowship in 1929.

One common issue I have seen many times is that students who have practiced Ujjai pranayama during asana practice to the exclusion of other types of pranayama have habitually conditioned the throat muscles, larynx, and glottis, to the degree that they have actually lost mastery of the breath rather than improving it, which is what pranayama is intended to do. In order to gain mastery of the breath, one must be adaptable to changes and variations in how we use our body and breathing to affect energy. What I have seen in many circumstances, when conditioning has occurred from repeated and excessive use of Ujjai, is that when a person tries to practice another technique, such as Kapalabhati or Bastrika, they do not relax the throat. They basically combine both techniques and then do not really receive the benefit of other forms of pranayama.

This is a common scenario. It is easier to teach someone how to do asana and pranayama properly from scratch than to teach someone to undo something that has been conditioned for some time. This is one of many issues associated with the commercialization of yoga. The importance of the historical points that I have referenced here is to foster greater balance between the scientific incentives of the West and the metaphysical spirituality of the East, and potentially to rescind the separation between mind-body and spirit consciousness that has occurred globally.

The Roots of Consciousness and Healing

The relationship of consciousness and healing is eternal and epitomized as Shiva and Shakti in the Tantra yoga system. The model of healing that we refer to now as mind-body medicine is tied to the relationship consciousness shares with healing. It is the most sacred relationship of life on the planet, and, as I have previously discussed, it demonstrates how the sun-moon, male-female, and passive-active concepts can be unified to establish living in a transcendental fashion. There exist two sides to the practice of asana that comprise the two main aspects of practice: austerity or tapasya and wisdom or buddhi. These make asana a sacred practice and not merely a form of physical fitness.

What distinguishes yoga asana from any other system is its focus on attaining stillness. This begins with cultivating the discipline and strength to still the body in any asana. It ultimately culminates in attaining stillness in Padmasana or lotus posture or one of its variations like Suhkasana, as mentioned in the scriptures. The *Hatha Yoga Pradipika* and the *Hatharatnavali* both list four poses as the most important. "Siddhasana, padmasana, simhasana and bhadrasana, these are the four main asanas. Always sit comfortably in siddhasana because it is best."[88] Siddhasana is the posture of perfection, Padmasana is the lotus posture and is sometimes called Kamalasana, Simhasana is the lion pose, and Bhadrasana is the gracious posture. These are all basically slight variations of a cross-legged position. Siddhasana seems to be the most practical and best posture for all types, and was even endorsed by Swami Sivananda. Vajrasana is an excellent pose for practice of pranayama.

The symbolism behind the sacred relationship of Shiva extends into mountains, body, asana, seat, stillness, awareness, and *sat* or truth. The symbolism behind the sacred relationship of Shakti expands into rivers, breath, prana, oxygen, blood and the interconnectedness of all organs, systems, and elements. The three bodies—physical, astral, and causal—are all linked by the creative power of Divine Mother. This Divine energy transports us from place to place and connects us to all of life.

Holding an asana expands the consciousness and level of awareness through observation and concentration. Asana is a way of becoming "seated" in consciousness, so that the postures are executed with the intention of uniting body and mind and eventually transcending them, as occurs in the relaxing state of Savasana. This practice, when repeated, gradually deepens the effects of pratyahara, thereby preparing the yogi for the sublime practice of meditation.

This is one reason why I strongly emphasize in my classes the importance of learning to attain stillness in the asana, and avoid constant, restless adjustments. The therapeutic value of asana comes through a flow of grace from knowing that the Divine feminine powers are, as Yogananda would say, "the nearest of the near and dearest of the dear." This requires acceptance of our capacity to practice and allow the flow of energies, fluids, and hormonal secretions to take place, by letting the asana work for you, rather than by you working for the asana. Even though asana utilizes the body rigorously, the sadhaka must find ease and learn how to surrender into each posture. Otherwise, the practice will always be a physical struggle that leads to nowhere.

Surya Namaskar has existed from ancient times, and continues in many lineages. Indians have always considered salutations to the sun, combined with Vedic chants, as a vital practice of healing through the higher consciousness symbolized by the sun. The sun, as the most visible planet in the sky, is like the decorative bindi worn on the forehead, which is symbolic of the spiritual eye. Traditionally, salutations to the sun are done without attachment to the

---

88 *Hatha Yoga Pradipika*, chapter 1 verse 34

fruits of the action and are performed with a selfless adoration, acknowledging the sun as the source of all life on earth.

Men and Women in Yoga Asana Practice

There are many important considerations women must make when integrating yoga practice into their lives. Yoga has proven to be an effective means for balancing hormones, increasing fertility, and regulating menstruation. Unfortunately, over the years I have seen yoga have a negative effect on women for two reasons: the approach to or type of yoga, and the modern lifestyle.

For women, yoga is based on feeling, and many seem to be drawn to it for its intangible sensibility. It can become a very personal and sacred ritual. In the Western world, more women practice yoga than men, because a woman approaches making choices and cultivating a lifestyle based on feelings and how those feelings can migrate into the emotional body. In general, the female body has less muscle and more fat than the male body. Because of the female body's unique endocrinology, women may find that yoga can bring them greater hormonal balance. They discover that connecting to something within the body can take them beyond it. It's a journey towards surrender, a sacrifice they are willing to take to get to that special place.

Holding yoga poses stretches the body, moves energy by increasing circulation of blood, and induces hormonal secretions from the pituitary and pineal glands, which govern an array of physical functions.[89] For women, the brain, nervous system, and endocrine system all work together and are directly impacted by yoga asana. The practice helps improve moodiness, enhance sleep, increase libido, mitigate the effects of menopause, increase estrogen, manage weight, reduce fear, and relieve anxiety. It also reduces the risk of breast cancer, fibroids, and infertility, as proper function of the thyroid gland influences the metabolism.

For men, asana influences the brain, nervous system, and digestive system, strengthening metabolism and increasing appetite. Of the hormonal secretions produced by yoga asana, two are vitally important and relevant to both women and men. Dopamine is key to brain function, motor-organ operation, and lactation. It influences the function of the nervous system, kidneys, and pancreas. Serotonin is found mostly in the gastro-intestinal tract, regulating

---

89   Breast-milk production, blood pressure, body growth, water balance/retention as controlled by the kidneys, body temperature, sleeping cycles as controlled by the pineal gland, the function of the thyroid gland, which controls metabolism and how food nutrients are converted into energy, and much more.

its movements. Serotonin is released in response to positive events and can affect our relationship with food.

The way in which a woman approaches the science of yoga on the whole is more conducive to progress physically, mentally, and emotionally. I am not saying that the male gender does not have the right capacity, but that they have to work away from the outer mind, which can keep their awareness externalized. Feelings have no limitations. They can open one door of energy and creative expression that naturally leads to another. Men in general tend to reason with yoga and validate it through the intellect. Such structured thinking and becoming fixed on a concept of finite end goals can create limitations and prevent the process of continuous exploration.

I feel that one of the keys to success with a science such as yoga is to embrace its devotional side or bhakti. Bhakti Yoga is Divine love born from the motion of the moon. Devotion softens the mind and awakens and sensitizes it by attunement to the finer energies within us. Our society teaches us to look outside of ourselves when doing anything and, worst of all, for answers to life's problems. We look to doctors to heal us, teachers to guide us, the police and insurance policies to protect us, astrologers to tell us everything about our future, and psychotherapists to help us understand how bad our relationships are and how to fix them. All of these externalities put us on a wheel that keeps us continuously turning away from ourselves. The design of yoga is to look within, to turn our awareness inward to solve our problems, and to answer the most mysterious of life's questions: Who Am I?

Yoga without devotion becomes heady jargon filled with intellectual equations and formulas that keep the mind and body attached to each other or, in some cases, very separated, because the body is looked on as an asset or entity. Devotion is a motion of consciousness that originates in the heart, allowing our consciousness to transcend bodily shape and form, time and space. It can become a very powerful vehicle for healing both mind and body. The skin and endocrine system rule the emotional body, and can trap us in an endless cycle of lack of fulfillment unless we can learn to bridge these sensations and feelings with the mind, freeing ourselves. In other words, the mind is a necessary tool. We must use discrimination to move beyond external sensations. It is fine to have such sensations but what we do with them is the factor that matters most. Otherwise, they are just another emotion, a story in the head, a physical sensation with nothing to direct it.

Women and Hatha Yoga

There are two main factors that influence the impact yoga has on a woman's body. In the Western world, with the commercialization of yoga, what we find is a physical-fitness approach to practice, devoid of spirituality, devotion, and any understanding or consideration of the natural laws yoga is aligned with.

Cosmic intelligence *(mahat)* takes form in creation as the five elements. It is responsible for the manifestation of the individual constitution or prakriti, and influences the cycles of the twenty-four hour day and four energy shifts of the year known as seasons. When yoga asana is fragmented from its counterparts, pranayama or breathing techniques and pratyahara or relaxation techniques, it becomes excessively heating, raising the agnis to levels no longer beneficial. How this affects each person will vary depending on their prakriti and vikriti or imbalances. This leads to a number of potentially chronic health issues that, for women, largely affect the endocrine or hormonal and the nervous system.

The other major issue with women practicing yoga today is the modern life-style's stress levels. You would think that yoga is something that would relieve stress, and it is. The problem has more to do with the pattern created where the mind-body complex is in a repeated a cycle of intoxication, through stress and lifestyle, then elimination by exhausting the body with yoga. The cycle repeats, never allowing the mind-body relationship to attain equanimity. Both the emotional body and nervous system experience what I call the yo-yo affect.

This is another peril of fragmenting Hatha Yoga away from proper diet, individual constitution, and an integral lifestyle. The term "yoga" implies wholeness, to unify, integrate, and transcend. By integrating Hatha Yoga with the balanced lifestyle that Ayurveda provides, the sun-moon-earth relationship can again find harmony. On a grander scale, it is through this sacred reunion of practice and wisdom that humanity will experience joy in life and all the beauty and abundance it encompasses.

The challenge of having a stressful lifestyle and trying to use yoga to balance it is not limited to women. The difference is the specific responses of the female anatomy and physiology. Yoga asana in general is a rigorous use of the body, and if a woman comes to it with stress, irregular sleep patterns, poor diet, and lack of alignment with other lifestyle principles, yoga may release some stress in the short term, but in the longer cycle of months and years it depletes the body.

Women should use caution in practicing asana during menstruation. They should also be cautious if, as is the case for many women these days, their lifestyle is not well suited to maintaining the ojas necessary to practice yoga for gaining energy rather than becoming exhausted from it. This becomes one of the main reasons the menstrual cycle becomes irregular. Excess heat in the body wears down the strength of the dhatus or tissues and drains the ojas that sustains them. It taxes the adrenal glands designed to fight off stress by secreting cortisol and estrogen. Both of these steroid hormones are necessary for homeostasis, but if the adrenal glands are weak and depleted, the physiology begins to react unfavorably. In vata types, this would create amenorrhea and, in pitta types, painful menses or dysmenorrhea, which can lead to uterine fibroids, infections, and even excessive bleeding or menorrhagia.

In such cases, I find the physiology is simply revolting at incongruous behavior affecting the mind-body relationship. The basis for a healthy endocrine system in a woman's body depends largely on estrogens. If these hormones, such as estradiol, are deficient, infertility can result. I have seen many cases over the years of women having lost their period and unable to get pregnant, with too much intense vinyasa asana to blame. This was not the right approach for these women, given their prakriti, lifestyle, and mental attitude.

Nancy was a student at Dancing Shiva for years, coming to my classes very regularly and consistently three to five days per week. She was a married woman with no children at the time, but was thinking about starting a family. She worked long hours and had a very stressful job. Worst of all, she was not really content with the work she was doing. It seemed to lack a purpose.

After consulting Nancy about her lifestyle, I learned that she also ran three to five times per week, in addition to the intense yoga classes she was attending. She had not had a period for many months. Then, suddenly, they would come back, and then disappear again. This went on for years. She wanted help and said to me sincerely, "I want to have children." I believed her and asked her why she was doing so much exercise. She never gave me a good reason, except that she loved coming to my classes and enjoyed the feeling she got from working her body.

Nancy was a pitta prakriti and vikriti. Those with fire as the main mind-body type are more susceptible to imbalances of that element, because it is the most predominant. She was also experiencing digestive hyperacidity and had an all-or-nothing personality. I tried to guide her to become aware of the way she approached things, because if I had just said "do this and that," without having her understand why, that would not have been an organic approach to removing the causes of her imbalances.

After I gave Nancy a number of examples of how her lifestyle paralleled the approach she took to both yoga and running, she began to realize the pattern of her excesses. The first thing I had her do was reduce yoga by 50% and replace running with jogging and walking intervals, as well as to reduce its frequency by 50%. This would give her system time to restore. By reducing heating practices, I could get her to focus more on lunar balancing practices, such as Savasana, meditation, cooking, and other Ayurvedic practices that involved massaging the body with oils. I also gave her a simple Ayurvedic herbal formula that included brahmi and shatavari.

After a few months, I stopped seeing her at class every week. Eventually, I did not hear from her for many years. What happened after the sessions we spent discussing how she was to go about implementing these changes was quite interesting. It is something I have never forgotten. I began to realize that she had to let go of how she was doing things in her life. Initially, this may have been disappointing, because yoga and running brought her so much pleasure. These were an escape, a great physical release, and a chance to meet up with friends. I almost had to tell her not to come to class if she wanted to be able to achieve the health results we had discussed. Many years later, she walked into the lobby of the center. I was quite surprised because she looked a little heavier. In fact, she looked great. I asked, "Where have you been?" She said, "I did what you told me to do. It was the hardest thing in the whole world, but it worked! I have two beautiful children and I am very happy."

Asana and Adrenaline

I have mentioned the importance to immunity of the vital energy called ojas throughout this book. I want now specifically to address a few things that I feel are fundamental to a balanced life with respect to this vital energy, which sustains the body. I want to discuss ojas both from a more mystical perspective and how it figures practically in our daily lives.

The first thing we need to understand is that life exists on borrowed energy and the human complex operates on the same laws as nature. Life can be seen both as a gift and as a search for a higher purpose. Seeing life as a gift assumes that we are given an opportunity to explore, enjoy, love, and potentially discover that life is a beautiful mystery, a type of crossword puzzle that can bring us all that we seek, if we can discover the source. The design of life is rooted in compassion through the law of karma and rebirth. This gives us endless chances to learn how the world operates and find joy in life.

The energy that sustains our heart and inspires our quest to overcome obstacles and to love derives from ojas. All of these things require vitality. The system of yoga asana is a type of body prayer that can keep us in touch with this vehicle, the earth, and the mind, all of which are fueled by ojas. These spiritual gestures require energy and attention. I have repeatedly mentioned that the mind-body relationship is intrinsically connected to our health and spiritual evolution. However, if our lifestyle diminishes the energy we have by looking for fulfillment externally, through materialism, the practice of asana becomes a struggle and can reduce our health. Life and health become a perpetual struggle if the searchlight is always turned outward.

The practice of asana relies on ojas, which keeps the mind-body relationship intact. The body transports us into sensual pleasure, and the body is also our sacred temple. It is the vehicle for creating the events and experiences that define our lives. The Bhagavad Gita, as explicated by Paramahamsa Yogananda and such disciples of Lahiri Mahasaya as Swami Sri Yukteswar and Swami Pranabananda Giri, provides deep insight into this profound spiritual ideal. Krishna and Arjuna ride a chariot symbolic of the *Sarira* (body). They ride into the battlefield together, with each of them symbolizing one of the two aspects of mind: Krishna of the higher intuitive mind, and Arjuna of the sensory or externalized mind. The horses are the five senses and Krishna, having the great power of discernment derived from buddhi, holds the reins, demonstrating mastery and control over them.

The story is a vital metaphor. First, the battle is still going on today right within our own minds and all the time. Second, we must develop mastery and discipline over the senses, or else the horses run wild. In order to maintain an asana practice, we must learn to preserve the ojas through mastery over the senses. Otherwise, we will discover that our vehicle no longer serves to fulfil our higher life purpose.

Another factor in preserving ojas is *satmya* or immunity, and relates to our capacity to habituate to a particular lifestyle. The capacity individuals have to adapt to different diets, environments, asana practices, and climates are all a measure of their immunity. Hypersensitivity to varying conditions is typically a good indicator that immunity is low or weakening. The manner in which we live and adapt is a good indicator of the level of ojas. One of yoga's core principles for sustaining sadhana and avoiding *ojakshaya* or diminished ojas is the practice of **brahmacharya** or celibacy for single people and sexual moderation in marriage. All of these aspects are important measures to consider before launching into an asana routine. This is why yoga is considered a lifestyle and not merely a system of exercise.

Basic Qualities of the Five Elements

Air (Vata) – Its **qualities** are *dry, cool, rough, light, and moving.*

Fire (Pitta) – Its **qualities** are *hot, sharp, a bit oily, and transformative.*

Water (Kapha) – Its **qualities** are *heavy, stable, oily, smooth, and supportive.*

Yoga Practice Guidelines for the Dosha Types

Vata Dosha in Yoga Practice

The greatest struggle for vata types is the ability to focus and concentrate. The other is to hold still. Whether in a posture or during breathing exercises, the body is usually restless and the eyes are wandering from person to person and gazing around the room or out the window. Vatas seek attention and interaction to satisfy a short attention span, and often need some form of entertainment like engaging instruction or dialogue. Vatas can lack flexibility and strength and seem to stay on the dry side, perspiring very little. Generally, they are not flexible in the sacrum and coccyx or hip region, as this is closely located to the large intestine, the seat of vata.

Often in postures, vata types will over-adjust themselves, never really settling into being still. In pranayama, they tend to start breathing too quickly, and can struggle to maintain a steady tempo. With asana, they often anticipate the next pose before it has been decided by the teacher. In Savasana or corpse pose, they usually keep their eyes open and need time to relax and internalize their awareness. They are sensitive, especially with floor poses, and often require additional padding to hold a pose comfortably. They are also sensitive to cold temperature and benefit from a warm room and a heating practice. These days, the majority of individuals, regardless of constitution, have some form of vata imbalance, usually on the mental level.

Pitta Dosha in Yoga Practice

Pitta types enjoy asana, as they are physically very capable. With a medium and symmetrical build, they can balance well and have a strong will when challenged with more complex postures. It is common for pitta types to push into positions, when they should be easing in. A pitta type tends to pulse or bounce slightly while in a pose, feeling more is being gained by doing so. They are usually relentless in difficult poses and struggle with having to stay even-minded while practicing. They have a tendency to tense up in postures when the intention should be to release and expand. They have such great concentration that it can be intimidating and involve interesting facial expressions. In breathing exercises, they can be aggressive and overly forceful, especially in bellows breathing (Bastrika) or nasal exhalation (Kapalabhati), where they shrug the nose and tense the brow and forehead. As the dosha of fire, they begin to sweat very quickly and profusely, but this usually does not endure. They often become fatigued through over-strenuous effort in every aspect of the practice, and finally disengage or surrender from exhaustion in corpse pose. These pitta characteristics are most commonly seen in men between 20 and 40 years of age.

Kapha Dosha in Yoga Practice

Kapha types enjoy doing floor postures, where excess body weight is not such a burden. They tend to tire quickly, especially in balancing postures, but can have good stability. They can move slowly and are often a bit behind the class. As the dosha of water, they are generally very flexible and enjoy stretching on the floor, where they can leverage their weight. Like pitta, kaphas sweat very well. Perspiration is usually slow to start but endures for some time. Kaphas benefit from heat, which promotes sweating and helps to reduce fat tissue or medas. They are the best breathers and benefit from strong and quick breathing techniques. Kaphas, who breathe deeply, find refuge from a fluid vinyasa approach in sets of breathing that can be performed in between the postures or sequences. They are notable for stability and strength and an excellent ability to relax deeply, especially in Savasana, where they often fall asleep.

Generally, it is important to analyze all aspects of your life and find parallels to your yoga practice. In eating, talking, working, and speaking, you can begin to see characteristics that may reflect air, fire, or water. Ideally, we want to embody a balance of all three elements, and be able recognize when our behavior may be in disaccord. The practice of asana, pranayama, and pratyahara benefits all dosha types, but they have varying degrees of influence on each dosha. The idea is not to limit individuals to one or two of these limbs, but to learn how to practice them in a way beneficial to the person's constitution and level of experience.

Asana as an exercise is a very effective way to reduce kapha, as postures raise the body's digestive fire, jatharagni. The Ayurvedic approach to weight reduction is to increase the body's metabolic rate, which is commonly slow with kapha body types. The rigorous nature of yoga postures raises body temperature and promotes sweating, which is helpful in the reduction of fat. When sequences or inversions are combined with fast and strong pranayama like Kapalabhati, the lungs are activated, removing phlegm and clearing the sinuses. Maintaining a strong and clear respiratory system and good digestion are primary principles in weight management. Everyone can benefit to a certain degree from heat, sweating, and a stimulating yoga practice, but kaphas generally benefit the most. It is important to understand that, while everyone can benefit from a stimulating kapha type of practice, such a practice may aggravate both vata and pitta types, especially if done repeatedly for an extended period of time.

Pitta types will receive the greatest benefit from learning moderation. Pratyahara is a great experience of relaxation that balances pitta dosha. In pitta types, the fire is always on, so to speak, and pratyahara teaches the individual how to turn it off and let go.

There is no stronger theme in yoga and metaphysical teachings than the concept of "letting go." All great teachers profess this, in different languages and many ways. A yoga practice that consistently gives short periods of passive rest will teach pittas how to disengage. During the practice of standing or balancing postures, rest and relaxation can be taken in a standing position. During kneeling-type positions and sequences, rest can be taken seated upright on the feet (Vajrasana), and, with floor postures like cobra (Bhujangasana) and camel (Ustrasana), restoration can be taken in the lying position (Savasana). These moments of rest should also be taken after pranayama exercises or bandhas (energy locks).

Our society is learning the hard way that being fast, persistent, and forceful is not the best way to get things accomplished. Pittas are often reactive, so, when they are given a challenging posture or complex sequence, they sometimes respond in a competitive manner. The teaching of pratyahara becomes learning not to react but to observe and surrender. Observation is a powerful tool for self-analysis and necessary to avoid making mistakes.

Balancing vata goes hand-in-hand with proper breathing, as pranayama directly involves control of the air element. There are many techniques to control the prana, but making a simple note to keep aware of the breath during each position is especially helpful. Specific techniques should be performed slowly and with attention. For vata, the breath is the link that connects the body and mind. When I see a restless room of students, I usually start them with alternate-nostril breathing (Nadi Shodhana), a variation explained in the pranayama section. The experience of feeling balanced and grounded deepens when postures, breathing techniques, and periods of relaxation are combined. The ultimate experience comes when the sacred link of posture, breath, and restoration is maintained. The intention of adhering to an integral model is in achieving *samatva,* a balanced state of mind.

Summarizing Dosha in Yoga

Vata (Air) – The key word for vata types in yoga sadhana is *balance*. Postures should be approached or moved into carefully and slowly, while maintaining a gentle attitude. Keep the intention of connecting to the earth to cultivate a feeling of being grounded and stable in each pose. Place major emphasis on setting up and settling into each posture. One should never rush. Try to avoid over-exertion or quick movements that may create a loss of balance. When holding the poses, try to deepen and expand the breath by breathing through the nostrils only. *The aim is to release tension from the hips and the lumbar spine, where vata has a tendency to accumulate.*

Pitta (Fire) – The keyword for pitta types in yoga sadhana is *moderation*. Practice in general should be soothing. The primary intention should be to moderate the effort exerted in each posture. Become aware of tensing the body, and especially the face, and try to "let go" in each pose, knowing that the benefits come without tension. Identify the pitta energy as it commonly appears, as a pushing force. The idea is to hold the asana in a way that is relaxing and somewhat soothing, but still physically effective. Never force your practice, but find a steady rhythm that is moderate in effort. Take rest when necessary and try to practice even-mindedness. At times when the practice is intense, it is important to alternate breathing between the nose and mouth to keep from over-heating. *The aim is to release tension from the mid-abdomen, where pitta tends to accumulate.*

Kapha (Water) – The keyword for kapha types in yoga sadhana is *motivate*. I like to call this approach "kapha busters." The heavy quality of water requires strong stimulation and quickness in order to balance kapha. Do more than is preferred to heat the body properly and create a good sweat. Most postures should not be held long, except for balancing poses, which are excellent for exercising the lungs and heating the body. Rest between asanas should be short and breathing should be done more rapidly so to keep momentum up. *The aim is to open the chest and lungs, where kapha tends to accumulate.*

Asana and Pranayama

Yoga postures and breathing practices are inter-functional, like our hands and feet. Asanas are a vehicle to transport us towards a more prepared state for practice of pranayama, which is the more subtle practice that allows us to direct and control energies within the entire field of the body.

Asana and pranayama work together very effectively to address various regions of the body that are affected by the dosha and require energy-balancing. The practice of asana alone without any direction or intention becomes no different than an aerobics class at a fitness center, resulting in a tiring and mindless experience. When asana is combined with pranayama, the practitioner develops a balance between cultivating the outer and inner being. Physical exercises are an outer experience. For the athlete, it is about winning the game. For the yogi, it is about solving the mystery of life.

Pranayama can be a good tool for improving our health, as it can specifically target certain mind-body issues. There are many breathing techniques, and each can be performed in a unique way to stimulate the organs, affect the body, and treat the doshas. Postures affect the doshas, spine, and internal organs differently. It is the same with pranayama but on a more subtle level.

I have seen many people whot do a lot for their bodies by way of asana but have very poor breathing habits. When they became more conscious of breathing in daily life and integrated pranayama into their yoga routine, their mind-body relationship changed. There are various techniques for breathing that can be much more effective when practiced in conjunction with a specific asana program. Later in the book, I discuss various ways in which breathing exercises can be integrated into an asana practice, so as to make yoga more valuable.

Asana and Age

The best time to begin practicing asana is at a young age, when discipline is a necessary part of balanced development. In Vedic times, asana and other austerities were integrated during what was called the brahmacharya phase of the four *ashrama* periods or life-stages. From an early age, children are taught the value of the mind-body relationship. Asana becomes a useful practice for children to develop strength and flexibility in the body, coordination, and good concentration skills. Asana is excellent for osteogenesis or the development of bones and joints, and promotes muscular elasticity. The practice of asana from an early age can prevent stunted growth and actually increase the height and prevent the shrinking of the body as it ages into the vata or last stage of life.

Ideally, the practice of asana and pranayama should be aligned with and follow the life cycles of the doshas. A strong and more rigorous practice should occur during youth and the young adult phase, which is characteristic of kapha predominance (ages 0 – 16). More moderate practice should occur during the mid-age period, which is characteristic of pitta predominance (ages 16 – 50). Then, eventually, there should be much gentler practices during the vata period, after 50 years of age. It is always beneficial to include inversions during all phases of life because of their unique effect of massaging the inner anatomy. Overall, asana is something that everyone can benefit from, and even more so when approached with the right intention.

Chapter SEVEN

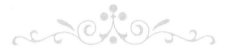

The Art and Science
of Postural Yoga

A cotton thread can cut an iron bar if passed over it daily.
If you work on Yoga, Yoga will work on you.
Baba Hari Dass

Creating the Right Intention

Before beginning asana, it is important to set the right intention for practice. We should ask ourselves what our needs are, how we are feeling, and what we need to do to get into the stillness and reflective quality of sattva guna, a state of calm. Sattva guna is the primal essence of yoga, which aims at purifying the mind. The gunas are an important measure of the mind's quality, and one of the prime teachings of the Bhagavad Gita. The Gita states, "One may know that sattva is prevalent when the light of wisdom shines through all the sense gates of the body."[90] When the right attitude towards our practice is established, all the senses can become purified, allowing the light of wisdom to guide us.

The rajasic or very active person is likewise attached to activity in yoga asana, and struggles to transcend the senses. The tamasic person, beset by inertia, dwells in miscomprehension and negative thoughts. The concept of a vehicle is central to the entire Vedic-Hindu pantheon, which recognizes that all forms of energy require a container in which to be transported. This concept originates in the subtle essences of prana, tejas (vital power), and ojas, which are the positive qualities that recharge the soul.

Ojas, as primal essence, provides energy for the heart while the body is resting during nightly sleep. It supports immune functions and gives us the inspira-

---

90   Bhagavad Gita; Verse 11, Chapter XlV From God Talks With Arjuna: The Bhagavad Gita by Paramahansa Yogananda (Self-Realization Fellowship, Los Angeles, Calif.).

tion for life. Without a good level of ojas, the light of tejas and flow of prana cannot exist.[91] The essences are of key importance in Ayurveda, which aims to correct imbalances of the doshas. The yogic tradition of vehicles as carriers of energy is depicted in Lord Shiva and Nandi, his bull, who is always near him and represents ojas, strength, and power.

The idea of a consort or partner is similar and demonstrates the distribution of power and creativity as seen in the sun-moon relationship. Krishna and his foremost devotee Radha reflect this as eternal lovers of the Divine, as do Shiva and his wife Parvati. The vehicle of the body serves as a means for invoking the Divine qualities hidden within us, all of which can help us attain the right attitude for yoga practice, so that it can diffuse into our lifestyles.

Part of the disciplinary effect of yoga is established by a warrior attitude. A warrior attitude is reflected in one who can remain unchanged as the senses deliver fluctuating signals, who is steady, calm, and unmoved by personal preferences.

In the Bhagavad Gita, the warrior is symbolized by Arjuna, who rides in a chariot along with his counselor and guru, Bhagavan Krishna, to fight the battle of his life and discover his dharma. The warrior or the *kshatriya* caste, as determined by birth, is a powerful yogic symbol that reveals the capacity certain personality types have with respect to discipline and mastery over the five senses. The warrior, known as a "virabhadra,"[92] is created not by birth, but by choice. One must cultivate this attitude through yoga sadhana and the grace that comes with taking on a yogic path. Asana can help to produce a virabhadra attitude and inspires us to create a balanced mind-body relationship. This mind-body synergy is enhanced through a process of selecting the proper vehicles (asanas), the ones you find best suit your needs and level of yoga practice.

---

91   Tejas is the positive fire that gives the body its attractive qualities and the mind its insightful capacity. Prana (subtle ether-air) is the life force that propels our thoughts, produces words and manifests actions. While the doshas also have negative or disease-forming capacities, prana, tejas, and ojas are positive aspects of the elements of air, fire, and water respectively.

92   Virabhadra is considered one of the most revered Avatars of Lord Shiva. In a heroic deed performed in Hindu mythology, Virabhadra stepped in to destroy a yagna (fire sacrifice). Daksha had several daughters, including Dakshayini, who wanted to marry Shiva. Dakshayini jumped into the sacrificial fire because of her father Daksha's lack of support for her marriage. An enraged Lord Shiva beheaded Daksha, trampled on Indra, and broke Yama's staff.

ASANA INVOCATION SERIES

Virabhadrasana (Warrior/Four Poses)

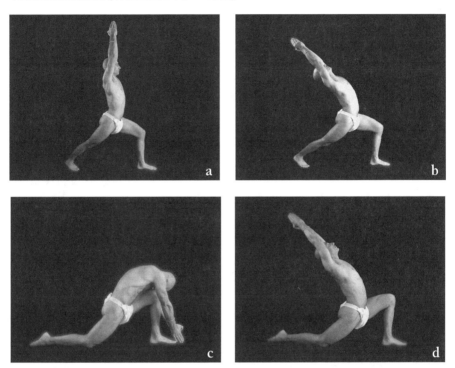

General Description & Symbolism:
This is a simple series of leg stances to warm up the body and invoke the warrior or hero (*vira*) within. Yogis can develop their warrior-like qualities and sensory control through asana and energy control. The practice consists of a forward lunge, followed by a forward lunge with a backward bend. Then, there is a transition into a kneeling forehead-to-knee position, as a gesture of reverence and humility, followed by a kneeling backward bend. Then switch legs and repeat the other side. As you advance in this series, the length of the hold can be increased gradually. Be careful to limit the range of movement in the backbend while the body is still warming up.

Therapeutic Benefit:
This series increases circulation in the legs and improves flexibility in the hip flexors. It strengthens the quadriceps muscles around the knees and creates a good foundation for balancing poses.

Ayurvedic Benefit:
This series is tri-doshic, as warming up is an important practice for all types.

Spiritual Benefit:
It has a centering effect on the samana prana (prana of transformation) as it works with the energies of both apana (downward-flowing) prana in the lunges and udana (upward-breathing) prana in the torso and arm extensions. Mentally, this series of simple positions helps create tapasya (discipline), kindle agni (fire), and increase concentration.

Level: Beginner

ASANA WARM-UP SERIES I

Surya Namaskar (Sun Salutation/12 Poses)

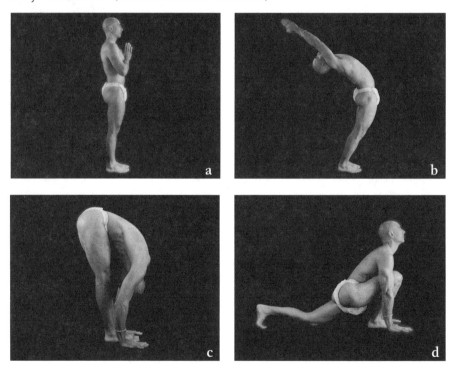

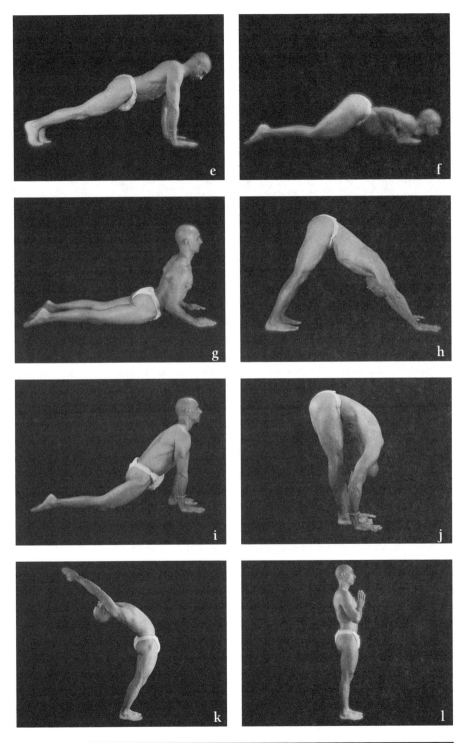

Surya Pranam

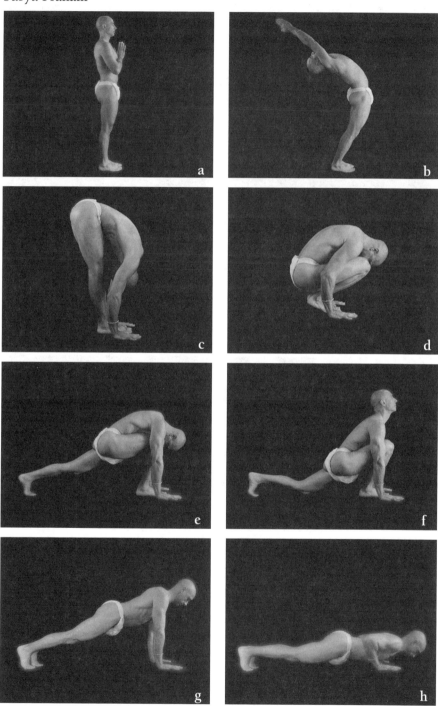

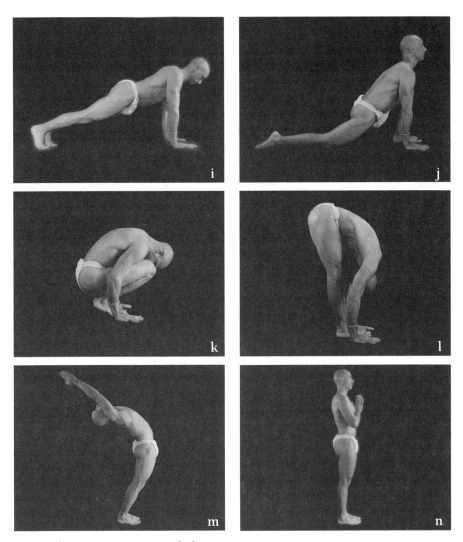

General Description & Symbolism:

The Sanskrit word for the sun is *surya* and the term also appears in the Rig Veda. Although the most recognized series of poses in yoga asana, the sun salutation does not appear in Hatha Yoga texts and seems to be a development of the modern yoga revival. Although the sun has always been revered and considered as father of the solar system, its powers and qualities were commonly invoked in through mantras and prayer rituals. The sun as the soul in every living being inherently guides human beings to seek, reflect, and discover.

While the Hatha Yoga system continues its evolution, many variations and forms of the sun salutation already exist. Regardless of the form you practice, the sun salutation is an excellent warm-up for an integral yoga practice, and when practiced alone, it serves as an excellent system for keeping the spine supple and strong. As a symbolic gesture of the soul's longing for something beyond the world, the series is ideally practiced at sunrise to precipitate its inspirational affects. In the most popular form, the twelve positions represent the months of the year and twelve signs of the zodiac. In the Bengali yoga asana tradition, there is a similar sequence called Surya Pranam, which is virtually unknown and has some slight differences from Surya Namaskar, although it is also considered good preparation for holding individual poses.

Therapeutic Benefit:
The combination of back-bending and forward-bending brings great flexibility to the spine and hips. The plank, crouching tiger, and cobra positions strengthen the arms, lumbar spine, and trapezius muscles. The push-up variation in the Bengali salutation builds chest and arm strength. Both versions, by the repeated action of compressing and extending the spinal vertebrae, balance the hormonal system and promote harmonious systemic function and improved circulation. The series gently strengthens the jatharagni (metabolism) and promotes blood circulation and lymph purification, improving heart function.

Ayurvedic Benefit:
This series is tri-doshic, as warming up is an important practice for all types. It is particularly beneficial for vata types, who can have a restrictive range of movement in the hips. The lunging action releases apana and stretches the hip flexor and buttock muscles. Overall, the sun series has a moderate tone to it that is good for pitta types. The forward bends also release pitta bound in the mid-abdomen. The standing backbends are strong and heating poses that benefit kapha types.

Spiritual Benefit:
Saluting the sun is an acknowledgement that Divinity is our birthright and increases yearning for the "One" all-encompassing love, peace, and contentment we seek to discover in our hearts. Overall, it enhances the flow of prana. As it improves flexibility in the hips, it prepares them for seated positions like Siddhasana and Padmasana, the main positions used in meditation. Salutations improve flexibility in the spine and prepare it for the Raja Yoga practices of mantra, pranayama, and meditation. If the spine is stiff and contorted, it will lack the feeling and subtle sensitivities necessary for yoga meditation.

Level: Beginner-Intermediate.

WARM-UP SERIES II

Chandra Namaskar Series (Moon Salutation/14 Poses)

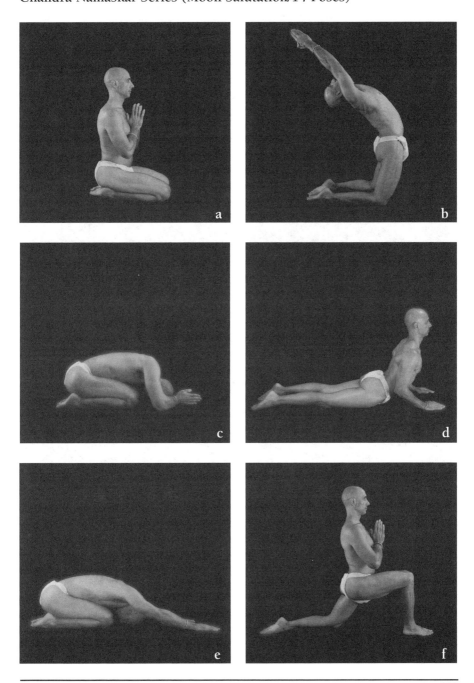

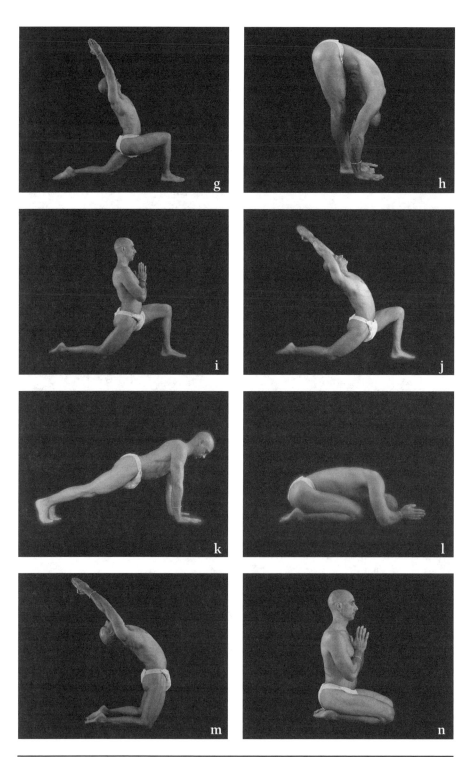

General Description & Symbolism:

The Sanskrit word for moon is *chandra*. Like the sun salutation, the moon series does not specifically appear in the Hatha Yoga texts, but seems to have developed through several lineages emphasizing Tantric wisdom. A similar prostration exists in Tibetan Buddhist traditions. The intention of the moon sequence is to invoke a more restorative quality, which teaches us to embrace the grace and kindness of the moon. The moon imbues us with qualities of kindness for all living things, creativity, fertility, endurance, love, and greater affinity to the Divine feminine. It can be a powerful aid to balancing the fire element, as the moon is closely related to the air (waning moon) and water (waxing moon) elements.

Therapeutic Benefit:

Moon salutations have an overall soothing quality on the tissues and help to build strength in the dhatus, mainly the muscle, bone and nerve tissues. They help improve mental balance mentally, and are grounding and calming if issues related to vertigo are present. They are especially important for nervousness, anxiety, and spinal-related issues such as kyphosis or hunching of the back. Like the sun salutes, they are also good for opening the hips and releasing tension in the gluteus maximus and gluteus minimus. They gently improve digestive irregularities or flatulence. The two most therapeutically beneficial positions are cobra and child's pose.

Ayurvedic Benefit:

Spinal mobility and muscular strengthening are both improved, and these are key areas for working with vata dosha. Cobra position and child's pose both directly benefit the lower back muscles, kidneys, and colon. Sciatic nerve issues can be treated with a gentle emphasis on back-bending positions. Moon salutes are good for intense pitta types because of their soft and soothing action. Because they are done so near the earth, they have a cooling quality. Yet they are also very grounding and help reduce restlessness, a common characteristic of vata types. They are excellent for increasing concentration.

Spiritual Benefit:

Concentration on the qualities of the moon is necessary for attracting soma or nectar-like qualities. Moon salutes kindle the bhava (feeling or emotion) of bhakti, devotion, and are an excellent preparation for mantra, pranayama, and meditation practice. They bring a clearness of vision, insight, and alertness of mind that fosters sattva guna or calmness. In essence, they are a physical means for purification of the mind and its desires (*vasanas*).

Level: Beginner-Intermediate.

STANDING POSES

These are postures practiced with both feet on the ground. Many of these stances were influenced by the temple dance traditions (*deva dasi*), part of classical Indian artistic traditions and the martial arts.[93] The variety of standing postures is extensive and many provide similar therapeutic effects on the body. I have chosen to list select postures mentioned in classical texts such as the *Gheranda Samhita, Hatha Yoga Pradipika*, and others.

Uthkatasana (Chair)

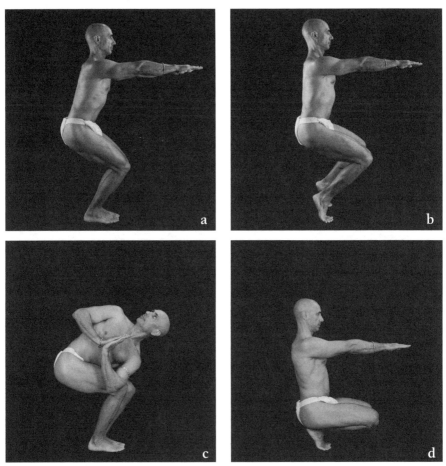

---

93 *Dhanuveda* (martial arts) is derived from two words, *dhanushya* for bow and veda for knowledge. Dhanuveda is one of the four Upavedas, along with *Gandharvaveda* (study of music and sacred dance), *Ayurveda* (science of health and well-being) and *Arthasastra* (dealings of military science, governance, and economy).

General Description & Symbolism:

Asana is the first stage of Hatha Yoga and the third limb of Patanjali's Yoga Sutra model. The chair pose is a primary positioning of the hips, knees, and spine, which provides a good foundation for practicing many other poses. In Sanskrit, *uthkata* means awkward, as it often feels awkward when holding this asana. This can also be broken into two words: *ut* meaning upward or raised and *kata* meaning hips. There are several variations of chair as shown, some with feet close together, and another with feet about hip-distance apart. Another variation is practiced with the knees and feet together and fully bent until the soles of the feet are perpendicular to the floor and the calves and thighs kept parallel to the floor.

A twisting variation can be added, where the feet are together and the hands joined at the heart in prayer gesture. There are additional variations of chair, which involve fully squatting down to the ground so that the heels are fully raised and holding the position while keeping the spine upright. The arms can also be extended forward and the eyes closed as a practice for attaining inner balance. There is another variation mentioned in the *Gheranda Samhita*: "Let the toes touch the ground, and the heels be raised in the air; place the anus on the heels: this is known as the Uthkatasana."

Therapeutic Benefit:

This is probably the best asana for strengthening the calves, legs, buttocks, and lower back. It also increases circulation in those areas. The second and third variations, with the heels raised, strengthen the tibial and peroneal areas of the feet, which support the arches. This helps correct foot placement distortions created from years of poor alignment while walking or doing other physical activity. It is good for those that have flat feet, as the knees lose muscular support when there is little or no arch in the foot.

Interestingly, the pose improves a sense of balance and promotes a feeling of being grounded. When practiced with eyes closed, the optic sense perceptions are shut out, which improves the cerebellum function that coordinates body equilibrium. The heart muscle is also exercised, as heart function and rate are increased the longer the asana is held. This simple pose provides excellent cardiovascular conditioning, especially when the posture is repeated several times.[94] The twisting action has both structural benefit to the thoracic spine, mainly in the mid-area, and internal anatomical benefit to the ascending and descending colon, as well as the stomach and liver, which are also massaged.

---

94 See: *Self-Realization* Magazine, November/December 1957 (Self-Realization Fellowship, Los Angeles, Calif.).

Ayurvedic Benefit:
Chair and its variations are best for vata-type issues, which typically include a lack of thigh, buttock, and back strength. It helps build muscle and strength specifically in the quadriceps, buttocks, and lumbar muscles. Overall, it is also good for pitta and kapha types, depending on the length of hold and related factors. The twisting-chair variation is excellent in promoting digestive regularity, detoxifying the liver, and removing kapha build-up in the stomach. The twisting variation of chair is excellent for removing excess pitta, which tends to accumulate in the small intestine, tightening the thoracic region of the spine. For pitta-related conditions, this is one of the few twists that allows for a great release of tension in the mid-spine, and also massages the internal digestive organs.

Spiritual Benefit:
"Posture is half the battle," Paramahansa Yogananda used to say, and this posture is one that prepares the entire spine for meditation. Chair builds the muscles around the low- and mid-back to support the spine from slumping, especially during longer practices of pranayama, mantra, and meditation. The increased circulation during the practice of chair pose allows the legs and lower spinal nerves to relax more fully during seated meditation practice and improves the depth of practice.

Level: Beginner-Intermediate

Padahastasana – (Hands to Feet)

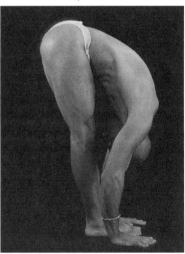

General Description & Symbolism:
This standing forward bend joins the upper torso with the upper thighs and

benefits the back, shoulders, and rear thighs. It is important to sandwich the body completely. If necessary, the knees should be bent so that the both halves of the body come together. In time and with gradual practice, the palms of the hands will begin to press flat against the floor on either side of the feet, and the knees may eventually completely straighten.

According to Samkhya philosophy, the hands represent the instrument of touch, related to the air element, and the feet are correlated to the element of fire. Both are instruments of action. The practice of Padahastasana symbolizes the combined practice of both the paths of yoga and Samkhya through the union of the hands and feet, and of the torso and thighs. There are requirements for reaching the ultimate state beautifully described in Vedanta: "Samkhya teaches that renunciation of all actions is necessary in order to gain Self-knowledge. Both practice of Sankhya and yoga teach how to attain Brahman."[95] Yoga is the path of discipline and Sankhya that of wisdom. Their balance brings true empowerment.

Therapeutic Benefit:
As a standing forward bend, this pose provides a good stretch for the lower back and hamstrings, (which I also like to call the "leg biceps"). It is also a partial inversion and provides effects similar to full inverted positions. The benefits specifically include bringing circulation to the lungs, head, and brain. The posture releases pressure in the lower back sometimes related to sciatic-nerve discomfort. The gentle pressure on the abdominal nerves has a soothing effect on digestion and general stomach issues. The pose is effective for treating diabetes and sinus issues, and helps to increase the length of the spine.

Ayurvedic Benefit:
Due to the extension of the spinal vertebrae, the posture has a cooling and diffusing effect for pitta types. The inverted position helps bring circulation to kapha issues, particularly those of *avalambhaka kapha* (kapha located in the heart, chest, and lower back). Vata types benefit from stretching the lower back and legs, areas where they usually lack flexibility.

Spiritual Benefit:
The extension of the spinal vertebrae has a key benefit of enhancing meditation, which requires being seated and can often create tightness in the back. Releasing the muscular tension in the lower back and legs, and improving clarity in the mind, enhance relaxation and stillness.

Level: Beginner

---

95   Quote taken from *God Talks With Arjuna: The Bhagavad Gita* by Paramahansa Yogananda (Self-Realization Fellowship, Los Angeles, Calif., 1999), specifically the commentary on Chapter XVlll verse 13

Ardha Chandrasana (Half Moon)

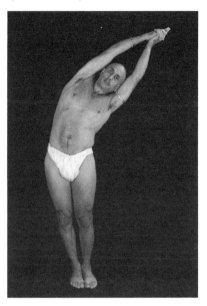

General Description & Symbolism:
In Sanskrit, *ardha* means "half" and *chandra* means "moon." This posture entails bending the body and spine sideways while keeping both feet together. It is practiced in two different directions, one a lateral position that stretches the sides of the torso, and the other a full back-bending position. Both are very beneficial for the spine, although the back-bending position is much more difficult and heating.

Therapeutic Benefit:
This posture increases the flexibility of the spine, particularly in lateral range of motion. It strengthens the abdominal muscles and wall, due to the support and engagement required while practicing the pose. It stimulates function of the liver, spleen, and kidneys. It tones the latussimus dorsi, external obliques, and rectus abdominis, and reduces excess fat around the shoulders and back. The back-bending action is excellent for strengthening the lower lumbar muscles, expands the lungs, and increases cardiovascular function.

Ayurvedic Benefit:
Depending on the length of hold and intensity of practice, this posture can be beneficial for all dosha types. Lateral stretches such as these are excellent for pitta types, because they are not overly heating and provide a necessary and unique stretch for the spine. With its effect on the liver, spleen, and kidneys, it is anatomically beneficial to both pitta and vata.

Spiritual Benefit:
Most all standing postures require focus, motivation, and endurance, important factors in developing mastery over the body and the senses. Standing postures require rajas (outward energy) that can help to remove tamas (stagnant energy) and lead us into a state of sattva (stillness and clarity) for higher meditation.

Level: Beginner-Intermediate

Trikonasana (Triangle Pose)

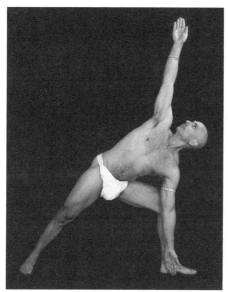 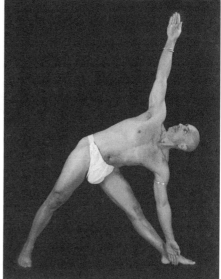

General Description & Symbolism:
Triangle pose is another of the few poses that bends the spine laterally. Some lineages teach the pose with both legs straight and legs wider apart. In the Bengali lineage, the pose is practiced with one of the legs in a bent or lunging position, and the stance is approximately two to three feet wide, or half the length of the body. No weight should be placed on the leg that is being held straight, or on the hand that is reaching down towards the floor. The shape of the triangle is created with the base as the distance between the feet, the extended arms as one side, and the straight leg as the other. The triangle is directly associated with the yantra or geometric designs of the Tantra tradition, which are used for chanting mantras and meditation. The upward-pointing triangle is related to Shiva and the downward-pointing to Shakti.

Therapeutic Benefit:

By placing all the weight on the lunging thigh, all the thigh and buttock muscles are strengthened. With the lateral placement of the torso and abdominal wall, blood flow increases and circulation in the entire thoracic region is stimulated. One side of the trunk is being stretched, while the other is being engaged in an opposing action. This energizes the lateral organs on the right side (liver, right kidney, and ascending colon) and the lateral organs on left side (spleen, left kidney, and descending colon).

The lateral stretching action of triangle brings increased flexibility to the lateral muscles in the lower back region and creates additional space in the tissues of the intervertebral discs between the vertebrae. Trikonasana massages the abdominal aorta, which supplies blood to much of the abdominal cavity. This begins at the 12th thoracic vertebra, and runs parallel to the inferior vena cava, which is located just to the right of the abdominal aorta. These are important arteries that improve blood supply to the kidneys, aiding in the elimination of waste and toxins. Triangle is also important for the nerve bundles in the lower spine and the sympathetic ganglia that lie parallel to the spinal column. Although the positioning is similar to that of half-moon pose, triangle pose provides greater internal benefit, as the lateral positioning of the spine is much deeper.

Ayurvedic Benefit:

As triangle places much emphasis on the lower spine and legs, it greatly benefits vata dosha and its related organs and systems, the kidneys and nervous and digestive systems. It improves digestive strength and regularity. It can be a very heating asana if the position is held between 30 seconds and one minute. Because of its capacity to increase blood flow and improve kidney function, the pose is restorative and can greatly increase the balance of both prana and ojas. This is the case if the posture is not practiced excessively, and is combined with a Savasana, where the benefits are ultimately attained. The thoracic nerves of the sympathetic ganglia deliver information to the body about stress and impending danger, and are responsible for the familiar fight-or-flight response rooted in fear, which is characteristic of imbalanced vata.

Spiritual Benefit:

The increased vitality that triangle brings affords the yogi much of the inspiration necessary for the practice of meditation. The soothing and strengthening effect on the sympathetic ganglia is essential to calming and settling the vata mind, enhancing the quality of concentration, and increasing the capacity for expanded awareness.

Level: Beginner-Intermediate

BALANCING POSTURES

These are postures practiced with one foot on the ground. Their focus is leg strength, stamina, and balance. In general, balancing postures require abdominal support for lifting one leg off the ground. The abdomen plays a major role in the capacity one has to be able to stay balanced in a posture, as the abdomen supports the lower back.

Natarajasana (Dancing Shiva Pose)

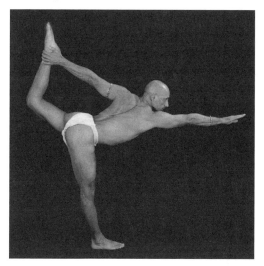

General Description & Symbolism:
This is one of the most auspicious postures, as it specifically refers to Lord Shiva as King Dancer. It could be considered the king of all stances. It is awakened prana shakti that inspires Shiva to dance and perform his *ananda tandava* or dance of bliss. This is a metaphor of what comes with the dissolution of the ego. Shiva is part of the Hindu trinity and represents the destructive force of creation, while Vishnu is the preserving, and Brahman is the creative. Practice of this posture invokes the all-consuming power of Lord Shiva.

Therapeutic Benefit:
This is a full-body pose that stimulates the entire body through the respiratory system and strengthens all the muscles in both legs, the torso, arms, and shoulders. It both strengthens the quadriceps muscles in the legs and stretches the rear hamstring muscles. It tones and strengthens the entire abdomen as well as the shoulders in the area of the trapezius and deltoids. It is one of the best postures for improving respiration and removing stagnation of excess phlegm by expanding the lungs. When held for periods of 30 seconds to one minute, it can increase metabolic rate and strengthen the jatharagni.

Ayurvedic Benefit:

Practice of the posture on both sides allows for a full opening of the chest and increased respiration. The slight compression of the lower back muscles that occurs while balancing on one leg makes it excellent for kapha and related issues. I have probably integrated this pose into my clinical healing practice more than any other posture, particularly during programs focusing on detoxification and weight loss. It works well with pranayama techniques practiced separately, like the double breath, Kapalbhati, and Bastrika. Its practice increases the function of all the agnis, including seven dhatus (tissues), panchmahabhuta (5 elements), and jatharagni (digestive fire).

Spiritual Benefit:

This posture promotes udana vayu, the upward-moving prana necessary to bring the mind into sattva guna or calmness. During its practice, we can become connected to the power of the King Dancer within us, who frees us from the ego's limitations, allowing us to rise above the fluctuating circumstances of life. As a balancing pose, it strongly develops concentration on the mind-body relationship, purifies the mind from restless and disturbing thoughts through single-point focused attention, and brings great balanced flow of apana and udana. This eventually seats or settles the prana in the form of samana vayu, accumulated energy that is now balanced in the navel and abdominal region, that is, at the *jiva* (soul) in the *hridaya* or spiritual heart.

Level: Intermediate-Advanced

Vriksasana (Tree Pose)

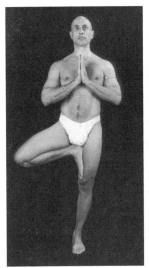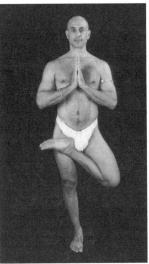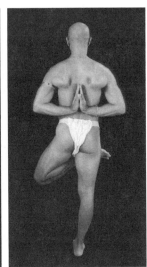

General Description & Symbolism:
The tree posture involves standing on one leg while placing the foot of the opposite leg at the top or origin of the inner thigh. Those yogis more flexible in the hip and knee joints can alternatively place the foot on the front top of the upper thigh, with the bottom of the foot facing upwards. The spine is symbolic of an upturned tree with its roots of receptivity at the top of the cervical vertebrae or, more specifically, at the medulla oblongata. The roots of our energy come from the thousand-petal lotus at the top of the head. Through yoga sadhana, including tapasya (effort), svadhya (self-analysis), and ishwara pranidhana (commitment to the divine), we gradually allow the prana-soma to fill the roots of the nadis throughout the body, producing higher states of consciousness.

Therapeutic Benefit:
Physically, the tree pose gently increases flexibility in the major muscles of the hips (the tensor fasciae latae, iliacus, and psoas major), which are important for releasing tension and tightness that builds up in the lower back and gluteal muscles. It strengthens the main leg muscles (quadriceps) and also the major muscles in the feet and around the Achilles tendon. As the brain is "cross-wired," with the left hemisphere controlling movement on the right side of the body, and the right hemisphere controlling movement on the left side of the body, the tree posture helps bring balance to both sides.

Ayurvedic Benefit:
Overall, tree pose can help vata types as long as they are not struggling to maintain balance while holding the pose. As it targets the legs and spine and balances the brain, vatas can receive much benefit from this posture. They should start with short holds and then gradually increase the length, or practice tree pose with arms extended to the sides. The pose can be practiced standing near a wall for occasional support if desired. The pose can also be helpful for pitta types with extremely developed muscles in the hips, gluteals, and thighs. If held for extended periods (5-15 minutes), the pose can be good for kaphas.

Spiritual Benefit:
Tree pose can inspire us to aspire and direct our ambitions to the highest goal of happiness through inner contentment (*santosh*) and self-realization (*samadhi*). As we practice yoga consistently, we can grow like the tree does, with regular exposure to sunlight and water. Our yoga practice needs the sunlight of optimism and discipline and the fluid qualities of patience and acceptance, which enable us to transcend to greater awareness.

Level: Beginner

SPINAL POSTURES

Sacred spinal postures directly affect the energy and functional quality of the vertebrae. Ancient and modern sages like Yogananda have always emphasized the importance of revitalizing the spine with life-force energy, physical strength, and straightness, so as to facilitate the ascension of prana shakti. Some of these positions compress the vertebrae to produce various therapeutic benefits. Others require a forward-bending action in the spine, which has distinct effects on the internal anatomy.

Spinal-rotation (twisting) postures are limited in number, but the main one practiced in a seated position offers a multitude of benefits, physically and spiritually. A strong and upright spine is not only important on the physical level, but has a major influence on our psychological attitude. Yogananda spoke of the perils of bad posture, saying, "It is slow but sure suicide." Physical health begins with a healthy spine, and awareness of the spine affords us spiritual wealth. The two are the keys to the kingdom of well-being.

BACK-STRENGTHENING POSTURES

Bhujangasana (Cobra Posture)

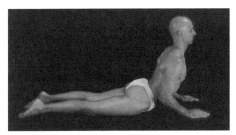 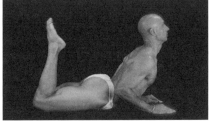

General Description & Symbolism:
Cobra pose is probably the most popular of asanas because of its name, symbolism, its connection to the lower spine, and its capacity to shift prana. In cobra, the lower spine is compressed, creating concentrated muscular pressure and energy flow. This is one of the major energetic seats of prana or apana, which influences downward-flow and elimination processes. Cobra is one of the key postures of the famed sun salutation series, but can also be practiced individually with great benefit, especially for those suffering from weak lower backs.

The cobra is symbolic of the kundalini energy that lies coiled at the base of the spine, an area stimulated by the practice of this asana. The key point is to keep the navel pressed against the ground while lifting the chest up and pressing back against the back muscles and vertebrae. It is important to remember that the back muscles should be doing most of the work, while the arms provide only minimal support. This is an auspicious pose connected to Lord Shiva, who wears the snake as a garland. As the great Mahadeva, he is the master of asana, pranayama, and the sacred agni.

While the elbows are kept bent in cobra posture, there is an alternative variation known as Mahabhujangasana in which the arms are almost completely straightened. This requires much flexibility between lumbar vertebrae three and four. Working up to this, with regular practice of asana to condition and tone the muscles and avoid straining, is recommended.

Therapeutic Benefit:

This is one of the best postures to begin to strengthen the vertebrae in the lumbar region and all the supporting muscles. It also strengthens muscles higher up the spine, like the rhomboids, trapezius, and latissimus dorsi, and also gently tones the serratus inferior muscles. Due to its neurological effects on the spinal cord and spinal nerve pairs,[96] it provides relief from abdominal pain and other discomforts associated with digestive disorders such as constipation, gas, or distention. For women, it is has a balancing effect on the overall menstrual cycle, as it increases blood circulation to the ovaries.

Cobra is an excellent pose for those that do not have good posture in general, a slouchy spine, or kyphosis. Regular practice can even alleviate neck pain and headaches. One way to increase both therapeutic value and subtle pranic flow is to start by tensing the lower back muscles while in the position and then releasing the tension. Repeat this so you can learn how to isolate the muscle groups as you work all the way up the spine from the lumbar to the trapezius. Each tensing and releasing motion should not take more than two to four seconds.

Cobra pose is very beneficial to the housekeeper organs of the body, the liver and kidneys, which receive an abundant supply of blood. Thus it is a good posture for detoxification or when going through Ayurvedic pancha karma. The posture has a toning effect on the endocrine glands and thyroid, as well as the suprarenal and reproductive systems.

Ayurvedic Benefit:

Due to its ability to bring focused energy to the lower spine, sigmoid colon,

---

96 Two long ganglionated nerve strands along the vertebral column, which are connected to each of the sympathetic nerves along the spine.

and lumbar muscles, cobra is highly beneficial for vata and related vayu (air or wind) disorders. According to Ayurveda, the digestive system is considered the mother of the body. Cobra pose is a bull's eye for improving the digestive balance necessary for vata issues related to the nervous system and psychological calming. Cobra has a moderate quality that pitta types can benefit from, as it diffuses excess heat, particularly when Savasana, equal in length to each cobra practice, is added.

Spiritual Benefit:
The cobra is sacred and symbolizes the expansion of consciousness and the capacity we all have to arise from the limitations of our ego and the fluctuating circumstances of life. The cobra dances to the prana guided by our breath and teaches us how to live as compassionate beings. The cobra can also represent the spine and the concept that with a good spine we can have a good life.

Level: Beginner-Intermediate

Salabhasana (Locust Posture)

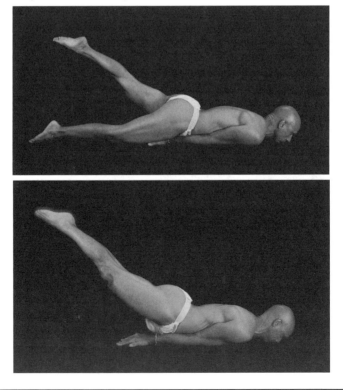

General Description & Symbolism:
Locust pose is practiced while lying face down on a flat surface, with extended arms and the palms of the hands and elbows facing downward underneath the abdomen. To reduce discomfort in the elbow joints, the elbows can be slightly bent. When the legs are lifted in this pose, the lower back muscles and arms, elbows, and shoulders take on high amounts of pressure. For those new to yoga, locust posture can be practiced with the mouth on the floor to avoid excess pressure to the cervical vertebrae. For the more seasoned, the chin can be placed on the floor. This increases pressure in the neck, so more flexibility is required. Those new to yoga can begin practicing this pose by raising one leg at a time (Ardha Salabhasana). This is much less strenuous and a good way to begin to build up strength in the lower back muscles.

Therapeutic Benefit:
Strong back muscles help prevent the vertebrae from slipping out of place and the common problem of pinched nerves. There is a general medical understanding that, if the spine is healthy, then the rest of the body will follow suit. This posture directly influences the spine and all the back muscles that support it. The anterior spinal artery is the main vessel that supplies blood to the spinal cord and also feeds the spinal muscles. Both are nourished by locust pose.

I often say circulation supports life and stagnation leads to death. In other words, locust pose helps keep our spines alive. In locust, the upper back and neck muscles are also strengthened because the entire upper and lower torso are tensed. This strongly reduces the flow of venous blood back to the heart, while the heart still actively pumps fresh blood into the arteries.

Here is where we experience the magic of yoga and the specialized benefits that tension and relaxation exercises bring. When the body is relaxed after a pose, there is an extra flow of venous blood back to the heart. A naturally occurring tension and relaxation technique like locust pose was also used by yogis to release energies into various channels and marma points throughout the body. Like bow pose, locust quickly creates accelerated breathing and heartbeat. It enhances cardiovascular function, but only for those who have had some prior conditioning should practice the posture. The pose also detoxifies the liver, digestive glands, and adrenals.

Ayurvedic Benefit:
Locust posture requires major ojas. Otherwise, it can be very taxing energetically. Kapha types really benefit from the heat created in this posture, and vata-related issues are also treated by its impact on the entire spine. This posture creates

a connection to the spine and has a tremendous psychologically grounding quality for vata. It has a relaxing or surrendering quality for pitta, because afterwards one really doesn't want to move much. The posture requires large amounts of energy and concentration.

Spiritual Benefit:

Locust is a great boon in increasing circulation and pranic flow into the entire spinal region, including the three areas of the vertebrae (lumbar, thoracic, and cervical), the supporting lumbar muscles, and the arteries. It releases back tension, pain, and discomfort. With regular practice, it enhances the straightness of the spine in meditation. Locust is a practical and robust way to get connected with the spine and reunite mind and body, as well as to enhance the links among mind, spine, and consciousness.

Level: Intermediate-Advanced

Dhanurasana (Bow Posture)

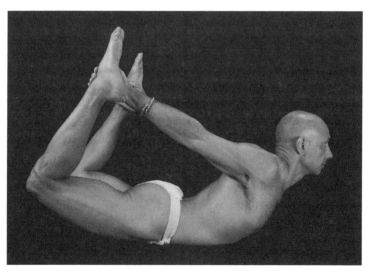

General Description & Symbolism:

The term *dhanu* means bow, and, as mentioned earlier, is connected to the warrior or kshatriya caste, which defends society. In Hindu mythology, King Janaka gave his daughter Sita up for marriage when Rama picked up Shiva's massive bow and broke the bow while stringing it. The bow posture is symbolic of the power that exists in a supple spine. It requires a certain degree of flexibility even to get into this posture, but it brings great strength to the entire spine.

The weight should be evenly distributed between the abdomen and the hips, while the hands clasp the outer ankles on each side, with the palms facing inward. By slowly engaging the muscles in the back, without any jerking action, the legs begin to rise off the ground. There is another variation with the hands clasping the insides of the ankles and palms facing outward, which allows for a greater range of movement. It is more important to find a good position to hold the bow pose and breathe naturally and mindfully than to try to lift the legs as high as possible.

Therapeutic Benefit:
In bow pose, the back muscles are fully tensed, and the leg muscles also tensed, while the shoulders, chest, and abdomen are simultaneously stretched. As a position that extensively compresses the vertebrae, bow can strengthen the entire spine and all supporting muscle groups, from the base to the neck. Cobra and locust postures can be considered good preparations for bow, which is more comprehensive.

As is the case with all back bends, breathing and heart rate increase quickly and substantially. Therefore, those with high blood pressure should take precautions. Unlike any other asana, the weight of the entire body is being directed entirely on the abdomen and pelvis, thus stimulating the liver, stomach, and transverse colon. It is excellent for those with flatulence, slow (*manda*) jatharagni, or constipation. The endocrine glands of the abdominal-pelvic area are nourished and the function of the adrenal glands, which sit at the top of the kidneys, and the pancreas, located very close to and just behind the stomach, is improved. The sexual glands benefit as well due to increased circulation. As a spinal asana, bow strongly invigorates the nervous system and, when combined with Savasana, provides a neutralizing or calming psychological effect.

Ayurvedic Benefit:
Bow pose brings a special quality to issues related to the primary pitta organs, the small intestines. It regulates pancreatic juice secretions and other important hormones, such as insulin and glucagon. Its great influence on the digestive and nervous systems also benefits vata-related issues. As previously discussed, bow is probably the best asana, along with seated spinal twists, for simultaneously targeting both the spine and digestion. It thus addresses two key areas that are the common root causes of many disorders.

Spiritual Benefit:
Practicing bow is likened to planting our spines like the roots of a tree into mother earth to receive her nutrients and powerful calming qualities. Practice

of bow pose connects us to our spine, which is the path of the sages or rishis. Raja Yoga teaches that our mind is essentially in the spine. A pose such as this one improves the mind-spine relationship, affording us once again connection to our Divine self. The spiritual eye and the spine represent the sacred doorway to the path of the light.[97]

Level: Intermediate

Ustrasana (Camel Posture)

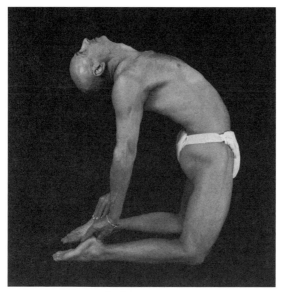

General Description & Symbolism:
Camel pose is another of the major back-bending positions that directly influence the spine. It creates symmetrical compression on all the vertebrae. It is distinguished from other back-bends done on the floor because it is practiced in a kneeling position. The camel as a species primarily inhabits the Middle

---

97   The Bhagavad Gita Chapter IV, verses 1-2. From *God Talks With Arjuna: The Bhagavad Gita* by Paramahansa Yogananda (Self-Realization Fellowship, Los Angeles, Calif., 1999). Yogananda specifically refers to Ikshvaku, as "symbolic of the astral spiritual eye of life and consciousness in man." He then explains how the soul descends from Cosmic Consciousness to human consciousness, and the steps one must take to reascend to God Consciousness. As described in Samkhya philosophy, the soul descends to operate through sense-perception channels known as *jnanendri-yas* and then flows into the physical senses of the body. Mankind becomes associated with these, and this is known as the *rajarishi*, or sense-identified state. Yoga practice helps us connect to the spine and relinks us to the light-source of our existence. Yogananda states, "Life force and mind are intimately associated, for in the body of man one cannot exist without the other."

East and Central Asia and is known to bear distinctive humps of fatty deposits on its back. The term "camel" is derived from the Greek and Latin (*camelus*), and also the Hebrew, meaning to go without or weaning. The camel pose represents ojas and tapas, as it requires endurance to hold this asana for any extended period of time. The key to its practice is to keep the pressure moving forward in the direction of the hips.

Therapeutic Benefit:
Camel pose turns the spine and body into the shape of a camel with its fatty humps. Its back-bending action creates a good deal of heat in the body. It is particularly beneficial for expanding the lungs and improving breathing in the upper respiratory tract, making it excellent for those with weak lungs who suffer from coughs, bronchitis, and even asthma. It helps remove excess water or phlegm build-up in the lungs, which travels up from the stomach, kapha dosha's primary site of accumulation. The pose has a weaning action on the internal respiratory channels, clearing them of excess residual deposits and toxicity. As the hips are pushed forward in this pose, it creates an expanding and releasing effect in this area, promoting the flow of apana (downward-flowing) vayu (wind) for grounding and elimination. With the shoulders, chest and head going back in the opposite direction from the hips, the pose promotes the flow of udana (upward-flowing) vayu. Thus, both opposing directions open the center or heart and balance the energy in samana (centering and transformative) vayu.

Ayurvedic Benefit:
Vata types benefit from knees on the ground, which promotes calm, as long as the pose is not held too long or beyond the point of discomfort. Each person, depending on various factors, including experience, constitution, and age, must measure the length of the hold according to their capacity. As back bends are heating and often expand the chest, camel pose is an effective position for maintaining balance of kapha dosha. It specifically addresses issues related to *avalambaka* (chest) kapha and *pranavaha srotas*.[98] Camel pose specifically heals and addresses issues related to these particular channels and kapha dosha.

Spiritual Benefit:
This posture teaches us to follow our heart, not our head. The back-bending action itself is a boon for opening the heart and becoming more accepting of

---

98 *Pranavaha srotas* is a comprehensive Ayurvedic anatomical term used to describe, but is not limited to, the respiratory system, as it is termed in modern medicine. This is in fact a broader region, with many other organs that require and support the flow of prana. These sets of *srotas* or channels play a major role in the proper function of the circulatory system. The organs related to the pranavaha channels are the heart, lungs, nose, pharynx, trachea, bronchi, pleura, alveoli, brain, and colon.

others and the variable nature of life. It tells us that body language speaks, and when we walk through life with a straight spine and confident chest, nothing will disturb us. When the shoulders are back and the chest is raised, avoiding psychological collapse, we will tend to focus on the positive aspects of life and continue to move forward through life with optimism. Our bodily structure and alignment can change our attitude and the relationship we have with our mind. Asanas like camel can reconnect us with our center of being in the heart.

Level: Intermediate

FORWARD-BENDING POSES

Sasangasana (Rabbit Posture)

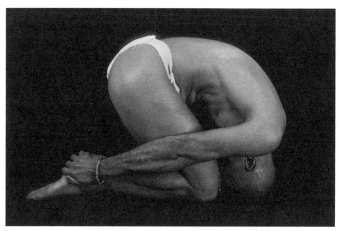

General Description & Symbolism:
The name of this pose comes from the Sanskrit word *sasa*, which means "hare." There are few Hatha Yoga postures that can fully stretch the entire spine, and rabbit is one of them. It is similar to Halasana (plow) and Malasana (garland) in its capacity to bring much fresh energy flow into the spine. Its practice requires that the feet and knees remain together. Once the spine is curled over with the chin, pressing into the chest, the forehead is drawn towards the knees if possible. Ideally the top of the head does not touch the ground, while the forehead touches the knees. If it is not possible to make contact with the knees, then one must be careful not to place too much pressure on the cranium when rolling the weight forward on the head. This can strain the cervical spine and muscles in the neck. With regular practice, the spine increases its length and it becomes much easier to bring the forehead and knees together

without contacting the ground with the head. Perhaps you have something to look forward to!

Therapeutic Benefit:

Rabbit is an extremely healing posture, as it resembles the fetal position and is very soothing to the intestinal nerves. When we are afflicted with stomach pain of any kind, the body naturally assumes this position. It is probably the most effective pose for drawing energy into, increasing the flexibility of, and releasing vertebral tension in the cervical region of the spine. It impacts the upper vertebrae slightly more than the lower ones, in an approximately 60-40 ratio. It targets an area as far down as the eighth thoracic vertebra up to the third cervical vertebra. The proper practice of rabbit pose effectively releases pressure in the 24 vertebrae of the spinal column, and stretches all the muscles along the spine. It improves circulation to the head and upper chest, making it very good for migraine headaches, sinusitis, insomnia, and amnesia. Due to the positioning of the cervical spine and respiratory changes, the pose produces increased activity in the thyroid, thymus, and pituitary glands, thus treating many related hormonal issues, as well as balancing menstruation.

Ayurvedic Benefit:

Rabbit is an excellent pose for all three doshas, with its comprehensive effect on the entire spine, and a soothing, massaging action on many internal organs such as the stomach, liver, colon, and small intestine. Rabbit pose releases stagnation in the upper torso, lungs, throat, and head, areas usually challenged by kapha. It releases tension and tightness along the entire spine and shoulders, where vata is commonly trapped. The forward-bending action releases pressure on nerves that send a heating or activating signal to the liver to produce bile, thus supporting balance of pitta dosha. This posture combines well with pranayama practices like Kapalbhati and Bastrika, which, when implemented after completing the asana pose, powerfully enhance lung and heart function and strength. Pranayama in this particular configuration can also increase hemoglobin levels in the blood.

Spiritual Benefit:

Rabbit pose is a great asset to meditation, as it increases circulation of oxygen and prana to the upper spine and head. Additionally, it releases tension and tightness from the trapezius, rhomboid, and deltoid muscles, which can interfere with keeping a straight spine and relaxed muscles. If it is difficult to relax the muscles externally, it is also challenging to relax the mind internally, so rabbit pose is great before meditation or during breaks in a longer meditation practice.

Level: Beginner-Intermediate

Malasana (Garland-Rosary Posture)

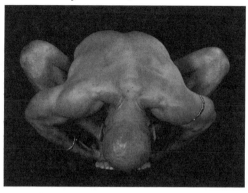

General Description & Symbolism:
Malasana is a posture similar in its effect on the spine to rabbit, as all the vertebrae are elongated. The key to effective practice of the garland is that the feet, including heels and toes, remain together. Once the spine is arched, the ideal position aligns the forehead or third eye with the base of the spine or *muladhara* region. As the forehead makes contact with the feet, the legs and arms become snug with the body. Initially, if the lower back is tight, the heels may not touch the ground. Eventually, regular practice makes the spine longer and the body taller. The garland is symbolic of the yogi's rosary or *rudraksha* (beads made from seeds) necklace, used for counting during mantra and pranayama practice. A garland of flowers is often given ritually to one's guru or a Holy statue (*murti*) during sacred ceremonies or auspicious celebrations.

Therapeutic Benefit:
While the rabbit pose targets the upper vertebrae, garland focuses more on the lower spine. It impacts the lower vertebrae slightly more than the upper in a 60-40 ratio. It targets the area from the lumbar vertebrae 3 and 4 to the upper thoracic vertebrae 6 and 7. The simple practice of squatting with the feet together and allowing the thighs to open and come apart is very effective at releasing tightness in the hips and gluteal muscles. The garland pose gives somewhat less benefit to the internal organs, as the internal pressure is reduced in this position compared to rabbit. As the pressure around the gluteal muscles is released, so are the nerve bundles in this area, especially the sciatic nerve. It can be a good pose for alleviating sciatic pain, although caution must be taken to make sure the body has been warmed up and there is good circulation before practicing this pose. It should be practiced only after some asana such as Surya Namaskar or other standing poses, so blood is circulating properly.

Ayurvedic Benefit:
Garland targets the vata zone of the body and promotes the healthy flow of apana vayu (downward-flowing wind). The colon gets a good push of apana,

opens up, and relaxes, reducing constipation and gas. As a forward, bend, garland also benefits pitta dosha by diffusing rajasic influences and promoting greater stillness and calmness in the mind.

Spiritual Benefit:

Garland is good for those looking to transition their meditation practice from sitting in an armless chair to such traditional seated positions as Siddhasana and Padmasana, as it helps prepare the hips and knees. Such seated positions really only seem advanced to us now because culturally we avoid sitting on the floor. Sitting on the floor was considered lower-caste once the British Raj expanded its rule throughout the world. Stereotypes developed in such a way that sitting on the ground was considered uncivilized and discourteous behavior.

One of the first things I say to those with severe tightness in the hips and knees is to begin eating and reading while seated on the floor. Even short intervals of seated mantra and meditation are great ways to increase flexibility in these sometimes challenging areas. On a more subtle level, garland promotes a balance of the two main directions of prana, ascending (udana) and descending (apana). This is calming and promotes elimination. Balance of these two opposing forces is the key to centering the prana at its source in the heart, where we can realize the higher Self. The *Siva Samhita* states: "In the heart, there is a brilliant lotus with twelve petals adorned with brilliant signs. The prana lives there, adorned with various impulses, accompanied by its past works, which have no beginning and are connected with egoism (ahamkara)."[99]

Level: Beginner

Paschimottanasana – (Seated Forward-Bending Posture)

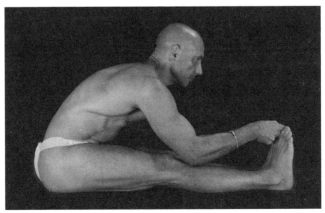

---

[99] Siva Samhita Chapter 3, Verses 1-2

General Description & Symbolism:

The *Gheranda Samhita* states, "Extend the two legs on the ground, stiff like a stick (heels not touching) and place the forehead on the two knees and catch with the hands the toes." The term *paschima* means "posterior or west" and *tan* means to stretch. In nineteenth-century America, the popular statement "go west young man" was symbolic of the idea that agriculture and other opportunities could solve the nation's economic problems. In yoga, we say "stretch west" to stretch the western part of the body, the back.

This seated position is similar to the standing Padahastasana (hands to feet), although it is more challenging because the weight of the upper torso cannot be leveraged to stretch over the legs. It is important the spine remain extended with the chest lifted while reaching for the feet, to avoid collapsing the chest. If one cannot perform the pose in this manner, then Padahastasana is recommended for an extended period, until more flexibility is attained.

Therapeutic Benefit:

Paschimottanasana is another key pose in the spinal series, which not only benefits the spine as a whole, but the nervous system as well. As a seated posture, it has a calming effect that is good for treating anxiety and nervousness. It allows for consistent stimulation and benefit to the nerves in the legs and buttocks (apana), through the nerves in the lumbar region, and also to the nerves that feed the shoulders and arms (vyana vayu: heart and lung prana that circulates throughout the body). Ultimately, Paschimottanasana targets the sympathetic nervous system, strengthens the muscles of the abdominal wall, and improves circulation to the entire pelvic region. When held for more extended periods of up to one to three minutes, it improves the function of the kidneys, bladder, and prostate (vata organs), and the liver, pancreas, and spleen (pitta organs).

Ayurvedic Benefit:

As previously mentioned, both vata and pitta receive much benefit from this posture. It is also an excellent counter-posture when combined with poses that compress the spine, such as cobra or camel. It increases suppleness in the spine and supporting muscles. It connects our awareness to the feet when they are flexed and the hands wrap over them, as is done in Padahastasana.

Spiritual Benefit:

Seated bends connect us with the spine and move prana upwards. Paschimottanasana is a good preparation for meditation and can also serve as a break during longer sadhana. This is one of those postures we can probably do for our entire lifespans to complement our spiritual evolution.

Level: Beginner-Intermediate

Janushirasana (Head to Knee Posture)

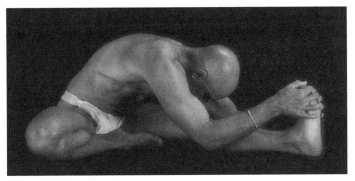

General Description & Symbolism:

The literal translation of this pose comes from the Sanskrit words *janu* for knee and *shira* for head. In its complete form, the pose joins the head and knee. This posture benefits almost everyone because the hamstrings ("leg biceps") naturally tighten from lack of mobility, being seated, from any type of exercise, and as the body ages. As a seated posture, it combines well with Paschimottanasana (seated forward bend) and Ardha Matsyendrasana (spinal twist). In a more advanced variation, the foot that is usually pressed to the inner thigh is placed on top of the thigh of the extended leg near the hip flexor, with the top of the foot facing downward and the bottom of the foot facing upwards, as in a half-lotus position (Ardha Padmasana).

The posture is not recommended for those who are chronically stiff or suffering from hip injuries, as it can be difficult to leverage the weight forward over the extended thigh from a seated position. The hip may also not be prepared for this level of stretching. Typically, for those with severe tightness, I recommend standing positions like the Virabhadrasana (warrior) series or Surya Namaskar (sun salutation) series to increase hip-flexor flexibility.

Therapeutic Benefit:

Janushirasana requires neither a great deal of balance nor strength. The spine both bends forward and stretches in a lateral direction, creating a subtle twisting action that infuses the thoracic vertebrae and sciatic nerves with increased blood and pranic flow. When held for periods of a minimum of one to two minutes, it can increase jatharagni (metabolic power) and treat urinary problems related to the bladder and other issues related to the kidneys and adrenal glands.

Ayurvedic Benefit:

This floor posture predominantly benefits vata and pitta-related issues, as it specifically targets the legs, lower back, and digestive organs. It relaxes and soothes, allowing pitta types to increase flexibility without much risk of over-heating. Kaphas can benefit by taking the more advanced variation, placing the foot on top of rather inside the thigh. This variation is also good preparation from those working towards achieving Padmasana (lotus posture).

Spiritual Benefit:

I consider Janushirasana an excellent prerequisite for meditation, as it relaxes the hips and the nerve bundles in the gluteals and lumbar spine, and also loosens up the knee joints for those who wish to meditate sitting on the floor rather than in a chair. With its soothing side-stretching action, it releases much of the tension that builds up along the sides of the back, including the serratus anterior, the external oblique muscle of the abdomen, and the outside of the latissimus dorsi. These key muscles have a compressing action on the spine, and, when tight, they pull the energy in the muscles and spine downward. Therefore, the pose supports the rise of prana-kundalini to the higher chakras, promoting a sattvic or calm state of mind.

Level: Intermediate

INVERTED POSES

The inverted postures are iconic of the entire Hatha Yoga practice. Hatha Yoga originated from ancient Tantric rituals and practices developed mostly during an age of consciousness and culture that was craving a new sense of direction and new relationship with the body and mind infused with natural creative forces, which had been lost. It could be said that classic inverted asanas like headstand and shoulder stand are symbolic of the strong desires of certain individuals and groups to attain higher consciousness.

Although it seems like an elementary matter to turn the body upside-down so energy ascends the vertebrae, the postures were bold gestures to invoke the Gods and increase the capacity for awakening dormant kundalini in the spine. This represented a return to the body and a reconnection of the eternal, sacred mind-body relationship. These were courageous gestures from renegades in Indian societies, who were in many ways rebelling against mainstream religious and social practices. During the 6th and 7th centuries AD, Hatha Yoga was counter-cultural and practiced in mountains, caves, and other secret places.

Keep in mind that Buddhism was the predominant religion in India during these times. It had gained popularity as an alternative to Brahminical Vedic practices that had apparently lost understanding of the pure and original Vedic teachings. Siddhārtha Gautama, later known as the Buddha, was born in the 5th century BC. He started his monastic order when he was about thirty-five years old.

Yogis Goraknath, Matsyendranath, Swatmarama, and Gherand began revitalizing the Tantric teachings about the 6th century AD, after over a thousand years of Buddhist prevalence. Much of Buddhist practice was directed to attaining mental freedom through the practice of **vipassana** and **anapanasati**[100] meditation. Later, in the 12th century, expansion of yoga remained constrained by the development of Islamic rule, which culminated in what became known as the Mughal Empire. Islam, however, never gained dominance in the northern Himalayan regions of India, such as Himachal Pradesh and Uttarakhand, two areas populated with yogis and sages.

Of the eighty-four asanas mentioned in the original Hatha Yoga texts, the inversions have the greatest impact on shifting the flow of vital energies in the body. They are essential precursors of the most auspicious posture, Padmasana or lotus pose, and provide a medley of therapeutic benefits presented in more detail below.

Halasana (Plow Posture)

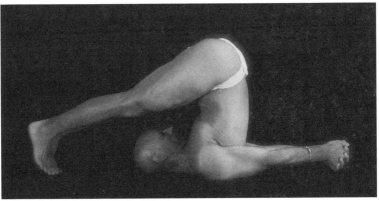

General Description & Symbolism:
Halasana means plow (Sanskrit: *hala),* which joins rabbit and Malasana as the most powerful spinal-stretching postures. The pose is started while lying on the back, but it is very important to have warmed the body up, so as to avoid injury from extensive pulling action on the entire range of spinal muscles. The

---

100   *Vipassana* – To perceive the true nature of existence as its three marks: impermanence, suffering, and non-self (non-duality). Ānāpānasati – mindfulnesss or awareness of the breath, which is embraced throughout the Tibetan, Zen, Tiantai, and Theravada schools of Buddhism.

plow is not advised for those with any type of back injury, and most specifically of the cervical region, as there is a great amount of pressure there during the practice of plow. The pose should be done on a mat or a slightly padded surface with a consistent contour, supporting the spine and shoulders, which are pressed by the weight of the body.

Plow can be considered the first stage of inverting the body, the second stage being Sarvangasana (shoulder stand), and the third Shirasana (headstand). The level of difficulty increases with each stage. It can be practiced in a variety of ways. In the initial position, the hips are in front of the torso, which may require supporting the back with the hands if the abdomen is not strong enough. Alternately, the hips can be placed above the abdomen and chest, or even, in the extreme form of the posture, above the face.

Therapeutic Benefit:
The most evident therapeutic benefit comes from stretching the spinal muscles, such as the erector spinae, and the bundles of muscles and tendons that extend from the lumbar, thoracic, and cervical regions of the spine. Some of these fibers are connected into the gluteus maximus and these provide release of tightness in the buttocks. Plow is excellent for elongating the spine and eliminating neuralgia (nerve pain), such as symptoms of sciatica and lumbago (low-back pain).

The pose is effective in reducing the onset of rheumatism, not only in the spine but in connective joints like those in the pelvis and pectoral or shoulder girdle. Over time, it can improve postural issues such as common kyphosis (shoulder-hunching), which is caused by cramping the upper thoracic and cervical vertebrae.

Plow massages all the internal organs, revitalizing them and improving their flow in the nerve pathways so they can function better together. As plow deals with the spine and central nervous system, it can improve overall health and well-being both physically and psychologically, creating calm and peaceful mindfulness.

It is important to note that during practice of the plow posture, blood pressure increases by approximately 25%. Therefore, those suffering from extreme hypertension or very high blood pressure (HBP) should avoid this asana. For those with moderate levels of HBP, the plow can be practiced at short intervals of 15 seconds to one minute, combined with relaxation in Savasana for equal lengths of time. This combined practice can be repeated multiple times, as inserting Savasana prevents blood pressure from reaching high-risk levels. As is the case with all inverted positions, women should abstain from the practice during menstrual periods.

Ayurvedic Benefit:

Halasana is a tri-doshic posture due to its strong impact on the spine. Through the spine and nervous system, all vata-related issues benefit. Its massaging action on the liver and heart and stimulation of the thyroid and parathyroid glands are important for pitta-type conditions. The inverted action kindles the otherwise sluggish digestion typically related to kapha dosha. Something I have done in my clinic to complement this posture and enhance its benefits is to massage warm mahanarayan oil along the spine for few minutes prior to holding plow for two to five minutes. Sesame oil can also be used. You will find that using oil has a stronger sedating effect on the nervous system than the asana practiced alone.

Spiritual Benefit:

The spine is the altar of the Spirit, and practicing plow helps keep the altar clean so that energy can flow through the spine more easily. When we improve our mind-spine relationship through postures like plow, we realize that the body is not sustained by bread alone.[101] There is a life force that carries and distributes fluids, blood, oxygen, and nutrients throughout the body. This prana enters the body through the medulla oblongata at the top of the spine in the back of the head. Plow is a godsend for assisting prana in feeding the tree of life, bringing us health, vitality, optimism, and sustained spiritual aspiration. The medulla is the real *asana* or "seat" of man's consciousness, whether ego-bound or enlightened. The practice of plow does not directly influence pranic flow. However, indirectly, it supports optimal purification and revitalization of the spine and all related tissues, organs, and nerve bundles or ganglions, enhancing our spiritual evolution. Yogananda says, "The yogi is busy withdrawing the life force into the spinal centers. When he succeeds in this work, the astral body with seven astral plexuses becomes visible to him through the spherical astral eye of intuition."[102]

Level: Beginner-Intermediate

---

101   Matthew 4:4: "Man shall not live by bread alone, but by every word that proceedeth out of the mouth of God."

102   *God Talks With Arjuna: The Bhagavad Gita* by Paramahansa Yogananda (Self-Realization Fellowship, Los Angeles, Calif.) This is the commentary on the Bhagavad Gita, Chapter VI, verses 3-4.

Sarvangasana (Shoulder-Stand Pose) & Viparita Karani (Reversing Action)

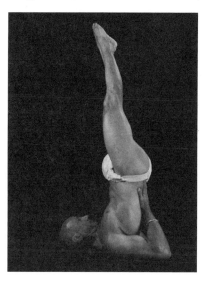 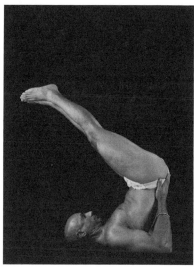

General Description & Symbolism:

As a second phase inversion, shoulder stand distinguishes itself from plow because the legs are raised upwards above the torso. This increases blood pressure by another 25%, because of the weight of the legs and the increased amount of blood moving from the thighs into the thoracic or chest cavity. Its name is appropriate, as the entire weight of the body rests upon the shoulders. With asana in general, one should abstain from food for at least three hours prior to practice, but this is especially important with inversions, as food can literally weigh the body down. Inversions benefit the body most in the morning, as after a night's sleep the energies and blood have become stagnant. Inverting in the morning is better than a cup of coffee.

Viparita Karani mudra is a slight variation of Sarvangasana mentioned in the *Hatha Yoga Pradipika,* where it is regarded as a seal (mudra), meaning it has the capacity to prevent energy from escaping. The *Pradipika* states, "With the navel region above and the palate below, the sun is above and the moon below." In Viparita Karani, the angle of the back is somewhat in the shape of a banana, at approximately 45 degrees. Such a position allows for space between the throat and chest, so that blood flow and circulation to the brain are increased. Often Viparita Karani is a more practical option for those not yet prepared to practice shoulder stand in its complete form. I often call this banana pose, a term much easier for students to remember. Women should abstain from the practice of these inversions during menstrual periods.

Therapeutic Benefit:

Inversions like shoulder stand mainly work on the cardiovascular system, as much of the body's blood ends up pooling in the upper thoracic cavity. Its most obvious effect is increased venous circulation in the heart and major blood vessels. This inverted action creates an interesting special effect on the lungs and heart, because they are also relieved of pressure and thus bathe in a fountain of youth. Bathing the lungs and heart in freshly circulated blood has a major anti-aging effect, promoting immunity as well as longevity. Both Sarvangasana and Viparita Karani increase pressure in the supra-cardiac veins, delivering fresh red corpuscles that provide oxygen, sugars, and many other nutrients to the cells. This also has a cleansing and detoxifying effect on the blood.

In my clinical practice, I have combined both of these postures with clients undergoing pancha karma (five cleansing actions) treatments combined with special oils on the skin and around the chest to promote bodily purification. Such a combination has astounding effects on respiratory issues and for improving blood and skin conditions. During practice of these inversions, both the thyroid and pituitary glands are stimulated, which promotes secretion of hormones that control a number of physical functions, like growth, especially vital for children, lactation, and glandular function in the gonads (sex glands) and thyroid.

The postures are very beneficial for those suffering from thyroid issues and digestive problems like constipation and sluggishness. They also help overcome premature ejaculation. Shoulder stand stretches both the cervical spine and sciatic nerves in the legs due to the pressure it places on the breastbone. When the neck is bent in this position what is called Jalandhara Bandha is created. This is one of the three bandhas or locks that help direct and lock energy in the spine.

The cervical spine is the most sensitive area of the spine, as it houses the phrenic nerve vital to breathing, which originates in the fourth cervical vertebra. The phrenic nerve is crucial to life and balanced physical function, because it contains motor, sensory, and sympathetic nerve fibers also linked to parasympathetic nervous function. This region in the cervical spine leads to the "holy" medulla oblongata, which, as I have mentioned, is the doorway of the prana distributed via the 49 main vayus or pranic channels and on into the many thousands of nadis throughout the body.

The medulla oblongata is the most sensitive and critical area of the body. If it is injured, instant paralysis in part or most of the body ensues. Knowing this, it is safe to say that shoulder stand, which promotes an intense flow of fluids and oxygen to this area, revitalizes the entire body. Regular practice of shoulder stand recharges the body with fresh energy, increasing ojas and prana, the body's highest foods.

Ayurvedic Benefit:
As we can see, the therapeutic benefits are extensive, touching on organs and functions related to all three doshas, vata, pitta, and kapha. As floor postures, they are very beneficial to vata. Both the entry into and exit from the posture have a grounding affect. Typically, anything that stimulates flow is beneficial for kapha types, as they commonly deal with sluggishness.

In general, inversions are done slowly to induce a greater sense of inner relaxation. They are therefore excellent precursors to Savasana and meditation. The effect of Jalandhara Bandha in shoulder stand is directly connected to key sites of kapha and its sub-doshas: *avalambhaka* (lung and heart), *bodhaka* (mouth), and *tarpaka* (brain and spinal cord) kapha. The poses mainly stimulate the form of pitta that is located in the brain, operates throughout the nervous system, and is known as *sadhaka* pitta. To summarize the broader effects of shoulder stand: It improves three key systemic operations in the body directly correlated with the three doshas. The nervous (vata), endocrine (pitta), and cardiovascular-circulatory (kapha) systems are all balanced through practice of this asana.

Spiritual Benefit:
As inversions, both Sarvangasana and Viparita Karani profoundly calm the neuromuscular system. The poses specifically target the area of the heart, drawing more flow of energy to the spiritual heart, which, in meditative terms, is where the mind must eventually dissolve. One of the key themes of Vedantic meditation is merging the mind into the spiritual heart. The heart chakra represents love and compassion, essential qualities to living a life filled with humility. Real, everlasting peace comes from the heart; the mind follows. Our spiritual practices teach us to follow our hearts for inner guidance, balance, and surrender to higher Divine forces. It may not always be the case that bodies need to be turned upside down to connect us to our heart, but poses such as these can enhance our overall well-being and provide great support for our spiritual discipline, They are valid forms of tapasya that help us develop greater fortitude on the path to self-realization.

Level: Intermediate

Shirsasana (Headstand Posture)

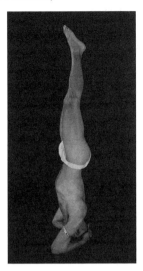

General Description & Symbolism:
Headstand is considered the king of all asanas for its profound therapeutic and spiritual affects. The pose could also be called the asana of the kings, as it is associated with a famous Indian monarch, King Janaka, who was an enlightened yogi. King Janaka lived an exemplary life and balanced both his material and spiritual actions. He was referred to in the Bhagavad Gita for this reason.[103] The Gita states: "By the path of right action alone, Janaka and others like him reached perfection. Also, simply for the purpose of rightly guiding mortals, thou shouldst perform action." Quite boldly, the Gita endorses the importance of taking action and shaking up the world through fulfilling both our material and spiritual responsibilities.

The headstand is symbolic of this stirring up. Even if it means turning our outer world upside down, we must not ignore our spiritual obligations. Headstand is strong metaphor for yoga asana, which teaches us to see the world upside down, released from appearances. The yogic concept of maya or illusion reminds us that we are not of this world and all things have a temporary existence.

The name of the asana originates from the Sanskrit word *shirsa,* meaning head. It places considerable pressure on the head and shoulders, which also support some weight. Headstand is not a posture for beginners and much preparation should be taken prior to its practice. The risk of injury can be very high without proper instruction, as it increases blood pressure and may cause blood vessels

---

103   Bhagavad Gita, Chapter lll Verse 20. From *God Talks With Arjuna: The Bhagavad Gita* by Paramahansa Yogananda (Self-Realization Fellowship, Los Angeles, Calif., 1999)

in the brain to rupture. It is contraindicated for those who are obese, have glaucoma, tendencies to detachment of the retina, high blood pressure, and chronic cardiopulmonary disease. Women should abstain from the practice during menstrual periods because it reverses the flow of bodily fluids.

Headstand places the majority of the body's weight on the upper part of the shoulders, neck, and skull. Therefore, those with injuries to these areas should re-examine practicing this posture and consider other inversions such as plow, which give many of the same benefits. In many cases, a simple standing forward bend like Padahastasana creates a substantial inverted effect that can benefit those not yet prepared for headstand, the "king inversion."

Other considerations should be taken by those who have osteoporosis and infections of the blood, lungs, heart, and teeth, as these can create brain abscesses. A proper headstand requires wrapping the hands around the head, but for many it can be difficult to hold the posture in this position. An optional variation is the tripod headstand, which involves creating a triangle position, with the hands flat on the floor and the head at the top of the triangle. For many, this variation gives more balance, although pressure on the top of head is increased.

Therapeutic Benefit:
Sirshasana has a great number of physiological benefits, although thoroughly warming up the body is necessary if such benefits are to be received. Headstand is the zenith pose for massaging the inner anatomy. Overall, headstand provides the utmost relief from the degenerative effects gravity has upon the organs. Headstand enhances circulation of blood through slightly more increased arterial than venous pressure, benefiting the lungs and left chamber of the heart. Enhanced venous flow improves the function of the right ventricle of the heart, while allowing the body to maintain safe levels of blood pressure, even while holding the posture for one to five minutes.

The action of blood flowing upwards during entry into headstand and the subsequent flow of blood while exiting the pose have a flushing and cleansing action on the intestines. This helps remove excess undigested food waste or ama that build up on the interior walls of the digestive tract, disrupting the balance of the doshas. This action increases the body's digestive and metabolic strength, a key factor in maintaining health, weight management, and cholesterol reduction. As an inversion, headstand promotes increased blood pressure and heat in the body. This is another key factor in promoting perspiration and detoxification of the dhatus, as ama can eventually find its way into the tissues and disrupt their proper function.

Yogis have known the positive benefits of headstand for thousands of years, but only recently has modern medicine recognized the positive effects of inverting the body. The Trendelenburg[104] position was named after a German surgeon who discovered that, when the feet are placed above the head, the abdominal organs shift upwards towards the diaphragm, allowing better access to the pelvic organs, since they are pulled away from the pelvis. This has become a standard position for abdominal and gynecological surgeries, to relieve abdominal hernia and hypotension (low blood pressure), and to prevent formation of varicosities.

The internal shifting action on the internal organs being uplifted away from the pelvis in headstand is almost equivalent to the yogic techniques of Nauli and Uddhiyanna Bandha, both of which involve engaging the abdominal muscles and lifting them upwards into the rib cage. These actions specifically push on and improve the function of the transverse colon, liver, and stomach.

It is interesting to note that the human fetus remains inverted throughout most of pregnancy. Each of the trimesters represents a phase of human development, beginning with the soul entering the mother's physical womb, followed by the mind during the second trimester. The body then develops most thoroughly during the third trimester. The head-down "fetal" position during pregnancy fits the shape of the pelvis like the yin-yang symbol, with the lumbar curve providing a kind of slide for the fetus to exit the womb.

Ayurvedic Benefit:
The king asana is tri-doshic and can be practiced differently by each dosha type. Both vata and kapha types can benefit from regular and consistent practice of headstand, especially in the morning, as headstand gives kapha types with a sluggish metabolism a morning boost that can last throughout the day. Headstand in the morning has a psychologically calming effect that helps vatas keep focused.

The pressure on the top of the head has a unique quality in the marma system[105] of Ayurveda, one of whose key points is at the top of the head. This is the *adhipati marma*, located directly where the head lands in this posture. This key point deals with the entire nervous and sensory system, and helps balance prana in the brain. Stimulation of adhipati marma in headstand improves alertness and the function of the pineal gland.

---

104   Friedrich Trendelenburg, May 24, 1844 – December 15, 1924, also had many other medical techniques named after him.

105   Ayurvedic medicine recognizes 108 marma points throughout the body, which are specific junctions of prana. These are pressed to address various doshic issues. Oils are also sometimes used. These points are related to the acupuncture points of traditional Chinese medicine.

Headstand requires a counter-pose like rabbit or child's pose to transition the energy properly. Long holds can disturb prana in the mind if it is not re-directed properly afterwards. Vajrasana (thunderbolt pose) can be taken afterwards to settle the energies and direct prana to the spiritual eye. *Shambhavi mudra*, gazing upwards towards the third eye, can be added to intensify the effect further. Savasana can be also be used for deeper restoration.

Headstand is a great posture to combine with pranayama, which benefits the respiratory system, strengthens the lungs and heart, and increases hemoglobin levels. The combination of breath work and relaxation afterwards is important for vata, pitta, and kapha. Rabbit pose releases much of the pressure on the cervical spine, increases space between the vertebrae, and cools the body down. It is as important to reap the benefits of headstand during practice as it is to transition the energy properly after the pose is complete. This is where counter-poses and pranayama come in.

Spiritual Benefit:
Headstand is an incredible asset in raising prana if used properly. Otherwise, the pose would not be much different from gymnastics. There needs to be structure, direction, and intention to reap the benefits. As the headstand moves energies upwards away from the pelvis and genitals, it provides support for the principle of brahmacharya.[106]

When, through the law of karma or the accumulation of toxins and sensory attachments, we create unbalanced sexual desire, ojas can be reduced in the body, thereby weakening the entire system. Headstand can help reverse the effects of such poor habits temporarily and balance urges that exceed the need to procreate. In other words, when our energies are balanced physically, mentally, and emotionally, the desire for sexual activity is reduced. This is supported by a proper lifestyle that includes the right foods, herbs, and practice of yoga meditation.

Asanas function mostly on the physical body, but can penetrate much deeper when the prana is directed spiritually. This is the quandary with recommending yoga to people these days, as there is much offered on the physical level, but few schools understand the importance of spiritual and energetic transcendence. Asana can shift the energy around, but the mind must be trained in how to unify prana. Otherwise, the dilemma of the separation of mind and body continues. The body should be used as a means of transitioning beyond the body. This is what makes yoga an effective transcendental system.

---

106 Brahmacharya is one of the five niyamas in Patanjali's *Ashtanga Yoga Sutras*. It endorses the importance of transmuting the sexual urge for spiritual enhancement. It does not necessarily mean abstinence, as has been widely misconstrued.

The idea with headstand is that we stand on our head to get out of it, to break away from the prison of thought, or "I" ness, into Oneness. We can receive this freedom when we return to the seat of our consciousness at the top of the spine.

Level: Intermediate-Advanced

ARM BALANCES

Kagasana (Crow Pose) / Bagghrasana (Tiger Pose) / Hastasana (Handstand)

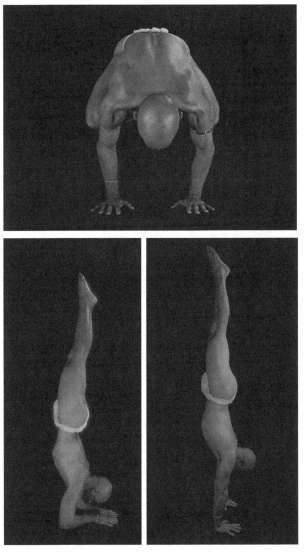

General Description & Symbolism:

One of the key aspects to practicing arm balances has to do with the placement of the hands, which control how the body weight shifts. Crucial to suspending the entire body off the ground is opening the hands to create as much space as possible between the fingers, which provides a good platform for balancing the energy. Another aspect that is commonly forgotten is the breath. While many try to grunt their way into inversions, this defeats the intention of Hatha Yoga, which is to maintain an ease and calmness of mind regardless of the challenge upon us. Arm balances require a good distribution of both apana and udana vayu. The former roots the body and the latter uplifts it.

The practice symbolizes the importance of courage and fearlessness in overcoming "I am the body" consciousness. Arm balances also teach us to be light and float above the trivial and often overly engaging dramas of life. This is felt in the practice of crow, which creates a feeling of flying and can instill greater confidence in the body. This parallels the development of *titiksha*, rising above the body and its sense enticements. Arm balances can teach us to stay even-minded, calm, and at ease, even when in tricky positions.

Therapeutic Benefit:

Arm balances provide the utmost strengthening and building of the upper torso and arm muscles. This begins with the triceps and deltoid muscles in the arms and shoulders. Crow and tiger pose specifically work on the trapezius muscles, which support the head and give us the power to lift and hold things. The upper pectoral muscles are also strengthened and toned in crow and tiger. Aside from the arms and shoulders, the abdomen must be engaged to lift and support the body in these postures. This also supports easing the body out of the postures, as, without any abdominal strength, the entire body would just fall out. Due to the intensity of supporting the weight of the entire body on the arms, these poses are not held for long periods, as is the case in shoulder stand or headstand. Therefore, much of the benefit to the internal organs is reduced. The handstand is an excellent practice for athletes, as it builds the fast-twitch muscle fibers needed for competition. In this regard, rather than lifting into handstand and holding the pose, it is better to repeat entry into and exit from the posture. These arm balances require remarkable focus and sharpen concentration with regular practice.

Ayurvedic Benefit:

Arm balanceare effective at producing heat in the body and are good for kapha issues that benefit from sweating. They are the invigorating to the jatharagni, as they require effort and concentration. They also increase respiration and circulation in the upper body, chest, lungs, and heart, all key areas for managing kapha dosha. These arm balances are important for vata body structures that lack muscular strength and endurance. Tiger pose is quite useful for toning the upper body in general, including the shoulders and back, which are key areas where vata can be deficient.

Spiritual Benefit:

Asanas that involve the use of the arms in balancing are grouped together, as they primarily focus on outer forms of strengthening the upper body. These are the few postures that can help build muscular strength in areas that can tend to become lean and weak. The strength of the upper body is symbolic of the God Hanuman, the disciple of Lord Rama, in the epic Ramayana. Hanuman's strength allowed him to provide great seva or service to Rama in overcoming the evil forces of Ravana. When we can acquire the confidence and bodily power to serve others in life, the negative and crippling power of the ego is demolished. Weakness and disease in the body originate from a fractured mind-body relationship. These arm balances can provide us greater physical upper-body strength and the confidence and determination to fulfill the highest dharma in life, to serve our brothers and sisters. Inversions such as these provide pure invigoration and the inspiration to persevere. Inversions such as tiger pose and handstand also support the upper thoracic and shoulder areas, which slouch during longer meditations.

Level: Advanced

DIGESTIVE POSTURES

Ardhamatsyendrasana (Seated Spinal-Twisting Posture)

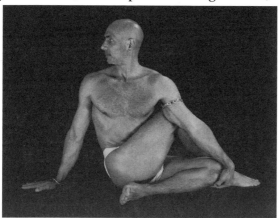

General Description & Symbolism:

The seated spinal twist is another classic Hatha Yoga position that rotates the spine unlike any other pose. It is the "twist of twists" and provides myriad benefits both externally and internally. The posture is named after the founder of the Nath cult, Matsyendranath, who valued the prerequisites of the purification of physical impurities prior to taking on the meditative practices taught in Raja Yoga. It can also be connected to Matsya, the fish-avatar, one of Vishnu's ten principal avatars, who saved Manu, the first man. The word *ardha* means half in Sanskrit. In this pose, the body is twisted half-way to either side. This idea of purifying the body before meditation practice developed during the 5th and 6th centuries AD, and aligns with the principles of Ayurvedic medicine. As I have mentioned, many of the purification practices of both yoga and Ayurveda, such as pancha karma and shat karma, are very similar, with some differences in their application and instrumentation.

Therapeutic Benefit:

The most obvious benefit of the seated spinal twist begins with the profound rotation of the thoracic spine. The twist elongates the spinal vertebrae, producing space between them to increase mobility and reduce the chances of spinal subluxation, which is when the vertebrae move out of alignment, creating pressure and irritating the spinal nerves. Beginning at the first two cervical vertebrae, the degree of rotation between the spinal vertebrae gradually decreases as the spine descends to the lumbar area. The twist is important in maintaining the spine's natural movement. This seated twist is critical to long-term spinal health, especially in modern societies, where more time is spent sitting in chairs and cars, and less time on active chores. Contemporary physical culture has found many creative ways to build muscles and stimulate the heart by the use of interesting-looking machines, but has lost sight of the value of flexibility.

This posture should be avoided during the second and third trimesters of pregnancy. Women should wait until about 21 to 30 days after birth to begin its practice, allowing the internal organs to readjust themselves.

Ayurvedic Benefit:

The most obvious benefit comes from the direct impact the seated spinal twist has on the three doshas and their operations in the digestive system. All three organs, the stomach, small intestine, and colon, benefit from major internal massage. The twisting action is almost equivalent to an Ayurvedic therapy called virechana or purgation. The twist purges excess pitta lodged in its primary site, the small intestine. It also relieves muscular tension in the mid-spine, which builds up in the erector spinae and even latissimus muscles. The unique seated position provides an expanding stretch to the gluteus maximus and lumbar spine, where vata dominates in the colon. One particular muscular benefit from the seated twist is that it provides much relief for illiotibial or IT-band syndrome. The IT band runs along the outside of the thigh from the pelvis and inserts just below the knee. The IT band, gluteal, and lumbar muscles are all connected to vata-related issues.

Spiritual Benefit:

The seated twist is a self-chiropractic position that keeps the vertebrae in alignment so that the flow of prana is not impaired. The twisting action on the spine is directly connected to the meninges, the membranes that envelop the central nervous system, and spinal nerves that influence the nadis or channels in the subtle body, particularly the solar and lunar channels that criss-cross up the spine. The spiraling of prana through the pingala (solar) and ida (lunar) channels is enhanced, as Ardha Matsyendrasana mimics this movement of the prana, thus ensuring its rise to the eye of Shiva or Oneness. Ardha Matsy-endrasana is mentioned in the *Gheranda Samhita*, with the recommendation of fixing the gaze between the eyebrows during the twist, indicating where the solar and lunar currents are to unify in order to dissolve illusion and duality consciousness. It is important that the neck region should also turn in accord with the rest of the trunk to promote upward-flowing prana. Perhaps we can all be as fortunate as Manu[107] and use this sacred and powerful asana to save ourselves from the floods of delusion that life pours through the spine and mind.

Level: Beginner-Intermediate

Uttana Padasana (Lifted-Leg Pose)

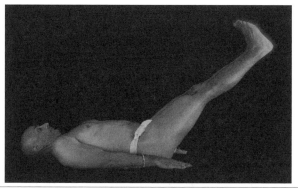

---

107   In the Vedic-Hindu scriptures, Matsya Purana Manu, the progenitor of man, is saved from a great flood by Matsya, the great fish avatar or aspect of Vishnu. Matsya is the first of the ten avatars of the Hindu God Vishnu. Vishnu is the preserving force that gives us birth and the ojas (energy) to enjoy life and its pleasures.

General Description & Symbolism:

This unique posture involves lifting *(uttana)* the legs *(pada)*, while lying on the back. It requires substantial abdominal and lumbar strength to start with, but can also be practiced with knees slightly bent to take some of the pressure off the lower back. In Uttana Padasana, the legs are extended outwards at whatever angle one is able to hold without strain. Another option is to synchronize the movement of the legs with the breath, beginning at a 90 degree angle with heels pointed towards the sky. As the legs are lowered down towards the ground, the breath is exhaled, and then inhaled as the legs are raised back up.

This pose can be held for 20 seconds or upwards of one to two minutes, depending on abdominal strength. A disciple asked his guru, "Guruji, how long should I hold this posture?" The Guru suddenly left the room. The disciple remained focused while holding Uttana Padasana, and waited patiently for his guru's response. Much later, the guru returned to the room and he said, "That's as long as I want you to hold the posture. Good job! Your focus and concentration were not lost by my delayed response to your query." The student offered *pronams* (bows) to his Guru for this valuable lesson.

Therapeutic Benefit:

This lifted-leg pose is excellent for strengthening the abdominals and reducing the excess fat that commonly accumulates in this area. Whenever the legs are extended in such a position, much back strength is required. This can develop with regular practice. It specifically targets the hip flexors, such as the psoas major and iliacus muscles, which support the flexing action of the hips. These muscles are strengthened, and provide support for the lower back.

Ayurvedic Benefit:

Digestive strength is enhanced through the lifted-leg pose because of the muscular stimulation on the nerves in the hip region connected to the sigmoid colon. This lower area of the colon is influenced by apana vayu and is usually an area of concern for vata types. When the legs are lifted and placed into motion by raising and lowering, excess wind is removed from the transverse colon, also an important region for vata types. Externally, the posture can reduce the excess medas dhatu (fat) that builds up around the waist and hips.

Spiritual Benefit:

One of most important aspects of meditation is the centering of apana and prana, so that the energy is balanced in samana. Deep and relaxed pranayama is essential, and this requires proper use of the diaphragm. When this is achieved, the resting heart rate is reduced and a calming and relaxed feeling is induced from within. When Uttana Padasana is practiced while taking a slow inhalation as the legs are lifted, and releasing a slow exhalation as the legs are lowered, there is an expansive effect on the lungs, arteries, and veins leading to and from the heart. This produces the effect of pratyahara in the nadis. Therefore, this asana indirectly provides the key benefit of withdrawing the mind from the senses, potentially enabling entrance to the breathless state in meditation. This is an exalted state where the sublime qualities of the soul are experienced.

Level: Intermediate

Mayurasana (Peacock Posture)

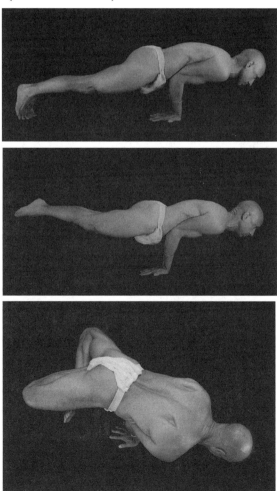

General description & symbolism:
Peacock is a classic pose mentioned in various Hatha Yoga texts, such as the *Gheranda Samhita* and *Hatha Yoga Pradipika*. It is performed with both hands on the ground, with the wrists turned outward and the elbows at each side of the navel. It is important to bend the elbows as much as possible, as the torso needs to mount on top of them with all of the body weight shifted forward, so that eventually the legs lift off the ground. Concentration should be placed on the solar plexus as the center of balance.

In a variation called Hamsasana or swan pose, the feet are kept on the ground while the torso is mounted on the arms. Another variation is to lift one leg at a time, to build up upper body and back strength. In a more advanced option called Padma Mayurasana (bound peacock), the pose is practiced while holding lotus posture. This has also been called Lolasana or swinging pose, because the torso swings slightly when the legs are folded.

The peacock's feathers are a very sacred symbol connected to Krishna, who wears feathers on his crown, which are called **sikhipincham** in Sanskrit. Symbolically, the eye in each feather represents the spiritual eye or **kutashta** of wisdom and intuition. Sri Krishna played his flute, causing the peacocks to dance in ecstasy for hours. The king of the peacocks was deeply indebted for this festival of bliss that Krishna created, so he offered him their plumage. Krishna lovingly accepted and placed the feathers on his crown.

The arms can be joined under the body, representing the spiritual eye seen in the peacock feather. The two arms come together to create a platform to rest the body on, so the legs can be lifted. The posture requires great flexibility in the arms and hands, as well as strength in the entire body. Structurally speaking, men will find such upper body postures easier than women, owing to their muscular strength in the chest and arms. Women will find leg postures easier due to their natural sense of groundedness and connection to the earth through the pelvis and legs. This posture is very ancient, with several references made in great yogic texts[108] like the Upanishads and *Yoga Yajnavalka*, aside from the descriptions in the *Hatha Yoga Pradipika* and *Gheranda Samhita*.

Therapeutic Benefit:
Mayurasana is a full-body asana that strengthens the entire muscular system and gives a major boost to the digestive system. According to the *Hatha Yoga Pradipika*, it can alleviate all diseases, balance stomach disorders, and kindle the jatharagni (gastric fire). Due to its intense focused pressure around the

---

108   Yoga Yajnavalkya (3:16,17), Sandilya Upanishad (3:12), Darsana Upanishad (3:10-12), Trisikhi Brahmana Upanishad (47).

stomach and digestive organs, it has great capacity for ridding the body of toxins built up by a poor diet high in meat, alcohol, greasy foods, and pungent spices. Interestingly enough, the peacock is unique in that it eats poisonous reptiles, such as snakes, and insects, without experiencing any harmful side effects, because of its strong digestive capacity to assimilate and eliminate such foods. Peacock pose strengthens the main abdominal-digestive organs (stomach, colon, small intestines, liver, and spleen) and has an invigorating effect on the lungs and heart. Swami Sivananda likens the pose to an injection of adrenaline, and it seems it could possibly be a good replacement for those addicted to coffee.

Ayurvedic Benefit:
The *Hatha Yoga Pradipika* states that peacock pose corrects imbalances related to all the doshas, vata, pitta, and kapha. It removes blockages of apana vayu through direct stimulation of the digestive organs, and at the same time enhances udana vayu by promoting the flow of blood through the inferior vena cava[109] into the entire upper chest and throat. The pressure of the torso on the colon removes flatulence and constipation, balancing vata. The massaging action on the small intestine and liver can alleviate chronic gastritis, and the acute pressure and massaging action on the stomach is helpful in eliminating excess kapha, which usually accumulates there. The increased flow of blood through the inferior vena cava also aids in removing kapha from the lungs and bronchioles (small bronchial tubes). Practice of peacock pose involves placing pressure on the abdominal region, as well as great mental focus on the solar plexus in order to balance. Both of these direct energy to the "mother of the body," the digestive organs, whose proper function Ayurveda sees as essential for health and wellness.

Spiritual Benefit:
When the peacocks were aroused by the melodious sounds of Sri Krishna's flute, they served him with a gesture of their plumage, symbolic of the one-pointed consciousness that appears in their colorful feathers. To enjoy the rainbow of colors that life has to offer, all sadhakas must establish a unified flow of prana and consciousness, whether it be on the breath as touted by hatha yogis, in focusing the mind as endorsed by raja yogis, on sweet devotion as practiced by bhakti yogis, or on the purest stream of knowledge undiluted by thought for jnani yogis. Peacock pose enhances our capacity to focus and concentrate our attention to balance the body and unite the body and mind.

Level: Advanced

---

109   This is a large vein that carries deoxygenated blood (blood rich in carbon dioxide) from the lower half of the body into the right atrium of the heart. The inferior vena cava enters the back of the heart through this right atrium.

Pavanamuktasana (Knee-to-Chest Pose)

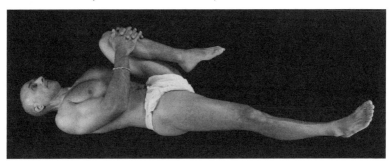

General Description & Symbolism:

Yoga is a spiritual science now known across the world. But the asanas have become more popular in the western world due to their healing effects on the body. Digestion is one of the most common health issues we have today across the globe, especially due to the variety of food in urban societies. With no real staple food, the stomach and intestinal tract are challenged by lack of habituation. The efficacy of this posture comes from its simplicity and gentle nature, as the thighs compress against the abdomen and the arms are wrapped around the thighs to keep consistent pressure. There is another variation that can be practiced by lifting a single knee to the chest, while the other thigh remains extended on the ground. It is usually practiced lying down on the back, but can also be practiced in a sitting position.

Therapeutic Benefit:

Pavanamuktasana plays a vital role in balancing the digestive issues of the colon, intestines, and stomach. These are the most sensitive organs of the entire body and the most abused, especially with the modern diet and the amount of mental stress people are carrying. The knee-to-chest posture is one of the gentlest ways to soothe an achy stomach. It is very effective at enhancing the pre- and post-digestive process for those who have weak digestions. The full position, with both knees to the chest, has the effect of broadly relaxing the nerves in the abdominal area. The word *pavana* in Sanskrit means gas and *mukta* mean to free. This is therefore also known as the gas-removing pose. The compression of the thighs into the abdomen creates intestinal peristalsis in the transverse and sigmoid colons, allowing trapped gas to pass through. The pose provides a soothing stretch for those suffering from lower back tightness or tension in the gluteals.

Ayurvedic Benefit:

When Pavanamuktasana is practiced with one leg extended, it controls the directional pranas in the ascending (udana) and the descending (apana) colon, which form during the final process of passing the stool into the rectum. In other words, this posture improves circulation and the function of the organs in the supra-colic compartment,[110] as well as the lungs and heart. Venous blood flow is shifted through the splanchnic nerves[111] and spleen, which holds a reserve of blood, to improve circulation through the lungs and the functioning of the heart. This is an important benefit both to vata types, who are shallow breathers, and pitta types, who are prone to hypertension and high blood pressure.

Spiritual Benefit:
Wind-removing pose is very relaxing and can be done before meditation sadhana or in the evening, prior to sleep. It is also a simple stretch that can be done in the morning to prepare the body slowly for a more challenging practice. Yoga does not always have to be difficult, and sometimes simple positions can go a long way to keep energy circulating and the mind from getting agitated by physical blocks. Pavanamuktasana is the kind of pose that can be practiced the evening period between 5 and 7 pm.

Level: Beginner

Nauli (Abdominal Massage)

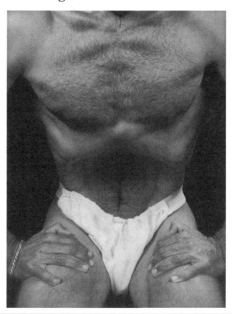

---

110   Liver, gallbladder, stomach, and spleen.
111   Sympathetic nerves serving the blood vessels and viscera in the abdomen.

General Description & Symbolism:
The Nauli exercise, according to the yoga texts, is considered a type of *kriya*, from the root word *kri*, to act or do. The term implies purification. Nauli is one of the shat karmas or six cleansing actions of the Hatha Yoga tradition. It combines well with Kapalbhati pranayama to remove excess waste from the digestive organs. It is an excellent exercise to do early in the morning just after rising, and should be done on an empty stomach. It can also be done in the evening time just before dinner.

Nauli is best done in a standing position, with feet hip-distance apart. The hands are placed on top of the thighs, with the torso slightly hunched over, so as to be able to engage and lift the abdominal muscles. The breath should then be exhaled through the throat until the lungs are completely empty. Finally, the glottis in the throat is engaged so as to seal off the breath. While holding the breath, the abdomen is undulated directly towards the center of the body as many times as is comfortable, in a slow and controlled manner.

With time, muscular control is increased and the muscles can be rolled from left to right (counter-clockwise), which is called Dakshina Nauli, or from right to left (clockwise), which is called Vama Nauli. When the undulations create more of a horizontal wave across the abdomen, there is greater therapeutic benefit to the digestive organs, as discussed below.

Nauli is basically a contraction of the vertical muscles in the abdomen. During practice, the muscles protrude outwards like reeds or tubes. In fact, the word *Nauli* originates from the term *nala*, meaning reed or tube. Some yogis call it Lauliki, meaning "to roll." I usually recommend it be practiced once the body is warm. Optionally, the abdomen can be massaged with some warm sesame oil beforehand. Women should avoid practicing Nauli during menstruation and pregnancy. Those suffering from heart disease and hypertension should also avoid it. The *Hatha Yoga Pradipika* touts Nauli as the "foremost of Hatha Yoga practices."

Therapeutic Benefit:
Nauli is the ultimate method of voluntarily and directly stimulating the digestive process. Yogis considered Nauli a practical means for purifying the bowels by moving the doshas from their respective sites, the colon, small intestine, and stomach. This is an area of the body we do not want to become hardened. The practice of Nauli keeps the abdominal muscles supple while at the same time strengthening the abdominal wall, thus preventing hernias.

Ayurvedic Benefit:

Nauli is a tri-doshic practice that massages the intestinal organs, increases jatharagni (digestive strength), and promotes bowel regularity. It is particularly beneficial for vata and pitta types, who are often challenged with excess sensitivity. Vatas, generally being lean, low in fat, and tight, tend to lack mobility in the abdomen, which can lead to different forms of neuromuscular twitching, poor breathing, and nervousness. Nauli can reduce such issues by stretching the muscles and relaxing the abdominal nerves.

Vama and Dakshina Nauli are more effective at releasing pitta from its typical site of accumulation in the small intestine. They also massage both the ascending and descending colon. Centered Nauli directs more pressure to the transverse colon, a problematic region for vata-type issues.

Nauli is an integral part of any detoxification program I customize for my clients. Sometimes I add Kapalbhati pranayama afterwards for kapha types, and recommend this be done in the early morning. I also recommend doing Nauli during abhyanga (self-massage with oil) for preventative health management. For vata types, I have recommended it along with basti (medicated enemas) and have always seen great results. Nauli has a vacuum effect on the pelvic floor and anus. In ancient times, yogis would perform basti with a bamboo shaft and would then do Nauli to create a water-vacuuming action to cleanse the rectum. It has such broad effects on the internal organs that the *Hatha Yoga Pradipika* states it corrects "all disorders of the doshas," including diarrhea, acidity, hormonal imbalances, urinary disorders, and sluggish digestion.

Spiritual Benefit:

Nauli has the capacity to stimulate and promote circulation in the venous spinal nerves and both the sympathetic and parasympathetic nervous systems. With its capacity to influence the endocrine system, it is helpful in control of the sex hormones. For those sadhakas on the yogic spiritual path, the practice of Nauli is effective in observation of brahmacharya[112] (sexual moderation), as this is the main practice for preserving the ojas (life sap). Ojas provides the strength, vitality and, endurance to support balancing the prana in the pingala (sun) and ida (moon) nadis, so it may rise and unify with the central prana

---

112   Transmutation of the sexual urge with spiritual intention. Brahmacharya has been misunderstood as complete abstinence, but its intention is to redirect the sexual procreative energy rather than to suppress it. Ayurveda does not recommend suppression of any natural urges, and neither does yoga, particularly for householders. However, *brahma* (creative) *acharya* (mastery), as a monastic vow, does require complete abstinence due to a lifestyle of intense austerities aimed at raising Kundalini Shakti and expanding consciousness. Ultimately, the practice of brahmacharya, whether for monastics or householders, is intended to catalyze human evolution.

in the sushumna nadi. Many do not realize the importance proper lifestyle plays on the spiritual path. For this reason, the sacred relationship between spirit and nature must be honored as the perennial Divine dance of life's four responsibilities or aims: kama or sensual affections and emotional balance; artha or vocation; dharma or purpose; and moksha or spiritual liberation. Our lifestyle must become an inspiring, rewarding, purposeful and spiritual relationship with the Divine. In this way, techniques like Nauli can confer comprehensive benefit.

Level: Beginner – Intermediate

Uddiyana Bhanda (Navel Lock)

General Description & Symbolism:
Nauli is considered a Kriya. Uddiyana differs in that it is called a bandha or lock, a means for controlling and directing prana to various areas of the body. The mechanical action is very similar in both, but there are some slight but important differences worth noting. What bandhas do is facilitate expansion of the prana in the three main energy zones of the body, the lumbar, thoracic, and cervical regions of the spine. The Mula (root) Bandha contains the prana at the lower region of the spine and the Jala (throat) Bandha holds the prana at the region of the throat between the heart and the third eye. *Jala* means water and refers to a jug-like capacity for holding the prana.

Although three distinct locks exist, Uddiyana Bandha is the most important, as it automatically engages both the root and the throat areas when the navel is contracted properly. Uddiyana Bandha creates a sucking action on the pelvic floor and anus area, making it much easier to engage and hold Mula Bandha. This specifically includes the perineum in men and the cervix in women. The positioning is the same as in the practice of Nauli, along with the complete exhalation of the breath. The complete practice of Uddiyana Bandha involves four steps: complete exhalation of the lungs, contraction of the entire abdominal region, relaxation of the abdomen, and lastly a slow inhalation. These four steps constitute one set and in practice these techniques can be stacked one after the other.

Therapeutic Benefit:
The main difference between a bandha and a kriya is that the former is a fixed hold, while the latter is an action. Although Uddiyana Bandha is a fixed con-

traction, it still creates peristalsis and stimulates the digestive glands, as does Nauli kriya. Uddiyana Bandha tones the muscles of the abdomen and relaxes the nerves and heart. With regular practice, the arteries and main blood vessels surrounding the heart expand and receive greater capacity for transporting blood and oxygen to the heart, lowering blood pressure and the resting heart rate.

Ayurvedic Benefit:

For vata dosha, Uddiyana Bandha can gently improve digestive strength and remove flatulence. It improves digestive regularity by relaxing the tension and tightness that build up in the abdominal area. This exercise is also excellent for removing excess pitta from its main site, the small intestine. It also massages the stomach, the source of many enzymatic secretions. This bandha helps to balance air and all vata-related issues, as well as fire (pitta). It combines well with Bastrika or Nadi Shodhana pranayama for raising the kundalini and suspending (*kumbhaka*) the prana in states of meditation.

Spiritual Benefit:

By stacking the four steps into series of sets, without pausing, one gradually increases the capacity to retain the breath in kumbhaka. I usually recommend beginning with three sets, and then gradually increasing the number, as long as the inhalation in the fourth step can be done in a slow, controlled manner. Control and mastery over the last step reflect the highest measure of practicing Uddiyana Bandha, as this represents a greater expansion of the lungs and regulation of pressure in the arteries and veins.

This breath control is a mystical form of pranayama that has also been misinterpreted in the ancient Hatha Yoga texts. Inhalation is *puraka* in Sanskrit; retention of breath is *kumbhaka*; and exhalation of breath is *rechaka*. Kumbhaka, as the physical retention of the breath, transforms the air element into its subtler counterpart, ether or *akasha*, connecting and awakening its even subtler form, prana, the life-force energy. Therefore, kumbhaka actually refers to suspension of the breath merged into prana.

The practice of Uddiyana enhances the shift of consciousness from an outer experience to an inner one, which gives the mind greater capacity to transcend the senses. Uddiyana Bandha becomes a potent technique for inducing pratyahara or sensory withdrawal, the fifth, mystical limb of Patanjali's Yoga Sutras. In essence, what Uddiyana does is harmonize prana and apana. I will expand on this further in the chapter on pranayama.

Level: Beginner - Intermediate

OTHER ASANAS

Ardha Kurmasana (Half-Tortoise Pose)

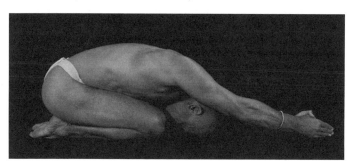

General Description & Symbolism:
This posture is known as half-tortoise or Ardha Kurmasana. It is done on the ground while kneeling, with the arms extended forward. The practice of this asana begins with the torso in an upright position, with arms extended up-wards, covering the ears. Then the torso is slowly lowered until the forehead touches the ground. The knees are kept together so that the torso can fold over the thighs to create the shape of the tortoise shell. Then, after holding the pose for about one minute, the torso is raised back up to Vajrasana (adamant or diamond pose). Another variation commonly taught is with legs extended forward and separated, so that the torso can fall between the thighs, with the forehead eventually touching the ground. However, this position requires great flexibility in the thighs and does not have as much internal therapeutic benefit.

Therapeutic Benefit:
The half-tortoise pose has a number of benefits obtained from the gentle ef-fect of the body resting on the thighs. Also, as the torso is lowered down and raised back up, the muscles in the back and along the spine are conditioned. When the spine folds over the thighs, there is a soft pressure to the colon and digestive organs, which relaxes the nerves surrounding the abdomen. For those lacking the strength to keep the arms extended forward, the hands can be brought into prayer gesture at the heart, reducing pressure on the back.

Ayurvedic Benefit:
Half-tortoise is an effective tool for treating various conditions of the digestive fire (jatharagni). Although the pose seems simple, it has a profound impact on the abdominal nerves, which influence the metabolism, assimilation of nour-ishment, and elimination of waste. Ayurveda teaches that the disruption of this process causes disease through the build-up of ama or undigested food waste.

The pose promotes functional consistency in both the neuro-anatomical and neuro-muscular systems. Through an effect on the crucial nerves in the lower spine and pelvis region, it treats *vishama* or the irregular function of the bowels often described as irritable bowel syndrome (IBS). Vishama agni is commonly associated with vata dosha and can take time to treat. This pose, like other vata-focused asanas, can be complemented by warm-oil massage to the lower trunk region prior to practice.

Practicing this asana will strengthen the jatharagni, as the body gets heated from increased respiration and circulation of blood. The gentle massage the intestines receive while in tortoise pose treats *manda* (slow or sluggish) agni. This type of digestive fire is common in kapha types, in whose stomachs food seems to linger long after a meal.

The opposite of this is the fast or aggressive type of digestion known as *tik-shana* agni, which is characteristic of pitta-related issues. This gentle forward bend creates space in the spine and is soothing to the spinal nerves, which can stimulate heat and over-activate the small intestine and liver. Floor poses like tortoise that have the feet turned upwards are also much more cooling than standing positions that have the feet turned downwards to the earth.

Spiritual Benefit:

The slow, gentle quality of half-tortoise pose teaches us that life has its flow and natural pace, to which we must all surrender. Such poses are also good reminders that yoga need not be aggressive or externally forceful to provide benefit. Ardha Kurmasana encourages us to breathe slowly and deeply, like the tortoise, which symbolizes longevity in Asian cultures, as some tortoises live over two hundred years. Poses such as this will need to play a more prominent role in our lives as stress continues to destroy the mind-body relationship, which is a critical bridge into the spiritual realm. The spiritual path is a life-long, slow commitment. It can often feel like we are trudging along with little progress. But like the tortoise, which keeps moving forward, we must each learn to embrace our own pace, which eventually will lead us to our home in the ocean of Brahman.

Level: Beginner

Vajrasana (Adamant or Thunder-Bolt Pose)

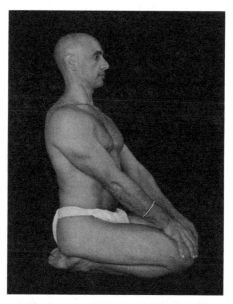

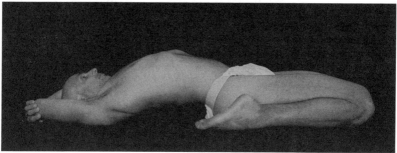

General Description & Symbolism:

The name of this pose derives from the fixed and tight positioning of the quadriceps muscles in the thighs. The Sanskrit root *vaj* means hard or adamant. This is also nicknamed diamond pose, as the diamond is the hardest gem stone, or the thunderbolt, connecting it with Indra, the Vedic God of lightning in the sky. It is first mentioned in the *Gheranda Samhita,* which says it gives psychic powers to the yogi who practices it. Other than this, not much explanation is given of the pose's deeper meaning. Other modern variations include sitting between the feet and reclining back into a supine position to expand the stretch in the quadriceps and hips. A variation with a single folded leg is also a good option to focus the stretch in each thigh separately. One may need to begin the pose in the seated position before even considering the supine variation. Those who have meniscus or patella issues should avoid this posture.

Therapeutic Benefit:

This pose is particularly beneficial for reducing excess tightness in the feet and the muscles in front of the tibia (tibialis anterior, peroneus longus, peroneus brevis, and extensor digitorum longus). These form a specific muscle group that, when tight, restricts movement and rotation of the foot. Supta Vajrasana, the supine variation, depending on level of flexibility, is the only posture that fully stretches the quadriceps and the longest part of the thighs, known as the rectus femoris. These muscles play a vital role in walking, running, biking, and all exercises involving the legs, as they play an indispensable role in stabilizing the knee joints and patellar tendons. Regular practice of this asana can reduce the risk of injuring the knees and straining the thigh muscles.

Ayurvedic Benefit:

Restricted flexibility in the hips and legs, as previously mentioned, is attributable mainly to vata dosha and most particularly apana vayu. The supine variation of this posture is especially beneficial, as the stretching of the rectus femoris, which extends from the pelvic bone to the tibia, releases tension from the trunk between the pelvis and clavicle. The position creates traction that directly pulls this area open. This entire region is vitally connected to proper functioning of the diaphragm during both normal breathing and pranayama exercises. During this process, the apana vayu is unblocked, and a calm and grounding feeling ensues. This action benefits the urogenital system, which includes the reproductive organs and urinary system.

This is one of the primary floor postures that directly targets most vata-related issues. One suggestion I make to new clients struggling to enter this pose is to sit on the floor and walk barefoot more often. Many shoes these days restrict the mobility in the feet, which also influences the function of the knees and hips.

Spiritual Benefit:

The supine variation has the capacity to increase blood flow. As blood is constricted in the thighs, it travels upwards into the organs and glands of the torso and head. This upward flow of blood promotes udana vayu. While balancing kapha-related issues, the pose brings greater awareness and lightness to the mind. Supta Vajrasana can be added to the list of floor postures that induce a calm and stabilizing state of mind in meditation. When both the upward (udana) and downward (apana) currents are unblocked, there comes a great feeling of being centered (samana) at the heart, individual soul, or jiva. Vajrasana can be useful tool for returning us to our true self and spiritual heart. The posture's open and vulnerable nature brings forth qualities ideal for expanding compassion and awareness beyond the level of body and mind.

Level: Beginner - Intermediate

Gomukhasana (Cow-Face Posture)

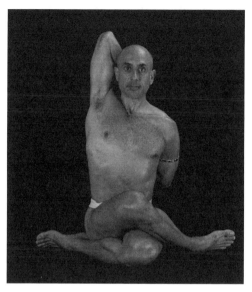

General Description & Symbolism:
The name of this posture derives from two Sanskrit words: *go*, meaning cow, and *mukha*, meaning face. The posture appears in recent yoga texts of the Nath tradition, but also in much more ancient Vedic texts,[113] indicating the antiquity of the cow-face pose. As with the majority of postures practiced on the ground, a substantial amount of flexibility is required. In Gomukhasana, the legs are crossed over each other, creating a strong stretch in the outer hips. Both the crossed position of the legs and the binding of the arms require much flexibility. However, the pose can be practiced without clasping the hands, and this may be required by kapha types, who typically have more girth in the upper chest and shoulders.

The cow is a gentle creature commonly connected to Krishna in his identity as Gopala, the cow herder. The cow is a very calm and nurturing animal that produces milk out of love for her calves, and lives a life of surrender and compassion for all. This unique posture braces the body and spine in an upright position, with the front of the body appearing like the face of a cow, which always looks ahead or upwards. The proper practice of this pose requires the lifting of homologous limbs, meaning that if you lift and place the right leg over the left, then the right arm will also be lifted over the shoulder to clasp the left hand behind the back. This practice brings much benefit to the entire torso, spine, and mind.

---

113   Trishikkhi Brahmana (36) and Sandilya (3:3) & Darsana (3:3,4) Upanishads.

Therapeutic Benefit:
The unique positioning of the legs automatically straightens the spine and is an excellent posture for correcting slumped shoulders, chronic kyphosis (hunchback), and issues involving forward projection of the neck and head, called trapezius syndrome. The posture strengthens the muscular area between the shoulder blades, and stretches the deltoids, pectorals, and latissimus muscles in the back. The spinal column is shifted slightly during the binding of the arms and crossing of the legs, and curves the spine into a stretched-out snake shape.

The practice of the posture on both sides with homologous limbs helps correct scoliosis issues, alleviating some of the tension and discomfort created by this type of distortion in the spine. The placement of the legs provides a tremendous pulling action on the outer side of the hips and thighs, with a particular focus on the illiotibial or IT band, which is usually tightened by athletics or long periods of standing. As a floor posture, it has a powerful capacity for calming the mind. Due to its deep pulling action on the hips, it is effective in releasing neuromuscular pressure, and helpful in treating issues related to neuralgia or nerve pain.

Ayurvedic Benefit:
During the practice of Gomukhasana, much emphasis is placed on the lifting of the chest to bind the hands properly. This lifting action increases respiration and blood circulation in the heart and lungs, balancing a region of excess kapha known as avalambhaka or chest kapha. This invigorates the entire respiratory system and can help reduce depression and laziness, which are common psychological traits of imbalanced kapha dosha.

The pose can help reduce issues related to bronchitis and chronic fatigue syndrome through increased flows of blood and oxygen, which are key factors in balancing kapha. I have a simple affirmation I often give to kapha types on the battlefield of life, "Let it flow and it will go." This is often the case, as circulation gives life, and stagnation brings death. When the shoulders slump and the ribs are compressed, the organs are constricted and can't function properly. Blood and oxygen are inhibited from flowing upwards and udana vayu or upward prana is blocked. Massaging the hips, lumbar region, and thighs with a warming vata massage oil prior to the practice of Gomukhasana enhances the treatment of vata and neuralgia-related issues in the back and legs. Alternately, massaging the chest area with diaphoretic and decongestant essential oils, like eucalyptus and peppermint in a sesame or mustard oil base, is excellent for increasing the pose's effects. Camphor mixes well with these oils and is also excellent in this regard.

Spiritual Benefit:

Although the mind is the ruler of the body, the body also has a voice that consistently feeds directly back to the mind and brain. This is precisely why the mind-body relationship must be established as a primary step toward wellness and spiritual development. Relative to the spine-mind relationship, one of the key assets to victory in life is not only a straight but healthy spine that remains erect during life's trials and tribulations. By focusing the mind's awareness on the spine, energy can be directed to it. This changes how the brain operates,[114] potentially liberating us from the egoistical patterning that destroys our well-being.

Gomukhasana brings the practitioner more in touch with the spine as the sacred pathway of consciousness. Hunching the spine is a slow death, bringing depression and lack of motivation. Gomukhasana is a great weapon for conquering the ego's trickery, and can give rise to greater confidence, courage, and perseverance over the fluctuations of manas.[115] Cow-face pose literally braces us up to confront life's challenges by keeping the spine straight and our heads up, so that one day we can look back and say, "Holy cow! How did I get to where I am today?"

A great disciple of Yogananda and resident monastic at the Self-Realization Fellowship, Brother Abhedananda, sums up the mind-spine-spirit relationship beautifully: "Ordinary people are conscious only of the surface of their bodies and of their senses. Beginner yogis become aware of their physical spine. More advanced yogis gradually become conscious of the flow of life energies and of the subtle centers within the spine. God-united yogis realize the spine and brain as the altars of God in the body."[116]

Level: Advanced

---

114   Clinical professor of psychiatry at the UCLA School of Medicine Daniel J. Siegel writes in *Interpersonal Neurobiology:* "Attention is the process by which energy and information are focused through the circuits of the brain. When we focus attention in integrative ways, for example, we can cultivate differentiation and then link these differentiated regions to one another. The neuroscientific saying 'neurons that fire together, wire together' reveals how the associated activation of neurons changes their linkages to one another. The process of using attention to change the activity of the brain-and therefore ultimately its very architecture-is a part of the larger process by which experience changes neural structure. This process is called neuroplasticity."

115   The aspect of the mind that operates through the five senses and develops the conditional and programmed habits associated with the ego.

116   "Yoga Postures for Health" by Brother Abhedananda (Self-Realization Magazine, September/ October 1960, Self-Realization Fellowship, Los Angeles, Calif.)

Siddhasana (Adept's Pose)

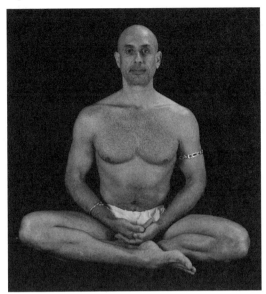

General Description & Symbolism:

This name of this seated pose originates from the Sanskrit term *siddha,* meaning one who possesses power or is a spiritual master. These powers are referred to as siddhis and Sage Patanjali in his *Ashtanga Yoga Sutras* describes eight of them. The immortal Siddha of the modern ages is Mahavatar Babaji, a figure first introduced in this era by Yogananda.[117] The pose appears in the *Gheranda Samhita,* which states that it "leads to emancipation." It is also described in the *Hatha Yoga Pradipika* as "holding the gaze steadily at the spiritual eye." This pose is unique in that it requires pressing the left heel into the perineum, the region between the anus and the genitals, while the right leg presses into the pubic area directly above the genitals. Lastly, the chin is lowered down to rest on the chest while the eyes are lifted upwards to the ajna chakra or "third eye."

Therapeutic Benefit:

Siddhasana on a physical level is a relatively easy position that anyone can do, although its subtle side, with the heel placed at the base of the spine and the chin and eye positioned as described, may not seem as therapeutic or profoundly beneficial as it in fact is. This posture can be used therapeutically to refine the subtle energies that affect the nervous system, spine, and mind. Other related issues that can be treated are constipation, gas, anxiety, and nervousness.

---

117   *Autobiography of a Yogi* by Paramahansa Yogananda (Self-Realization Fellowship, Los Angeles, Calif.)

Ayurvedic Benefit:

The perineum is a point used in the yogic technique of Mulabandha or root lock. It is also closely connected to a point called *guda* in the Ayurvedic system of marma therapy.[118] Guda marma controls the reproductive organs, colon, urination, and gas, and also stimulates the first or muladhara chakra. It is a powerful area for controlling the flow and balance of apana vayu, which governs all these functions.

The Shambhavi Mudra, in which the eyes are rolled upwards and centered on the third-eye chakra, has a subtle but powerful neurological effect on the optic nerves. Yogis say that during the subconscious state of sleep, the eyes drop down, during the waking state they are centered, and during the higher, sattvic, or peaceful states of mind, the eyes are uplifted. While the eyes are held steadily in this auspicious gaze, a subtle, triadic current is created between the two physical eyes and the one invisible eye. The triangular yantra created by the three eyes, two of which are physical and one astral, fires neurotransmitters that send signals to the brain, which slowly dissolve conditioned memory or samskara.

Spiritual Benefit:

This pose is very auspicious in that it combines three techniques that center the subtle pranic forces at the heart, which dissolve the mind into it. The pose's clear intention is to center the prana at the anahata (heart) chakra. It does so by sealing the energy off from escaping both at the muladhara and visshudha (throat) chakras. The pressing of the chin into the chest contains the prana inwards. The technique of pressing the heel into the perineum below the base of the spine is called Mulabandha (root lock), and that of the chin pressing into the chest is called Jalabandha (throat lock).

The gaze of both eyes is lifted in Shambhavi Mudra and unified at the ajna chakra to invoke the state of Shiva consciousness or *shunya* (blankness or empty space). This sacred gaze is symbolic of the three eyes of Lord Shiva or *Tryambakam*. Two eyes view the manifest physical world. One eye with intuitive vision transcends and destroys the world concept. Shiva is known as the destroyer in the Hindu trinity.

Practice of this three-eyed gesture is also symbolic of the three shaktis (powers) of the Goddesses. These three powers result from buddhi awakened in the mind field. They are known as kriya shakti, ichha shakti, and jnana shakti, and

---

118   108 prana power points exist throughout the body and are used in Ayurvedic clinical practices and originally in the Vedic system of martial arts or Dhanurveda.

are respectively managed by three Goddesses Durga, Lakshmi, and Saraswati. Durga, who rides a tiger, represents the power of protection needed during the formative stage of spiritual development to overcome the sensory habits and emotional identifications that keep us entranced by the force of maya or illusion. Lakshmi, who is depicted standing on a lotus flower, symbolizes the expansion of consciousness that arises from consistent tapas (discipline), yielding the virtuous qualities acquired on the spiritual path. Lakshmi grants us the inner qualities of abundance and prosperity. The last power is granted by Goddess Saraswati, who provides us the knowledge or jnana to float above the lake of life by means of reflection and discernment.

Level: Intermediate - Advanced

Padmasana (Lotus Pose)

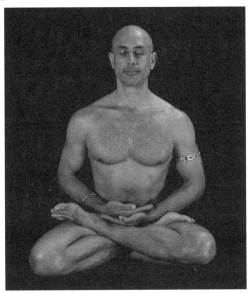

General Description & Symbolism:
The lotus posture is greatest of all yogic postures, as it represents the proper seat for meditation. It is the first of all the asanas that Lord Shiva sat in while in the Himalayan foothills. Padamasana represents the culmination of seated postures that a yogi aspires to attain after the other cross-legged positions, such as Swastikasana, Sukhasana (easy pose), Siddhasana (adept's pose), and Muktasana (liberation pose). These are all slightly different variations, and the *Hatha Yoga Pradipika* says there are different views on which is most the essential.

This is why Yogananda taught that what you do with your legs is not as important as how the spine is kept. A straight spine is the essential position for raising the prana to the higher spinal centers. Nevertheless, complex postures like the lotus pose do provide major benefits for advancing on the spiritual path. Initially, I recommend people to begin sitting on the floor more often, as a practical manner of preparing the hips, knees, and feet for the capacity of sitting in lotus. The name of the posture comes from the word *padma* or lotus and is sometimes also called Kamala. The original position is termed "full" lotus, while the variation of crossing one leg instead of both is called Ardha (half) Padmasana. The half-lotus is a good option for many of those still developing knee and hip flexibility.

Therapeutic Benefit:
This is a sacred posture symbolic of spiritual dexterity. Interestingly enough, Padmasana also benefits the mind-body relationship and has therapeutic value on a physiological level. As an advanced asana, its use in a therapeutic setting is limited. Padmasana is the most famous asana and is known as the "destroyer of all diseases,"[119] probably due to its capacity in raising prana. According to Ayurveda, diseases occur when prana is blocked and Padmasana balances the five directions of prana, naturally relaxing the heart.

The cross-legged nature of the position is one reason the heart works less. The heart does not have to pump large amounts of venous blood in the thighs upwards against the pull of gravity. If you check your pulse while holding the pose, you will notice your resting heart rate is lower than usual. The tiny red corpuscles in the blood are a vehicle for prana. Once the heart rate calms, the mind can more easily relax and release endorphins, chemicals produced by the central nervous system and pituitary gland, which inhibit the transmission of pain signals, producing a feeling of peace and contentment.

Full lotus has a tremendously stabilizing effect on the mind, for, by keeping the body very still and the spine straight, without any need for a cushion, the brain can release its internal healing medicines. Padmasana has a unique capacity to exhilarate and relax, stimulate and calm, at the same time. The pose redirects blood from the femoral artery in the lower limbs into the internal iliac artery in the pelvis, bathing the spinal nerves, reproductive organs, and bladder with fresh blood flow. This produces a transmutation of physical creative energy into the spiritual pranic energies commonly called kundalini. Matsyasana (fish pose) is also done with the legs in the lotus position, and is considered a powerful posture for purifying all impurities.

---

119 *Hatha Yoga Pradipika*, Verse 47, Chapter 1.

Ayurvedic Benefit:

Lotus pose brings benefit to all doshas through its pure and subtle effects on the prana. Any time prana is encouraged to rise and internalize, countering the tamasic and rajasic impulses of the senses, a positive impact on the doshas ensues. The term dosha means mistake or fault, and such "faults" typically occur because of a bodily imbalance in the agni and soma relationship. This means that imbalances of the doshas often occur due to stress, weak jatharagni, or low immunity. Both yoga and Ayurveda consistently stress the importance of balancing these forces if ascension of consciousness is to take place. Padmasana can be held for small intervals at a time after a proper warm-up. The other option is to practice the half-lotus variation, alternating between the left and right legs several times, until flexibility and mobility gradually increase in the hips and knees.

Spiritual Benefit:

During the golden ages of higher consciousness, the Satya and Tretya Yugas, when meditation was more commonly used to enter the hypnotic state of Savikalpa Samadhi, Padmasana was necessary to keep the body from tipping over. When the body and mind need to be balanced, it is necessary to feel grounded and connected to the earth, and the feet and hands of course enable us to do this.

The feet are connected to the element of fire and the sense of sight and the eyes. The hands are used to experience the sense of touch through the skin. Where we direct the hands and feet, there the energy goes. In Padmasana, both the hands and feet are turned upwards to increase the flow of prana upwards (udana), away from the earth's currents, to connect with the spiritual currents in the higher centers. This is why meditation must be practiced in a vertical position, to balance the horizontal gravitational forces connected to maya.

The whole intention of yoga is to raise the awareness beyond identification with the body. Yogic texts mention pressing the chin on the chest and gazing at the "tip of the nose." This also appears in the Bhagavad Gita,[120] a much older scripture, which says, "Let the yogi focus his eyes at the starting place of the nose." However, as Yogananda was taught by his Guru Swami Sri Yukteswar, one of the many misinterpretations of the dark ages was:[121] "Fix one's vision on the end of the nose."

---

120   Chapter 6, Verse 13

121   Kali Yuga. Four of the main texts (*Hatha Yoga Pradipika, Gheranda Samhita, Goraksha Samhita* and *Hatharatnavali*) on Hatha Yoga were produced during the tail end of the descending and ascending Kali Yuga, approximately between the 5th and 15th centuries A.D., the lowest point of human consciousness within the 24,000 year period. Commentaries on the more ancient Bhagavad Gita also began to appear during this time. Therefore the probability for misinterpretation was increased, and can also be seen in other scriptures that developed during those times, such as the Christian Bible and Islamic Quran.

Paramahansa Yogananda writes in his *Autobiography of a Yogi*, "This inaccurate interpretation of a Bhagavad Gita stanza, widely accepted by Eastern pundits and Western translators, used to arouse Master's droll criticism. 'The path of a yogi is singular enough as it is,' he remarked. 'Why counsel him that he must also make himself cross-eyed? The true meaning of nasikagram is "origin of the nose," not "end of the nose." The nose originates at the point between the eyebrows, the seat of spiritual vision.'"[122]

Whether we can attain the classic Padmasana posture or not, we must remember the pose is not the goal. It is more important to learn how we can best keep the spine straight in meditation, according to our own constitution. All people learning to meditate must find the position that best suits them and remember that meditation has nothing to do with the legs. "Spine and the brain are the altars of God."[123]

Level: Advanced

Savasana (Corpse Pose)

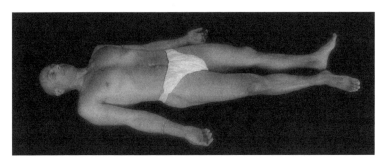

General Description & Symbolism:
Savasana, corpse or dead man's pose, is considered an essential and distinct component of Hatha Yoga practice. Asana is related to the sun, heating and stimulating. Savasana is related to the moon, cooling and soothing. On a physical level, this is symbolic of the meaning of ha-tha or sun and moon yoga. The posture-rest dynamic is the preeminent feature that distinguishes Hatha Yoga from all other art and fitness forms, as a sacred and scientific approach to attaining a unified state of consciousness.

122   *Autobiography of a Yogi* by Paramahansa Yogananda (Self-Realization Fellowship, Los Angeles, Calif.)
123   *The Great Light of God* by Paramahansa Yogananda (Self-Realization Fellowship, Los Angeles, Calif.)

Savasana involves simply lying on your back with heels together, but allowing the feet to fall to each side, with the arms to the side of the body. Two views exist with regard to the direction of the palms. The palms facing downward aid in calming the mind and promoting a feeling of being grounded, as the energy in the palms synergizes with the gravitational force. The palms facing upwards, as in Padmasana, aid in raising the subtle etheric energies upwards to lift the consciousness away from the body.

It is important to note that Savasana is not sleep or naptime, as many have misunderstood. During Savasana, a subtle awareness is maintained, with the mind shifting into a witnessing state. Traditionally, Savasana was practiced in between each asana, as postures in classical Hatha Yoga were held for much longer periods and required more rest than what we see today in the yogaerobics movement. Savasana was held for a period of time equal to the time the posture was held, and normally the longest Savasana is taken at the end of a practice. It seems to be rare these days if even two to five minutes are taken for relaxation at the end of class.

Therapeutic Benefit:
The essence of Savasana on a therapeutic level is restoration. The intention of yoga asana is not to exhaust the body but to purify while at the same time energizing it. It is a major practice to teach people how to relax and turn off the senses, which are bombarded by impressions all day long. Savasana slows cell function and also calms the heart. We breathe less frequently and exert less energy to pump blood. The posture is good for those suffering from hypertension, high blood pressure, anxiety, and nervousness. Savasana is very important for those experiencing adrenal fatigue or chronic fatigue syndrome caused by lifestyles that include excessive work, worry over unpaid bills, sensory over-stimulation, unhealthy diet, and medications. For such individuals, I prescribe a simple asana routine of three to seven postures, with Savasana after each, and then a longer rest at the end. The posture-rest dynamic eradicates the triggering aspect of e-motions as directed by the e-go. Savasana is an exercise that teaches us to "let go" and become more detached from the outer, changing world. Psychologically, it is the best posture for those who live in fear and frequently find themselves in the illusion of needing to be "in control."

Ayurvedic Benefit:
Usually, if the person falls asleep during Savasana, it indicates there is high kapha, or the body is afflicted with *ojashaya*, depletion of the physical "battery." Sleeping in Savasana also appears to be common with new yoga practitioners, who do not have a balanced lifestyle and suffer from adrenal fatigue.

So the moment they lie down, they fall asleep. When the body is relaxed, it can rest in an accelerated manner, unlike sleep, which sometimes takes seven to nine hours to produce a sense of being rested. Proper practice of Savasana throughout a yoga practice and for 15 to 20 minutes at the end of a class can feel like an entire night's rest.

Imbalanced pitta often "forces" rest by trying to find the perfect position and then keeping too much attention on the body, making it hard to relax. Vatas are challenged in Savasana with sensitivity to any sound. Initially, they are restless and sometimes look around, therefore requiring much more time to shut off. Because the body cools down in a horizontal position, it is vital they cover themselves with a blanket or put on extra clothing. The Ayurvedic shirodhara treatment provides an experience similar to Savasana.

Spiritual Benefit:
Savasana is critical to cultivating a witnessing mind, as it teaches one to detach from the sense-identified ego-mind. *Sakshi bhava* is a special esoteric sense that allows us to discriminate our body, mind, and thoughts from the real Self. The practice of Savasana is likened to what Sage Patanjali calls pratyahara, the fifth limb of the *Ashtanga Yoga Sutras*. The initial factor in experiencing this shift is stillness in the body and awareness of the breath. The "hum-sa" mantra can also be used to deepen the power of attention at the spiritual eye. A deep experience of Savasana serves to prepare the mind for meditation. Relaxation is the key to success in both Savasana and meditation. In each practice of Savasana throughout a yoga session, there should be a gradual deepening of consciousness, so that with each inward turn of the senses a greater purification takes place and the more subtle energy of prana can awaken the energy centers in the spine.

Level: Beginner - Intermediate - Advanced.

Clinical Yoga
One significant way to increase Ayurveda's efficacy is by including asana in any health and wellness program. Over many years of operating my own Ayurvedic clinic, I have been able to apply the wisdom of yoga therapy according to Ayurvedic principles. The relationship of yoga and Ayurveda is most important. This provides a synergistic approach that includes the tri-dosha system, the distinct dhatu layer system of anatomy, the channel systems or srotas, and the three-body concept of body, mind, and soul.

Ayurveda defines and views the physical body on the basis of energy-based laws, such as the five pranas, the force of agni, and the thirteen fires that sustain the entire physical body. Both prana and agni derive from a profound cosmology that links the physical body's operations with deeper mystical forces. This is precisely why yoga as a form of therapy must be aligned with Ayurveda. Obviously, allopathic medicine does not fit this mold.

The one area, I must say, in which allopathy has been very useful is diagnostics, such as blood panels, MRI (magnetic resonance imaging), radiology used to scan the body, functional MRI to measure brain activity, CT (x-ray computed tomography) scans, and ultrasonography (ultra-sound). These have made it much easier to diagnose health issues. However, I have also seen many cases where modern diagnostic tools are unable to discover the causes of instances where individuals feel that something is wrong with their bodies, sense being off-balance, and even experience certain sleep disorders, digestive irregularities, and skin problems.

There are a number of considerations when deciding how asana and pranayama should be applied to individual cases. These include:

1. Prakriti (constitution)
2. Vikriti (imbalance)
3. Nidana (causes of disease)
4. Rupa (signs and symptoms)
5. Length of time with issues
6. Ojas level (strength and immunity)
7. Dhatu (seven tissues)
8. Spine
9. Capacity or level of experience with yoga
10. Age
11. Overall health history
12. Culture and religion
13. Geography
14. Injuries, trauma, surgeries, etc.

These represent the main factors to consider. These can be looked at in much more detail, but such an overview is a good place to start. Yoga asana can be a very good system to help any new client better understand their body and capacities, as well as to instill discipline and prepare the body for detoxification. How a person does asana can tell you a lot about their health history and prakriti. It also exposes areas that are hidden and weak or for some reason may not have been discussed in an initial consultation. I have seen my understanding of a person change substantially when I see them in yoga practice. It forces me to review my intake notes and add new observations to those I have made.

One thing that really helps is actually seeing the body's physical contour, the skin, and the size of the ankle, knee, and hip joints. I have a saying I often share with regards to determining the dosha type: "What you see is what you get." This is true in most cases. However, this can get tricky, particularly when there is an issue of hypothyroidism, which usually slows the metabolism. A person's body weight can change, even though they never had excess weight before.

Recommending asana is an excellent measure for establishing discipline, and is vital to success in Ayurvedic medicine, a system that mostly depends on individual responsibility and effort. Asana, as discussed earlier, is a powerful tool for purification of the body. If ama or undigested food waste is high, asana will increase jatharagni to burn it out of the gastro-intestinal tract. If ama kapha has moved into the lungs, chest-opening postures like Ustrasana (camel pose) and Natarajasana (Dancing Shiva pose) are good for stimulating these organs. If ama has moved into the tissues, a variety of asanas and pranayama can be used to address each issue specifically.

Asana is applied according to vikriti imbalance with regards to how the postures affect the spine. Vata-related issues can be addressed with postures that target stretching the hips, illiotibial (IT) band, gluteals, and the abdomen in a clockwise direction. These types of poses should be done slowly, and if possible held for longer periods, especially when on the floor. Ayurvedic oils in a sesame base, typically including herbs such as bala, ashwagnadha, haritaki, dashmool, and tulsi, can be massaged into the lower lumbar region prior to the beginning of asana practice. The combination of these two modalities is a direct and powerful measure for treating vata dosha.

Massages with cooling and soothing oils, which include herbs such as amalaki, brahmi, and bitters like neem and manjistha, around the abdomen and in the middle of the spine, help release build-up of pitta dosha. Lateral stretching asana, twists, and forward bends all release tension and heat from pitta's seat in the small intestines and liver.

For kapha issues, warm, heating, and expanding oils, such as eucalyptus, camphor, peppermint, and herbs and spices like tulsi, cinnamon, and punarnava, an excellent herb-root expectorant, can be massaged onto the chest, upper shoulders, back, and neck prior to stimulating inversions, backbends, and strong

Kapalabhati pranayama. In general, it is beneficial for all doshas to massage warm oil along the entire spine, as the central nervous system influences the entire mind-body relationship and is a good area from which to begin. One of the greatest of such oil and asana combinations is massaging the abdominal region and practicing Nauli. I recommend this for general health maintenance and always include it in our pancha karma detox program.

To simplify the routine for new clients and those days when time is limited, I recommend massaging the abdomen and the lower spine and then performing Nauli. A happy belly can ensure a happy life, and a healthy spine can mean a healthy life. When simple therapies such as these are combined with some meditation, they become practical forms of preventative healthcare.

The best type of healthcare is that performed by ourselves, independent of any practitioner, government, or institution. Each year millions of people throughout the world die of preventable diseases and health complications. I am constantly encouraging people to understand that the only way to eradicate human suffering and reduce health issues is educating them on how to heal themselves. This is the highest responsibility of humanity. Ayurveda teaches us how to balance and heal the physical body. Yoga provides the mystical teachings for living with greater awareness and compassion. Astrology can teach us to surrender when we are supposed to. Again and again, the sun, moon, and earth teach us the boundless wisdom that exists in this universe.

Yoga and Athletics

The combination of yoga and athletics is of growing interest to many who want to improve their game. Professional athletes in sports all types, such as basketball, football, and tennis, are using asana to stay limber, as sports tighten the muscles.

The wisdom of yoga and Ayurveda can be integrated into all aspects of our lives, so that we can enjoy what life has to offer. Adaption is the key to success. Yoga and Ayurveda should be done in relationship with our lifestyles. These sciences teach us how to enhance the quality of our lives in all aspects: physical, mental, emotional, and spiritual.

Yoga asana has a number of specific benefits for athletes, including reduction of lactic acid build-up, increased agility, muscular flexibility, and mental efficiency and concentration. On the physical level, the most important consideration is to integrate yoga asana moderately, avoiding extremely deep stretches, jerking movements, and over-heating the practice room. Because of the wide physical contrast between yoga and sports on the muscles and joints, one must be careful not to over-extend the stretches, as this may stress the fibers and result in a tear. Most competitive sports involve fast-muscle twitch fibers and require keeping the muscles tight to maintain speed and acceleration. Asanas that stretch the legs and gluteals are essential to avoid cramping and straining of muscles.

Those persons that enjoy sports for recreational and health purposes probably utilize slow-muscle twitch fibers, particularly doing sports such as swimming, hiking, golf, bicycling, and others done at a more even pace. Lactic acid builds up[124] in the muscles and red blood cells when oxygen levels are reduced. The massaging of Ayurvedic body oils onto the skin before exercise allows the body to increase intake of fresh oxygen through the skin, improving circulation, and reducing the exhausting feeling that comes with intensive exercise routines. Oil massage done prior to asana practice can greatly benefit sports performance

---

124   Muscles produce a very similar compound called lactate, which is a link between anaerobic and aerobic metabolism.

Chapter EIGHT

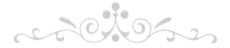

THE POWER OF BREATHING

One must be patient like the earth. What iniquities are being perpetuated on her!
Yet she quietly endures them all.
Sri Sarada Devi (1853 - 1920)

Understanding the Breath

The use of the breath, along with mantra, is one of the oldest forms of yoga. The two practices go hand in hand. Different forms of breathing practice can be found in many traditions: shamanic, qigong, Vedic, and, more recently, the holotropic technique that came out of the 1960s American counter-culture. The body is linked to breath and to sounds or mantra in order to enhance the mind-body relationship.

In any such system, the breath has always been considered the vehicle's power or energy, whether that vehicle is an asana, mantra, or creative dance expression. The flow of the breath makes it happen. The breath is the most powerful instrument we have, as it is our direct link to life itself, the five senses, and all the operations of the brain. According to yoga teachings, the breath can connect us to the world by calming the mind. Such techniques as alternate-nostril breathing can create greater awareness of both our physical and spiritual heart, the organ of health and center for experiencing love and compassion.

On the esoteric side, the breath can also disconnect us from the body, mind, and senses, and transition us into other domains of consciousness rarely understood except by advanced yogis. In the broadest sense, prana makes the ocean surge and allows the sun's rays to shine. It penetrates into the planet earth and influences the movement of the stars as the earth and moon revolve around the sun. Prana allows rivers to flow and gives valor to the mountains.

Prana is the sustainer of life and, in Ayurveda, the primary force behind the doshas, the formation of the bodily cells and tissues, and overall health. According to yoga teachings, the average person breathes about 21,600 times a day. If this pattern is sustained, a person will live 100 years, the standard life-span allotted in Ayurveda.[125]

I often repeat in my yoga classes that circulation promotes life and stagnation creates death, simply to remind people that breathing deeply will promote general wellness. For many people today, creating an intention for greater health and wellness should begin with awareness of the breath during all activities, not just in yoga class. This could be called "mindful" breathing or "heart" breathing, because it involves focusing on the heart or chest area with every breath. The seat of prana is the heart. This One heart influences four aspects of our human existence: senses (manas), intuition (buddhi), thoughts (chitta), and the ego (ahamkara). Breathing into the heart and learning to control the heart-breath is the essence behind attaining liberation or moksha in yoga. Therefore, pranayama, as an instrument of purification, increases our general well-being by promoting circulation of blood throughout the body, allowing it to operate optimally. Pranayama can help us feel more connected to the world, a fundamental component of stability and being grounded, calm, and clear.

It is important to recognize that pranayama exercises do not actually work with the prana directly, as the prana is different from the element of air.[126] The mind, senses, and body must be purified over time through proper lifestyle, diet, yoga asana, and pranayama in order for pranayama exercises to influence the prana in our body. Prana controls all movements and operations of the body and sustains it as long as its karmic code or destiny permits.

Breathing seems simply to involve inhaling and exhaling air. That is quite true, but yogic pranayama is much more than that. The science of yoga explains various techniques and exercises that can purify the body of toxins, elicit peace in the mind, and make us more efficient at the tasks we take on in life. As discussed below, breathing can also be recommended according to dosha type or to address specific imbalances.

There are three main forms of yogic breathing. When the breath is inhaled, it is called puraka. When the breath is exhaled, it is called rechaka. When the

---

125   *Charaka Samhita*, Chapter VI, verse 29. The text does mention that this lifespan is representative of "this age." This seminal text was written in approximately 200 BC, according to Professor P.V. Sharma of Bihar, India.

126   Brahma Sutras 2/4/9. *Na vayu kriye pritag-upadeshaat* is an assertion that prana is a separate principle and should not be identified with the element of air.

breath is held or sustained, it is called kumbhaka. The suspension of the breath is the most sacred form, as it increases the spiritual capacity to transcend the senses or ego consciousness, and also promotes longevity. In the yoga tradition, there has always been an affinity with retaining the breath, which I feel has been lost in the commercial Hatha Yoga movement. Asana is now mistakenly taught with the idea that one should first master asana or attain the perfect position before beginning the practice of pranayama. This is a foolish idea, and a reason why many do not progress spiritually. The breath and mind are left uncontrolled to behave like a wild monkey. As Sri Swami Sivananda said, "You need not wait for practicing Pranayama till you get full mastery over the Asana. Practice Asana and side by side you can practice Pranayama also. In course of time, you will acquire perfection in both."

Pure Mind for a Pure Breath

In the eight limbs of Patanjali's Yoga Sutras, pranayama is listed after asana, reflecting its connection to the body and ability to balance the prana. The term pranayama is composed of two words, *prana* meaning life force, the energy that makes up all living things, and *yama* meaning control or mastery. The combination of these two terms implies the discipline of controlling the breath. Pranayama is a technical practice that transports the energies in the body so that we can expand our consciousness beyond the limitations of both body and mind. The Raja Yoga path is focused on purifying the breath to aid in purification of the mind. Sage Patanjali explains that kriya is the main approach for doing this, and has three main components: tapasya or austerities, svadhya or study, and ishwara pranidhana or trust in God. These expansive principles make up the Kriya Yoga teachings brought to the West by Yogananda through the special dispensation of Babaji and Christ, so that many would awaken and hear the sacred vibration of the holy Aum.

Here are descriptions of the three limbs of kriya:

- **Tapasya:** Austerities of the body, like asanas, exercises, sattvic diet, and proper lifestyle. Vocal austerities: control of the tongue, words used to help not hurt others. Purification of the senses by reducing their use in solitude. Mental austerities like maintaining a relaxed mind, gentleness of heart, and verbal silence or not speaking. Tapasya as an austerity does not imply strain or painful exercises. Austerities must enhance the quality of the spiritual life and create a balanced mind and a greater overall sense of contentment in the sadhaka. The intention of tapasya is to enhance the mind's mastery over the body. Then, naturally, the breath follows suit, becoming calm, consistent, and deep. The breath is the link between the mind and the body. Mind-body synergy depends on breath control, awareness, and balance of the five pranas (see below).

- **Svadhya:** Study of scriptures, repetition of mantras as japa, that is, during acts of service or with a mala. With regard to the mind, the Gayatri mantra is best, as it is the mother mantra of the Vedas. Svadhya is like a type of satsanga or good association with the sacred texts of yoga, such as the Bhagavad Gita, Ramayana, and other uplifting spiritual books. Svadhya includes development of your inner association with your true Self through introspection.

- **Ishwara Pranidhana:** The most advanced of the kriya principles, as it encourages us to foster feelings for God. The intangible gifts of life can teach us to develop a trust and faith that, without any doubt, God upholds our entire life. There is a complete eradication of the doubting or tamasic attitude of mind. Such a level of mental quality requires the power of dispassion or vairagya, so the mind is not agitated by the ever-changing material world.

Spiritually speaking, the breath can be a powerful tool that allows deeper inner energies or shaktis to awaken with in us. The mind manages mankind's capacity of prana for expansion through the mechanism of the lungs. The manner in which they function is a direct reflection of the mind quality and can determine the depth of transformation, as well as the level of purification in our energy body. The nadis or subtle energy channels must be properly cleared and prepared for the flow of the prana if they are to produce shakti or occult powers (siddhi).

One of the main reasons I teach pranayama techniques like Bastrika, Kapalabhati, and Yogananda's double breath in small short sets, dispersed into an asana practice, is because they can have a strongly purifying quality on the organs, systems, blood, and even nadis. Without disturbing the mind, they can help clear the emotional body. The emotional body is largely misunderstood and even unexplored in today's world. Pranayama is the key to unblocking our emotional patterns, teaching us that we are neither our "emotions" nor our "thoughts."

The secret of yoga lies in its capacity to bring us into a state of awareness that is beyond the conditional patterning created by the thoughts and emotions we express and suppress.

When asanas are practiced, the obstacles of physical tension, blocked energy, and mental dullness are gradually removed. But in order to transcend beyond the physical, the subtler tool of pranayama is necessary. Our breath is also reflected in the quality or range of our speech or vak,[127] in accordance with our capacity to concentrate. With a good quality of breath, our capacity to communicate with others on the physical level is enhanced. Similarly, on the subtle energetic level, the power of prana empowers mantra to connect us with spirit and invoke the great powers of creativity and insight symbolized by the Goddess of speech, Saraswati.

Breath Therapy to Heal the Body and Mind

The essence of therapeutic breathing is captured in Hatha Yoga, which enumerates a number of breathing or pranayama techniques for a variety of purposes. The fact is that a poor quality of breath-flow, particularly through the nose, can affect sight, taste, smell, and even hearing, and delay the brain's operation.

When beginning any breathing practice, the initial task specifically involves overcoming resistance from the manas or sensory mind, which is linked to the ego or ahamkara, and can produce a feeling of malaise. As the practice is continued, the buddhi or higher mind is aroused from its slumber, enkindling the soul's sublime qualities. The breath is an incredibly powerful tool when used properly. When neglected, our mind-body wellness can be crippled.

The nose, the sense organ of smell, is one of the most important orifices in the human body and is commonly the most ignored. In these times, people take better care of their fingernails than their noses. I have often marveled that in some cities like Los Angeles there are nail parlors on every corner. I often think that, with all the dust and pollution, there should be nose parlors instead.

The Ayurvedic nasya treatment is considered vitally important for management of issues related to all the doshas. A powerful technique like Bastrika[128] gently stimulates various nadis or channels throughout the body, transporting prana to new areas and allowing for a deeper feeling of relaxation. Breathing techniques should not be rushed, but introduced in a gradual manner over time for best results. The inner anatomy of the arteries, veins, and organs

---

127   Correlated with speech and directly correlated with divinity. These "sounds" exist in four levels or tones, beginning with the audible, proceeding to the whisper, mental, and subconscious, and culminating in union with the supreme in a super-conscious state. Vak is also mentioned in the Rig Veda as the goddess of divine speech, who invoked great knowledge in the seers and rishis of the yoga tradition.

128   Translated as bellows or diaphragmatic breathing, this is a 50-50 exchange between forceful inhalation and exhalation without any gap between breaths.

must become adjusted to these new levels of energy and changes in systemic function. Obstruction of the nasal cavity can directly influence the function of the lungs and mind. In many cases, I have drawn a connection between poor nasal function and cardiovascular capacity. Blocked sinuses even create poor balance in yoga. Poor breathing can also be correlated with fear, depression, and low self-esteem. Collapsing shoulders disturb the expansion of breath-oxygen-prana into vital areas, reducing use of the diaphragm.

In yoga and Ayurveda, the use of a neti cup is recommended. This flushes the nostrils with warm saline water until they are cleared. Another great breathing technique, Kapalabhati,[129] is the best exercise for clearing mucous or kapha from the upper respiratory tract and sinuses. Kapalabhati translates as "skull-shiner" or "brain-cleaner" for precisely this reason. It affects the forehead and the frontal lobes of the brain or cerebrum, responsible for control of thought and speech.

The breath-brain functional relationship explains how pranayama co-operates with mantra and meditation as part of a sacred trinity that can create a harmonious balance of the doshas on the psycho-physical level. It also merges us with our own inner cosmologies, which include the destructive (air), creative (fire), and preservative (water) forces of existence. Various breathing exercises can be used specifically to stimulate different areas of the body and improve concentration. With an Ayurvedic perspective, one can gain specific knowledge of which direction the prana has been disturbed, and then use pranayama to balance out such disturbance.

What follows is a breakdown of the five pranas and some of the characteristics correlated with each, set forth so that pranayama can be applied effectively to areas that need balancing. Typically, when one of the pranas is blocked, the balance of the entire body is affected, because the circulatory and respiratory systems, the flow of fluids, and neuro-muscular operations are disturbed.

The Five Directions of Prana

The life force, which governs all actions of the body, moves in five directions. As mentioned in the Agamas[130] and the Vedas, the five pranas govern all aspects of the body, including the elements, senses, and motor organs. The

---

129 Short and forceful exhalations through the nose while keeping the lips sealed. Approximately 80% of the energy used in breathing is on the exhalation, while 20% is on the silent and short inhalation.

130 A dynamic knowledge of revelations directly imparted by Lord Shiva. There are twenty-eight Agamas rooted in the Shiva community of Southern India. Pranayama as part of the Kriya lineage is, according to scriptures, rooted in the Agama tradition and connected to a great siddha yogi who has initiated many recognized saints into the sacred art of breath mastery.

Shivagama states, "A more useful science than the science of respiration, a more beneficial science than the science of respiration, a greater friend than the science of respiration has never been seen nor heard." The life of the body is supported by prana, which moves in five directions to influence all physical movements, physiological functions, and the nature of the mind. It is important to understand how prana moves in the body. Inhalations are primarily cooling and influence udana, while exhalations are warming and affect apana. The neutralizing of these two currents supports the balance of samana, which has a more neutral vibration.

The five pranas are it follows:

- **Prana** - This is the energy that we absorb in our bodies and minds and that moves inward to impress the cells. Prana is essentially a molecular activity in the mind reflected into the body. Prana is taken in through our environment, air, foods, and people. Our ability to increase the amount of prana we can hold is equal to the quality of our life, the time invested in practice of yoga, and the level of purity of our cells. Good prana aids in transformation of food and other nutrients into new and healthy tissues.

- **Udana** – This is the energy that moves upwards. It relates to inhalation, speech, positive energy, vitality, and creative expression. Udana is the energy in the throat region above the heart. When obstructed, lethargy, depression and lack of confidence, weakening of the will power, and a slowing of the physiology ensue. The double breath is an excellent technique for increasing the flow of udana and propelling the mind forward, onward, and upwards. Alternate nostril-breathing or Nadi Shodhana is also very effective for increasing udana, especially when combined with retention (kumbhaka) at the top of the inhalation. The practice of the throat lock (Jalabandha)[131] is also recommended. Imbalanced udana can prevent the growth of bones and disturb the healing of organs, which takes place by means of the protoplasm of living cells.

- **Apana** – This is the energy that moves downward. It relates to digestive elimination, reproduction, and exhalation. Apana is the energy below the navel. When blocked, it creates insecurity, a feeling of being ungrounded, and anxiety. This can also increase the sensitivity of neuromuscular function in the pelvis and lumbar region. Constipation, bloating, gas, and the growth of tumors are common signs that apana is disturbed. The use of

---

131   Three types of bandhas (mula, uddhiyana, jala) are mentioned in the Hatha Yoga texts in terms of three areas of the body (perineum-cervix, navel-abdomen, and throat), where the breath can be contained for the purpose of expanding the prana.

the diaphragm is essential here. Bellows breathing practiced slowly and in short intervals is effective. The practice of root lock (Mulabandha) is also important.

- **Samana** – This is the balancing force that moves from the outer layers of the body inward, towards digestive balance in the navel area. It influences stability in balancing asana, and an overall sense of well-being and contentment. When disturbed, it creates irritable bowels and in some cases diarrhea and hyper-acidity. Lack of balanced samana produces frustration, anger, and urgency. Yogic cooling breaths, such as Shitali, Sikari, and Chandra Bhedana are excellent for soothing and stabilization. A good Savasana is one of the most essential poses for balancing samana, especially when followed by lying in a right-lateral position to activate the lunar channel through the left nostril. Poor samana creates digestive disturbance, such as the common irritable bowel syndrome (IBS).

- **Vyana** – This is the force that moves from the inside of the body outwards to the periphery and throughout the entire body. Vyana is the energy in the heart and lungs, which creates circulation and governs our emotions. Vyana strongly influences prana, as they are closely interlinked. When this vayu (wind) is blocked, a person may feel stuck or trapped due to ischemia or a lack of oxygen. A person may feel sensitive, emotional, and vulnerable when vyana is affected. Pranayama in general is vital for vyana, as it promotes circulation and lymphatic function. Buddhist walking meditation practice is very effective in this regard, as are yoga postures that open the chest, including back-bends like camel or Ustrasana. Poor or imbalanced vyana creates blood deficiencies, variable high or low blood pressure, anemia, and even leukemia if the imbalance is prolonged. Cold hands and feet or temperature sensitivities reflect a vyana condition.

The Royal Path of the Breath

The highest intention of all yoga dharmas[132] is to awaken the real mind linked to the soul's vibrant energy. Hatha yoga provides many devices for awakening the coiled energy at the base of the spine known as kundalini. All paths aim to achieve the blessed state of self-realization, whether the energy is stimulated through breathing techniques or the postural expressions of Tantra, guided by the serene mind of Raja Yoga, or cleared and purified by Ayurveda. Yogic practices endorse an integral approach that includes pranayama, mantra, and

---

132 The term dharma is associated with having a duty and living a path of higher purpose. However, it also describes the four-fold principles (kama, artha, dharma, and moksha) of Jyotish or yogic astrology for living a balanced life.

meditation, all of which are meant to awaken this sacred energy. In most of humanity, this energy is dormant. The consciousness is fogged, has a limited capacity to discern between right and wrong, and follows a lifestyle ruled by habits and conditions. When the consciousness is aroused and uplifted with the right intention in meditation practice and right attitude in daily living, the individual is empowered to think, speak, and behave with greater awareness and live life as a higher, conscious being.

The breath can serve as a powerful tool to bring energy to the spine, which in turn brings stable, unwavering inner contentment. Prana plays an equally vital role in Ayurveda and is considered a major aspect of balanced health. According to Ayurveda, all diseases are a result of stagnation, irregularity, or blockage of prana. Without balance of prana, the digestive fire cannot attain the proper continuity or strength. Proper circulation is essential to good health. When prana is returned to an injured area, healing takes place. Pranayama is yoga's most therapeutic tool, as it improves lung function, which in turn improves circulation throughout the body.

Poor cardiovascular function can be correlated to a breakdown in the digestive, endocrine, immune, and other main bodily systems. Atherosclerosis, hardening of the arteries, one of the major health issues today, is a result of poor respiration and blood circulation, which create blood clots and deposits fats and calcium on the walls of the arteries.

The heart becomes weak in individuals who do not exercise, but it still has to perform to give life to the body. The heart can be considered the most overworked organ in the body, as it is never really allowed to rest, unlike other organs. Although modern fitness practices are beneficial in reducing stress and improving heart function, some types tax the body and can deplete the tissues.

Pranayama exercises help lower the resting heart rate, reducing the burden on the heart and allowing it to pump blood through the arteries without stressing the body and its organs. Pranayama can also be considered a method of controlling the heart's functions. As Yogananda points out in his commentary on the Bhagavad Gita (chapter I, verse 10), pranayama practiced with meditation is the most powerful weapon for conquering the ego, because the breath is the cord that connects our individual consciousness to the body. It describes a specialized technique of breathing that leads to a suspended state known as kumbhaka: "Other devotees offer as sacrifice the incoming breath of prana in the outgoing breath of apana, and the out-going breath of apana in the incoming breath of prana, thus arresting the cause of inhalation and exhalation by intent practice of pranayama."[133]

Even though the yoga practitioner may not reach such an advanced breathless state, the process of merging the inhalation (prana) with the exhalation (apana) bountifully benefits the body, as it balances the nervous system, lowers the resting heart rate, and reduces blood pressure. Mentally, this form of pranayama improves sleep and detaches the mind from the ego. It makes individuals less reactive to the upheavals of daily life by promoting a witnessing quality of mind, causing them to be less emotional.

The breath can become a key to the kingdom of health and happiness. It brings us health as we learn to awaken and direct life force to various areas throughout the body. It can bring us everlasting fulfillment by connecting us to our true source, God. There are many different ways to work with the breath through the practice of pranayama to help develop concentration and improve the depth of meditation practice. As prana expands in the body, the quality of our whole being changes. The body becomes lighter, more energetic, transparent, and balanced. This quality is called sattva guna.[134] When, through the regular practice of breath control, we can reverse a certain amount of the energy that usually flows towards sensory function, we begin to allow cosmic intelligence or mahat into our state of being. The amount of energy that we are able to redirect gradually increases with continuity of practice.

Good Life for Good Prana

In order to create a life of balance, one must eventually embrace the attitude that prana is the essence of life and sustains all living things. Being healthy begins with healthy breathing and a relationship with nature. Two components create a "pranifying" lifestyle. Firstly, the breath itself is the link that bridges the mind-body relationship. Proper breathing, exercise, and pranayama are all effective tools for creating this sacred mind-body synergy. The other is to embrace the concept that nature is a Divine living domain of intelligence, which reflects our own existence and that of the five elements. Our lifestyle is not only a major factor in health, but reflects our true capacities as spiritual beings. Five main lifestyle components can increase prana: food, water, air, sunlight, and the breath. These provide all the necessary ingredients for health and vitality.

---

133   Bhagavad Gita, Chapter IV, Verse 29, *Apane juhvati pranam prane panam tathapare pranapanagati ruddhva pranayamaparayanah.* Other Hatha Yoga texts such as the *Hatha Yoga Pradipika, Siva Samhita,* and *Gheranda Samhita* concur with the Bhagavad Gita, referring to this practice as *kevala kumbhaka.* The technique of suspending the breath is a sublime experience not to be compared to simple retention of the breath as inaccurately taught in some commercial yoga schools.

134   Gunas:These are three prime qualities of nature also known as Prakriti. They are sattva (balance), rajas (activity), and tamas (inertia), and are the energies that govern the quality of life.

It all begins with food, as food provides the main nutrition for the body. The most important thing is to eat foods that are fresh. This includes vegetarian, whole, plant-based foods that are not frozen, canned, or over-cooked. Such foods are filled with prana. These should be eaten in smaller quantities over time, instead of being gorged in one sitting. This makes them easy to digest, and all their vital nutrients can be extracted. Pork and beef are filled with toxins and bog the stomach down.

Occasional fasting on warm teas and fresh fruit and vegetable juices is good for the body. Water holds prana and the best water is from natural springs that have not been damaged by industry. Such water, filled with minerals and prana, can be found in many different parts of the world.[135] Filtered water is good as long as it has not been overly filtered to the point where nutrients have been extracted. Ayurveda recommends placing water in a copper cup or container and allowing it to sit exposed to fresh air for several hours or overnight, as this both increases prana and releases the important dietary minerals of the respiratory enzyme complex responsible for hemoglobin production.

Fresh air is harder to find, especially for those living in cities. Man's connection to nature in the form of earth, mountains, rivers, oceans, and so forth, cannot be denied, as these are where good air can be found. However, the sacred techniques of pranayama, practiced by someone who has developed the capability, can take air of virtually any quality and convert it into the subtler prana.

Sunlight is the sole provider of prana for the entire planet. It is healthy to sun-bathe daily for short periods (10 to 30 minutes), depending on an individual's constitution and skin tone. Sunlight provides vitamin D and is responsible for calcium absorption, bone development, muscle function, and much else. Psychologically speaking, sunlight motivates and inspires us to be positive and go outdoors. It expands the mind.

The Bhagavad Gita says, "Other devotees, by a scheme of proper diet, offer all the different kinds of prana and their functions as oblations in the fire of the one common prana. All such devotees are knowers of the true fire ceremony that consumes their karmic sins."[136] Prana exists in different forms. However it is part of the "One" inner instrument or *antahkarana,*[137] the primary force of life. As mentioned in the Gita, diet is a practical part of an integral lifestyle that works with the prana. On the esoteric side, the fire of the breath can

---

135 www.findaspring.com is a free website that helps you find natural springs throughout the world.

136 *Apare niyataharah pranan pranesu juhvati sarve 'pyete yajnavido yajnaksapitakalmasah.* Chapter IV, Verse 30.

137 A term used in Samkhya philosophy and mentioned in the *Samkhya Karika.*

dissolve karmic patterns when the prana and apana currents are neutralized. Therefore, the cultivation of prana should be considered in its physical, mental, and spiritual aspects.

The Vibration of Food

Food (*anna*) plays a major role in the teachings of both yoga and Ayurveda. Our relationship with food must be spiritual, as anything born of the earth has a divine origin. In Ayurveda, food is of vital importance in building the body's tissues or dhatus. It is a means for balancing the doshas, which are influenced by the foods we eat.

Annapurna is the Goddess of food and symbolizes its sacredness and how, when eaten properly, it can bestow countless blessings. Annapurna, a form of Parvati, Shiva's wife, nourishes us and prolongs the gift of life, while Shiva destroys all that is toxic or negative in us, such as ama. For example, the fire of Surya Bedhana pranayama can burn up excess ama created by vata dosha and provide healing of rheumatism, colon cancer, and parasites.

With this in mind, we can see how the elements of earth, wind, and fire play a vital role in sadhana. The element of earth relates to the diet or foods that maintain our body heat or agni, and also support new cell growth. The element of air is the basis of a sound mind-body relationship. When in balance and invoked through the practice of pranayama, the element of air is transformed into the Holy wind or vayu that is the impetus for the fire element connected to the kundalini, which ascends and begins the process of channel purification or *nadi suddhi*.

Pranayama can open the chakras through the nadis only when the body is not bogged down with unsattvic or impure foods. This also involves moderation (*mitahara*). The Hatha Yoga texts state that half the stomach should be filled with healthy foods and a quarter with liquid. The last quarter should remain empty to allow for the movement of gas, leaving some energy and room in the stomach to appease God. The *Gheranda Samhita* says: "He who practices Yoga, without moderation of diet, incurs various diseases, and obtains no success."[138]

All the elements, earth, water, fire, air, and ether, are linked. However, earth, wind, and fire must work harmoniously for evolution to take place through sadhana. Our outer life must have balance in order to attain the inner union or *yoga* of the sun (pingala), moon (ida), and central (sushumna) channels.

---

138   *Gheranda Samhita*, Lesson Five, Verse 16.

The quality of food we eat influences the quality of the mind, and this state of mind governs the prana. While at a social gathering with some of his disciples, Ramakrishna once turned away food served him because the food did not have a pure vibration. Some of the main yogic foods considered pure or sattvic are fruits, vegetables, milk, ghee, cheeses,[139] grain cereals, almonds, mung beans, ginger, and honey. A yogic diet should also not be too rich, salty, or spicy. A balanced vegetarian diet creates energy and promotes lightness and longevity. With continuity of effort (abhyasa) in sadhana, such a diet allows the prana to flow in a spiritual or sattvic direction. In the yoga tradition, as cows are holy and seen as a form of Divine Mother sacred to Lord Krishna, milk is considered part of the vegetable diet, while eggs are part of the animal diet and have a disturbing or rajasic effect on the mind. As the capacity to hold prana increases, the need for food as sustenance decreases.

Prana and Feeling in the Heart

Feeling peace is more important than expecting some reward from our sadhana. Peace of mind is a sure foundation for creating abundance and attaining happiness, and the best indicator of progress on the spiritual path. Too often, both yoga asana students and teachers aim to produce tangible signs in the body as evidence of being spiritual or evolved. If this were the case, circus performers and gymnasts would be very advanced souls.

Prana has many vibrational qualities connected to various moods or feelings we experience, as taught in the Bhakti or devotional branch of yoga. These subtle moods are called *bhavs,* qualities of the spiritual heart. I first became aware of this sublime quality while in Kolkata, India. I was invited by a few devotees to a meditation gathering that takes place every Sunday evening. The idea of a deep meditation sounded great after a full day of the hustle and bustle of the Bengali metropolis. As we were walking down a narrow corridor between old and decrepit buildings, I was clueless as to where I was being taken. As we approached a small doorway, I could hear some faint devotional chants drifting through the scented balmy breeze.

The door opened and I followed as my host guided me into a small temple room. The feeling was so overwhelming, it seemed as if all my thoughts melted into my heart. The devotional chants from this group of about twenty meditators

---

139   Dairy products should be eaten with discretion due to commercialization of the industry and inhumane treatment of cattle. Look for organic farms that provide healthy, grass-fed environments enabling cows to produce pure foods from a happy state of mind. Dairy products or beef eaten from poorly treated cattle are permeated with vibrations of fear and anxiety, and this produces disease and ailments in humans.

continued with greater fervor. All my senses were drawn in towards my heart center. My body relaxed and I sat in a deep state of calmness and overwhelming peace. The inner mood I was experiencing was absolutely Divine, pure, sweet, and all-pervading.

I subsequently understood that my awareness was expanding. A greater understanding allowed me to see my guru as a doorway into my heart. I realized that pure devotion was a type of spiritual vulnerability. It was around the time of this experience that I began to integrate the *Ishta Devata*[140] or preferred image of the Divine into my sadhana.

As prana expands, so does our awareness. Devotion can be one method for developing this. However, the mind must have deep concentration so that the prana does not become dispersed, weakening its ascent into the heart. The seat of prana is the heart, and to expand the feeling of love and devotion requires a calm and receptive mind.

Vata disorders deal with the vrittis or oscillation of thoughts, and can be equated with having "monkey mind." For this reason, mantra can be a very subtle means of managing the mind-heart relationship. While pranayama techniques can influence both the mind and the physiology, mantra works more specifically with the prana of the mind. Either form can be used as a method for experiencing a feeling of peace and surrender in the heart.

Basic Types of Pranayama

Pranayama techniques are a vast and integral part of Hatha and Raja Yoga. Learning their subtleties requires much practice. Many forms exist and vary by lineage and tradition. Other approaches entirely outside the yoga system also exist. Listed below are several pranayama techniques described in Hatha Yoga texts, as well as some I have learned directly from Swami Jyotirmayananda.[141] Breathing techniques depend largely on use of the diaphragm, as its contraction increases volume in the chest and entire respiratory system. This volume of breath exercises a complete range of motion in the lungs and heart, and this ensures a stable breath potentially able to slow down enough to quiet the mind.

---

140 Selection of the Ishta Devata is an important aspect of japa (mantra) yoga, meditation, and prayer. Depending on a person's samskaras (mental impressions in the subconscious mind), one may have a stronger affinity to a particular God or Goddess, or alternately to the image of a Satguru. This can also be decided through analysis of one's astrology chart.

141 Swami Jyotirmayananda is the last living direct disciple of Sri Swami Sivananda of the Divine Life Society. He currently lives in Miami, Florida, and is the spiritual director of his ashram and International Research Foundation. His teachings are the purest form of integral yoga and follow the principles of Vedanta, Samkhya, and the yoga dharmas.

The idea is simply that breath control reflects self-control. In other words, as we manage our breath, removing impairment and improving quality and depth, we increase our capacity to manage the badgering of excess thoughts.

The following is a list of the most commonly used pranayama techniques, along with a basic description of their practice and effect on the doshas. For the most benefit, one should find a well-trained yoga teacher and Ayurveda practitioner and receive detailed instruction.

Alternate-Nostril Breathing (Nadi Shodhana)

This breathing technique is the most important for balancing the subtle sun (pingala) and moon (ida) channels along the spine in the astral body. It is excellent for balance of vata dosha and serves as a wonderful preparation for meditation. It is neither heating nor cooling. Using the right hand, the right thumb closes the right nostril, and inhalation begins through the left nostril. After a complete inhalation through the left nostril, close the left nostril with the ring and small finger held together, and exhale slowly through the right nostril. It is ideal to keep the inhalation and exhalation of equal length for effectively calming the mind. Retention of the breath at the top of the inhalation can be added to expand lung capacity and increase breath control. This is also sometimes called Anulom-Vilom Pranayama or Sukha Purvaka Pranayama.

Solar Breath (Surya Bhedana)

This technique is an alternate form of Nadi Shodhana, where inhalation and exhalation are repeated through the right nostril. This is heating to the body and can be used for management of both vata- and kapha-related issues. It is useful in destroying toxins and parasites, strengthening metabolism, weight loss, and addressing general nervous system disorders. The lunar form (Chandra Bhedana) is alternatively practiced in the same manner through the left nostril. It is cooling to the pitta body and relaxes the pitta mind, reducing anger and stress. It can also be used for reducing hyper-acidity and related conditions, as well as soothing the liver.

Skull-Shiner / Punch Breath (Kapalabhati)

A strong and stimulating breath technique, I have nicknamed this the "punch breath," as emphasis is placed on exhalation and the abdomen snapped inwards. It has a strong effect on the sinuses and is helpful in kapha-related conditions. It can also stimulate the function of the pituitary and pineal glands.

This technique has a shodhana effect on the body, promoting purification, circulation, and warmth. It is one of the six actions (shat karmas) mentioned for yogic detoxification in the *Hatha Yoga Pradipika,* one of the main texts on asana and pranayama.

Bellows Breathing (Bastrika)

Bastrika pranayama is most easily translated into "bellows" breathing or dia-phragmatic breathing, in that it exercises the entire breathing instrument. This breathing technique can be considered the most primary and vital, because it enhances the natural function of the respiratory system and promotes the grounding and balancing of vata and all the pranas. It is therefore an excel-lent place to begin the yoga journey. One must first learn the breath's natural synchronicity before increasing this technique's forceful quality, gradually in-haling and exhaling more deeply. As a youth, Yogananda mentions observing Nagendranath, "the levitating saint," perform this technique before entering samadhi and levitating several feet above his bed. Bastrika, as described in the *Pradipika,* has several forms that also involve the use of each nostril, along with retention. There is a more in-depth discussion of Bastrika below.

Chest-Purification Breathing (Urasthal Shuddhi Pranayama)

Breathing techniques in general promote circulation, reduce stagnation, and release phlegm or kapha from the upper chest, lungs, and throat. This meth-od is simple and begins by closing the right nostril with the right thumb and exhaling out strongly through the left nostril. Then inhale again through both nostrils. Close the left nostril with the pinkie and ring finger of the right hand held together and exhale with force out the right side. This is one cycle. On a more subtle level, this pranayama clears and opens the three main nadis required for increasing consciousness, the pingala (sun), ida (moon), and sushumna. These are the main channels from which pranic energy flows into the chakras.

Victory Breath (Ujjai)

Ujjai means victorious breath. It increases udana vayu and promotes breath management and control. This breathing technique has become popular in the modern vinyasa approach that came out of the Mysore yoga tradition, which links movement and asana with breath. Technically, it involves restricting the space in the throat by engaging the glottis to reduce oxygen flow, thereby creating the "ocean" sound it is known for. This pranayama technique is not recommended for extended periods of time, particularly for pitta types who become overheated very easily. However, such breathing is very good for vata types, as they benefit from warmth and from slow and deep breaths.

Cooling Breath (Sitali)

This very subtle pranayama technique is known for its cooling quality, and is best integrated at the end of an asana practice. It is basically done by curling or rolling the edges of the tongue into semi-tube-like shape. The breath is inhaled through the mouth, while feeling the cooling sensations across the top of the tongue. The exhale is done by closing the mouth and allowing it to release softly through the nose. This can be done for a few minutes while in Savasana to promote a deep and relaxing experience and to induce the restorative or rasayana affects brought on by the release of soma, the sublime energies of the moon. Since yoga asana is predominantly a solar channel or pingala nadi-based system, pranayama such as Sitali (pronounced "sheetali") serves to bring the sun-moon synergy into accord. This reminds us that the main theme of Hatha Yoga teachings is to balance the sun-moon energies in both the physiology and the mind.

Hissing Breath (Sitkari)

Sitkari is similar to Sitali in that it is cooling. However, it is practiced by clenching or biting down the teeth, somewhat as when smiling, while placing the tip of the tongue on the palate or roof of the mouth, and then inhaling like you are breathing through the teeth. This creates a soft, hissing sound. The exhalation is released gently through the nose without any force. Both Sitkari and Sitali are meditative, cooling, and promote restoration.

Long and Short Breathing (Deergha Shwas Prashwas Pranayama)

This simple practice involves a slow, stretched-out inhalation, followed by a slow exhalation, both equal in duration. The emphasis should be on continuity and steadiness of breath. Yogananda includes retention for the same length of time as the inhalation and exhalation. This form of breathing is an excellent introduction to pranayama and helps calm the mind. It represents the essential theme of yoga and Ayurveda, which prompt us to slow down, live in the moment, and enjoy the peace that comes from deep inner stillness. In the short form (Laghu Shwas Prashwas Pranayama), after inhalation, the breath is exhaled in 10-12 pulsations, until the lungs are empty. Then the same is done on inhalation. This variation promotes good circulation, strengthens the blood by raising the hemoglobin, and increases the energy level.

Humming-Bee Breath (Brahmari)

Yogis consider this pranayama to be a mind-cleanser, as its settles restless thoughts in the mind and is a good preparation for meditation. After a strong and quick inhalation, the auricle, which is the cartilage or visible, projecting portion of the external ear in front of the ear canal, is pushed with the thumb or index finger, and then the soft palate is lifted towards the pharynx. This produces a buzzing bee sound or vibration of the palate felt and heard in the medulla oblongata in the back of the head and the top of the cervical spine. I often integrate this in meditation to deepen the mind's focus on the ajna chakra or spiritual eye.

Dazed or Fainting Breath (Murchha Pranayama)

This pranayama, taught in the *Hatha Yoga Pradipika*, includes a chin lock or bandha known as Jalandhara. It is not mentioned in the *Gheranda Samhita*. At the top of the inhalation, the breath is held while performing the chin lock and gazing upwards at the third eye (Shambhavi Mudra). The intention is to create a state of "fainting" or feeling of expanding beyond the body. The other technique is to lift the head at the end of the inhalation, as if gazing up at the full moon and the third eye. This can be done repeatedly. The number of rounds can be increased gradually and integrated into a regular meditation practice. Pranayama that includes mechanical breath retention (kumbhaka), especially when repeated, should be avoided by new yoga practitioners. Such techniques involve raising awareness by improving attention or dharana and penetrating the prana into the higher energy centers or chakras.

Floating Breath (Plavini Pranayama)

This technique requires inhaling through the nose until the lungs are full, or gulping air into the stomach. Then you must swallow the air, a technique that enables the body to float on water. This can be practiced repeatedly and is done as a precursor to meditation. As it fills the stomach with air, it reduces hunger and is helpful in hyper-acidic conditions associated with pitta dosha.

Belly Undulations (Nauli)

Nauli is one of the best exercises for massaging the abdominal region and entire gastrointestinal tract. After taking a strong and quick inhale through the nose, exhale completely through a wide-open mouth until the lungs are empty. Abstain from breathing and begin drawing the abdominal muscles inward and upwards. Then push them outwards, repeating this motion 5-10 times, or until you need to breathe again. This should be done on an empty stomach and is best practiced early in the morning, before morning sadhana. After some time, the range of motion is increased and the abdominal muscles can be pulled up and inwards from the left to right side and from the right to left side, with something of a water-ripple effect.

Kevala Kumbhaka

This pranayama is the golden key of Raja Yoga techniques and opens the do-main of moksha (liberation) dharma. The Kevala pranayama technique can be equated to the Kriya Yoga technique revived by Mahavatar Babaji in the modern ages,[142] although it is described in many of yogic texts[143] with vague reference to its broader themes. The term "kumbhaka" has been often incorrectly defined as the holding of the breath. This has certain limited physical benefits. However, these are different from the end results of the true Kevala or Kriya Yoga technique. This technique extracts the prana or life force from the breath. As the inhales (puraka) and exhales (rechaka) are slowed, they are dissolved into pranic currents, eliminating any requirement for natural breathing. Such a technique is not about controlling the breath. It is a means of controlling prana with the mind. Practice of this type of pranayama requires a lifestyle in accordance with the moral and ethical codes of yoga, or yamas and niyamas, the tri-doshic health of the physical body, and the power of attention or dharana.

Bastrika Pranayama and the Doshas

Bastrika is the ideal pranayama to begin with, as it provides a dynamic use of the diaphragm and the entire respiratory complex. What I often see with new practitioners, or those who follow a fixed style of yoga that repeatedly imple-ments only Ujjai pranayama, is that in most cases there a lack of coordination between the belly and breath, in that the diaphragm is not operating naturally. This is due to the conditioning of the throat muscles, which become so fixed that adaptation to other forms of breathing becomes difficult. In any breathing exercise, the diaphragm should expand on inhalation, filling and expanding into something of a teardrop shape. On exhalation, the entire abdomen should contract inwards. The range of this action will vary according to the technique being practiced, but this is the basic motion.

Bastrika is the ideal pranayama for learning the tempos appropriate for each dosha, because it is an enhanced or forced form of the natural movement of

---

142   See Paramahamsa Yogananda, *God Talks With Aryna: The Bhagavd Gita*, commentary on Chapter IV, verse 20 (Self-Realization Fellowship, Los Angeles, Calif.)

143   *Siva Samhita, Gheranda Samhita, Hatha Yoga Pradipika* and the *Ashtanga Yoga Sutras*.

breathing. Initially, as one's yoga practice is beginning, one should start with lower repetitions. Count off, say, six to 12 breaths, followed by a rest. Gradually increase the repetitions to as high as 50 if you have practiced for many years.

Lower counts are beneficial for anyone wanting to improve respiration, circulation, mental alertness, and concentration, or to increase overall energy levels. In general, one should practice Bastrika at a slow pace to ensure proper technique and effectiveness.

Vata types generally have a low or shallow respiration, and often have a tendency to breathe quickly. When introduced to this practice for the first time, they commonly feel uneasy, nervous, and even lightheaded. In time, such resistance will disappear. For this reason, it is essential for vatas to breathe slowly and do short sets. This will obviously vary depending on many factors such as experience, constitution, and so forth.

The pitta tempo can be increased by approximately half a step. In this "medium" tempo, the breath is not too fast or too slow, but hovers between the two speeds. Pittas should also be careful to avoid tensing the body, face, and brows, and be careful with clenching the teeth while practicing this or any breathing exercise. Pittas are known to create interesting facial expressions during both pranayama and asana practice. All breathing techniques should be performed with a sense of surrender and relaxation.

Kaphas benefit from the forceful quality of Bastrika and a quick and more aggressive approach. The tempo for kaphas is a whole step faster than the vata timing. Practice should be done in shorter, repeated sets, or in one longer series if the yogi is experienced. One cycle of inhalation and exhalation is considered a count of one. In more advanced practices, I recommend a cycle of 50 - 60 breaths before taking a rest.

For more subtle purification, the doshas can also be addressed more specifically according to the predominant nadi or channel. The **fire** element (pitta dosha) can be balanced by breathing through the moon channel or ida nadi (left nostril) and closing the right nostril with the right thumb. The **water** element (kapha dosha) can be balanced by breathing through the sun channel or pingala nadi (right nostril) and closing the left nostril with the ring finger of the right hand. The **air** element will find balance by breathing alternately through both nostrils, as in the Nadi Shodhana technique.

Pranayama infused into a yoga practice promotes a deeper connection between the mind and body. Asana alone will only cultivate a certain level of body-mind relationship, but when Bastrika is infused, the yogi is brought into a deeper level of concentration, which develops awareness further than expected. Asana and pranayama together help build this deeper connection, which can help awaken the higher mind in a manner necessary to reach yoga's highest intention. The breath is a practical instrument to unify the body's and mind's fields of energy. When we can begin to merge the body and mind through the breath, our attention begins to dwell more in the present moment. This is one of the many rewards of the traditional yoga system. A fragmented approach aimlessly seeks to fulfill this intention through varying external means, but leads nowhere. Asana and pranayama must be united if we are to reach the deeper levels of our spirit nature.

Tempo of the Breath

What Ayurvedic wisdom brings to yoga is a consideration of the therapeutic value of a number of factors, such as the tempo or speed of the breath cycle. In general, yoga aims at establishing a slow breath, which can equate to a calm mind. There are two main points to consider relative to yogic breathing. As we have examined, yogis have devised a multitude of breathing techniques to purify the body on a physical level, and enhance and expand the prana flowing through us. This circulatory function affects our capacity to manage the doshas, improving our quality of health.

While some yoga practitioners may feel great benefit from one form of breathing, such as the punch breath (Kapalabhati), others may feel better doing another. A variety of pranayama exists so one may be able to find a technique that is helpful to their doshic type and level of spiritual aspiration.

With kapha being predominant in the morning, (6 to 10am), generally speaking it is more effective to practice breathing techniques that stimulate, heat, and promote circulation at this time. The midday period (11am to 2pm) is pitta-predominant and produces heat in the body, stronger digestive capacity, and increased will power. All of these can be managed with alternate-nostril breathing (Nadi Shodhana). In cases of pitta imbalances, cooling pranayama like Sitali and Shitakari should be used.

Vata dosha becomes predominant the remainder of the day (2 to 6pm), and requires slow, deep, and steady breathing. Alternate-nostril breathing can again be used in this regard. However, Bastrika is very effective, given its profound effect in promoting the diaphragmatic function necessary in working with vata dosha. The mind controls the breath. However, the breath can be used scientifically to manage the mind. While the intention of pranayama from a yoga perspective is to control the flow of prana, pranayama can be used from an Ayurvedic perspective to maintain balance of the doshas.

In Ayurveda, the rate at which something is performed is of vital importance, as each element reflects a particular vibrational frequency. When the intention is to balance a dosha, the opposite quality must be considered. Understanding the natural qualities of the five elements (pancha mahabhutas) is critical in using pranayama to manage the doshas.

As I pointed out earlier, asanas, as external postures, provide a type of symbolism and a framework that gives the prana a vehicle through which consciousness can transcend the senses. At the same time, the influence of the postures has a therapeutic effect on the organs.

On the other hand, pranayama, as a virtually formless practice, has the capacity of awakening prana and working with the directional forces in their five forms (prana, apana, samana, udana, and vyana). Earth-water, as kapha dosha, has a slow quality. Therefore, to balance it we must perform therapies such as breathing techniques with a quick or fast tempo. This can be difficult for a new practitioner who has not yet had enough experience to learn proper use of the technique and so must initially perform it slowly. The tempo can then be gradually increased without compromising technique.

The fire element or pitta dosha, having a sharp quality, needs to practice pranayama in a moderate and gentle manner. The air-ether element or vata dosha has an erratic or moveable quality, and so this requires slow and deep breathing. Regardless of the pranayama, it is not the length but depth of practice that makes the difference. The benefit of breathing deeply and completely extends to all types, as this helps lower the resting heart rate, which is essential to well-being and mind-body synergy. There is a strong view by many Ayurvedic practitioners, including myself, that psychological factors must be considered with respect to the intention behind or "how" yoga is practiced, if any real capacity for balancing the doshas is to be attained. The attitude must change in order to achieve success on any level, physical, emotional, or spiritual.

Pranayama Timing in Practice

Breathing exercises can be used at different times throughout a yoga practice. In this way, the techniques can be used to stimulate the doshas optimally and deepen the experience of a practice. Pranayama can also be adapted to different times of day to address the predominant energy of that period. There are many considerations in the practice of pranayama that can make your practice more specific and beneficial in the long run

At the yoga movement's current stage of development, the practice of breathing exercises can be a tedious experience requiring development of a certain level of concentration and understanding. Therefore, do not expect yourself to implement all aspects of these breathing exercises comfortably all at once. Begin by making subtle changes that feel right, given your physical capacity and current level of understanding. What we enjoyed and understood five years ago is substantially different from where we might be today. Below are six phases in which pranayama can be practiced according to your dosha type. One can also practice the full cycle to purify and balance each of the elements in the course of an entire day.

Warm Up Phase in Early-Morning Practice (Purva Prana)

This phase is characterized by preparation for early yoga practice through increasing the flow of the prana and the apana, prana's two main directions. In Kapalbhati, the forceful action on the abdomen pushes excess mucous out from the nasal cavity, creating a clearer pathway for the breath to flow in and out through the nose. Kapalbhati has a heating affect, which reduces kapha from blocking oxygen flow through the nose to the brain by increasing the flow of prana. This heating quality counters the coolness of the morning, and also stimulates downward flow or apana. In Surya Bheda, the heat in the body is gradually increased in a gentler manner than Kapalbhati. It can be practiced for longer intervals without exhaustion. Kapalbhati can have an exhausting affect if practiced for long periods.

Warm-Up Phase (Purva Prana)

With a predominance of vata dosha in the evening, circulation is much more active. The best pranayama to practice during this time is Nadi Shodhana or alternate-nostril breathing. This is an excellent way to begin a practice, as it can settle the mind and increase the power of attention. I teach a standing variation of alternate-nostril breathing that involves alternating use of the arms. When inhalation is being drawn in from the left side, the extended left arm simultaneously rises upwards in a half circle. The traditional mudra, making a circle with the thumb and forefinger touching, using the right hand, is useful when preparing to go into meditation.

Pre-Heating Phase (Purva Agni)

A proper yoga asana practice should follow a pyramidal structure. The intensity and level of the postures increase gradually, as the body and mind are purified and prepared. During the gradual ascent of a yoga practice, the heart rate should be raised slowly and incrementally to obtain the greatest cardiovascular benefit. This is done through a good warm-up period. During this heating or middle phase of practice, Ujjai pranayama can be integrated into a vinyasa sequence that combines various asanas linked with the breath. Ujjai is the only pranayama that can be practiced at the same time as asana, and was popularized by the Mysore yoga tradition of Krishnamacharya. Ujjai is heating, but its practice can create a balanced state of mind and a well-conditioned heart. It is unrealistic to expend energy trying to practice this pranayama when the heart rate is significantly raised, especially during a challenging sequence that combines balancing postures and movements. Ujjai is most effective during the phase of ascension to the peak of a practice.

Heating Phase (Agni)

This is the pinnacle phase of a yoga practice, when the heart rate is increased, the body is perspiring, and the practitioner has attained a greater level of muscular flexibility. At this point in the practice, Kapalbhati can be added into repeated sets, followed by a few moments of relaxation or pratyahara. Bastrika is also an excellent technique to integrate at this point, as the synchronization of the breath and thrusting abdomen mimics the already active function of the lungs. A tremendous feeling of vitality, heightened awareness, and intuition is developed with this practice. Bastrika stirs the kundalini at the base of the spine for all dosha types. Both Kapalbhati and Bastrika have a strong cleansing action on the lungs, strengthen the heart, and clear the mind, especially when used in this phase of a yoga practice. Integrating sets of pranayama into a yoga practice also helps vata types sweat, which can be difficult for them.

Pre-Cooling Phase (Pre-Chandra)

This phase of the practice is where cooling the body down begins. This is not limited to the physical cooling of the body, but reflects the intention of directing the energy of sun, which has been awakened and ignited in the practice, to transmute to the higher centers or chakras, where the lunar energies abide. These are also known as the soma or moon centers. This is likened to the waxing of the moon. Meditation is effective only if the practitioner can bring the prana into these higher centers of awareness.

Moon Phase (Chandra)

This phase extends beyond the asana portion of the practice. The final pose of the cooling phase is Savasana, which prepares the practitioner for meditation, also a very lunar experience. The light of the solar energies that were awakened in the lower spinal centers are now illuminating the higher centers of compassion, peace, and intuition. These higher centers reflect the qualities of the full moon. Any of the cooling pranayamas, like Sitali or Brahmari, can be used during this period. Truly, here is the greatest strength of an asana and pranayama practice, which brings purity to the physical body and clarity to the mind now awakened to experience the inner bliss of the heart.

The Three Power Regions of the Body

Both the yoga and Ayurveda traditions recognize three main regions in the body, which have a substantial physical and mental influence. These can be correlated to the spine for identification purposes. However, they are also associated with the doshas and impact the physiology.

Ayurveda, as the science of health and harmony of the physical body, recognizes the lower spine or area below the navel as being influenced by vata dosha. Particularly when vata is excessive and out of balance, it accumulates in these lower anatomical areas. The area between the navel and the bottom of the chest is influenced by pitta dosha, as this area is the center of metabolism and the womb of creation. From the chest upwards to the throat, kapha dosha is predominant, affecting respiration and often creating congestion.

Ayurveda protocols aim at addressing these regions with a multitude of therapies, which emphasize reduction of each dosha. Interestingly enough, the Hatha Yoga teachings similarly provide a three-tier approach for working with prana to promote spiritual transformation. In these three areas, the breath can be locked in a bandha, either on the exhalation or inhalation, with the intention of expanding the prana and consciousness.

Bandha is a mechanical process of working with the breath and oxygen to establish mastery over the subtler life force. At the space between the anus and the genitals (perineum) is the Mula (root) Bandha, which is contracted or engaged after inhalation or exhalation. At the navel, and pertaining to the entire abdominal region, is the Uddiyana Bandha, which is contracted inwards and slightly upwards after a complete exhalation. The region of throat is another vital area, known as Jala Bandha, through which the subtle body can receive prana.

Yoga also classifies these three areas as knots or *granthi*, which refers to blocks of energy in the sushumna nadi or sacred channel of the light body. These inhibit the flow of kundalini to the higher centers. More subtle yogic practices combining mantra and pranayama with concentration or dharana loosen these blocks. However, this requires a substantial amount of physical, tri-doshic balance attained by adherence to proper lifestyle and the moral and ethical codes of conduct as outlined in Patanjali's yamas and niyamas.

Overview of Pranayama

In the highest sense, the intention of pranayama is to balance the sun and moon forces (the pingala and ida channels) and awaken the kundalini so it can ascend to enhance our consciousness. In this process, identification with the physical body, senses, and disturbing thoughts of the mind is reduced. The breath itself can be redefined and correlated with the mind's capacity to feel inspired through inhalation and enjoy the power of surrender through exhalation. When we intuit a new idea, we access a domain of consciousness that gives rise to the radiant power of the sun that is our soul. When we observe the continuous evolution of life through surrender, trust, and love, we embrace growth and promote transformation of ego-consciousness to Divine awareness in a manner that keeps us alive and inspired by the mystery of life.

In summary, the breath and its versatile variations are universal and intrinsically linked to prana. We could say that yoga provides us with the techniques of working with the energy of the breath to enhance prana, and Ayurveda teaches us how create balance and healing through the energy of food, water, and lifestyle. Yoga pranayama can be practiced by anyone, anywhere, whether the intention is therapeutic or spiritual. Breathing exercises can be adapted into all forms of health and wellness. They can also be practiced traditionally, as part of a holistic system.

In general, any breathing practice, even outside of a yogic context, can facilitate mindfulness and the power of attention, reduce stress, and be a great complement to many aspects of life. The breath is the cord of life, and when we take a moment to truly breathe, it can foster a greater sense of peace, increase patience and understanding, and perhaps even create more gratitude for the life that we have to live and share with others. There is something very soft, yet very profound in breathing. In every inhalation, there is the possibility of birth, a new perspective, idea, or lesson. In every exhalation there is death, a transition beyond, a surrender, and an embrace of the sacred sun, moon, and earth relationship, which is our own.

Chapter NINE

Vedic Lifestyle

I believe in God, only I spell it Nature.
Frank Lloyd Wright (1867 - 1959)

Nature

Lifestyle is yoga and Veda or Yogaveda, the union of the two systems. There is a growing trend of people claiming to be "spiritual rather than religious." In fact, the mere term "religious" is now shrouded with an array of disparaging connotations.

The quality of our health is equal to the quality of our lifestyle. There is no doubt that maintaining a harmonious relationship with nature can have an extremely positive impact on our health. Living a balanced life is the foundation of the Vedic teachings as expressed in the four dharmas of astrology: kama, artha, dharma, and moksha. Ayurveda provides us with the wisdom to maintain an intimate relationship with the cycles of nature kept in motion by the sun, moon, and earth.

What yoga and Ayurveda teach us is simply that spirituality is not something separate from our lifestyle, like occasionally going to church or temple service or meditating. Being spiritual is defined by the relationship we maintain between our mind and body, the relationship we share with the people, places, and things in our environment, and the relationship we have with the Divine: truth, God, Brahman, or the vast intelligence that infuses the entire living world. All three of these principles play a vital role in developing the capacity to live in spirit. Sri Daya Mata conveyed this beautifully in saying. "God has a physical form -- this world. Let us decorate this form, His nature, with all that is beautiful, all that is good, all that is wholesome."[144]

These three aspects of life are cultivated in various manners to establish a lifestyle in accord with truth. Have we ever taken the time to consider what religion is? What it means to be religious? I think the word has been misconstrued and associated with specific practices and inventions based on the particular ideas and experiences of certain individuals. These are then followed indiscriminately by most of humanity, without regard for natural law.

Alternatively, the ideals of Vedic teachings are provided to humanity by the coexistence of mankind and nature. Man digresses from these if he becomes stupefied, lost, and confined to the narrow walls of geography, time and space, and thought and sense. To abide in truth is the origin of dharma or natural law, which is that of spirit and nature.

To experience these principles is one thing that relates to individual insight. To learn them is another, and related to *moksha dharma* or the notion that life's purpose is to find freedom from the world. This ideal is based in the true meaning of education. To be educated is to know how to live in truth. Rabindranath Tagore said, "The highest education is that which does not merely give us information but makes our life in harmony with all existence."

The wisdom of Ayurveda and yoga provide us with a very powerful framework to follow in attaining these virtues. The best way to know a person is to observe how they live, see how they care for their body and home, and the attitude they carry through life. A balanced life is founded on the routines we establish. The word "routine" is derived from the word "route." Thus the natural routines or roots of the day, month, seasons, and years are the pathways of a balanced life that connect us to the source of wisdom. Our lifestyles are the roots of the tree, our body is the trunk, and the branches and leaves are the many experiences that enrich our lives.

In general, routines help us direct our flow of energy outwards, while meditation, writing, and reading direct our prana inwards. Other sadhanas like asana, seva and cooking can be both external and internal, allowing us to perform an action outwardly while at the same time practicing concentration and witnessing our actions, breath, and thoughts. Many mis-define the idea of a routine as something fixed and rigid, but it is actually the opposite. Being

---

144   Sri Daya Mata, "Free Yourself From Tension," Self-Realization Magazine, Fall 1982 (Self-Realization Fellowship, Los Angeles, Calif.)

in a routine is about learning to adapt. Routines are constantly changing in that our attitudes towards them must adapt to the outer circumstances of our lives. Thus, a routine serves as a tool to uplift and transform our consciousness beyond the instability of the material world. There are many types of routines, cycles, seasons, and periods in our life, and we must constantly be prepared to adapt ourselves to the shifts of life to sharpen our power of attention.

When the mind is required to go from one activity, like self-care therapy, to another, like yoga, and then to go to a job, it is trained in how to develop and exercise strength of will. Without any will power, the capacity to concentrate ceases to exist. Most of life's problems are created due to lack of attention, distracting the mind and causing turbulence. Routines help us charge the dynamo of will power to learn how to function in a manner that promotes physical health and mental wellness.

Cheri Huber, a Zen teacher, friend, and guest lecturer at Dancing Shiva, once shared something that explains this point precisely: "The quality of our lives is determined by the power of our attention." This is why the saints and sages of many traditions have touted meditation for millennia, because of its effect on the quality of life. If the physical body is in a room, it does not necessarily mean the entire person is present. If you are performing a specific task, it does not mean you are fully present. Attention is much more than just focusing. It has a profound meaning related to having a spiritual relationship with God while in the temporary existence of a physical, sensory life.

Preventative Medicine

What Ayurveda values most highly is *svastha vritta*, the state of balanced health. It is very likely that this is Ayuvedic wisdom's greatest contribution to mankind. According to Ayurveda, health is defined as a state where the doshas (air-fire-water), dhatus (seven tissues), *malas* (excretions), and agni (digestive fire) are in *sama,* a balanced, functional relationship to one another. Svastha vritta also implies that one must follow codes of conduct for maintaining health. In order for a lifestyle to be healthy, it must contain some level of discipline,[145] so that the body and mind can release all that it has absorbed. Health is not something that is granted to us, but comes from establishing routines that we must work consistently to maintain.

---

145   Tapas or self-discipline is a key principle in the yoga tradition and mentioned in Patanjali's Yoga
       Sutras as one of three requisites of Kriya Yoga, in addition to svadhya or self-study and ishwara
       pranidhana, selfless surrender to God.

In my view, today's global health problems can largely be attributed to a lack of discipline and education. The body's main form of nutrition comes from food or *ahara*, but ahara also includes all the sense impressions we absorb. As the saying goes, "What goes up must come down." What comes into the body and mind must go out. The soul does not stay encased in the body forever, and neither do all the karmic impressions that we take in.

The Ayurvedic approach to lifestyle is based on *chikitsa* or therapies that enable the body and mind to release (*vihara*) all that they have taken in. Another name for Ayurveda is *kaya chikitsa* or healing of the body. There are two forms of this. One form is based on therapies that purify and cleanse the entire body and are categorized as shodhana. The other form is used when a person is not well suited to endure cleansing therapies that require a lot of energy and could therefore further complicate symptoms. Shamana or alleviating therapies are recommended for those suffering from chronic fatigue syndrome, acute bleeding, fevers, heavy-metal toxicity, and a weak immune system caused by excess prescription medications or drug addiction.

Shamana chikitsa has a more soothing and sedative quality meant to neutralize excess ama or undigested food waste, and increase digestive strength. Yoga exercise, time in nature to sunbathe and take in fresh oxygen, and juice cleansing are also often recommended. Herbal medicines and many specialized food preparations can also be considered a type of shamana therapy.

The most effective and recognized system of shodhana therapies is pancha karma (five cleansing actions)[146] and these are best combined with abhyanga (oil massage) svedhana (steam therapy), and shirodhara (warm oil streamed over the forehead). Pancha karma is best administered by a trained practitioner and includes a specialized diet called *kichadi*, herbal medicines, and lifestyle counseling.

A properly balanced lifestyle is the best system for preventing disease. The main issue is that most people do little to prevent diseases. When they lose their health, they do not have much education on how to treat themselves. In a majority of my consultations I find this to be the case. This is why I always ask my clients about their health history and routines. Do they exercise regularly? Do they keep to specific meal times? What is their diet like? Do they practice yoga asana or meditation, and, if so, what is the approach?

---

146 *Nasya* (nasal therapy), *vamana* (emesis therapy, which induces vomiting), *virechana* (purgation therapy), *basti* (enema), and *rakta moksha* (bloodletting).

If none of these factors are in place in clients' lives, the integration of Ayurveda is jeopardized and much discipline will be required. In such cases, I often focus on educating clients on daily and seasonal routines. If knowledge is at least available, the possibility of integrating lifestyle change and new habits increases. The success of any health practitioner is not in healing clients but in giving them the capability of healing themselves.

Can we teach people to live a healthy lifestyle that prevents diseases, giving them independence and not developing codependency on other people or institutions for healing? God's gift of health and wellness is the wisdom of Ayurveda, but we need to teach people how to implement it in their lives. This may take a little more time now, because there are so many misconceptions of what health and happiness are supposed to look like.

Dosha Day Cycles

The key to establishing health is knowing how the energies of the elements shift within a twenty-four hour period. The elements also shift in different periods throughout the life span. Samkhya philosophy teaches us how the five elements, as vibrations of consciousness, affect the physical body and mind. Life and health are all about energy and nothing more. We can actually feel how the elements affect us through our senses.

The 24-hour day is a miniature version of the 24,000-year yuga cycle. Chronology and the order of events occur within the cycle of time determined by the movement of the earth and its binary, the moon. Therefore, our sadhana is always in relationship with where we are standing on the planet earth. The earth's close relationship with the moon mimics the grander cycle of the sun and its partner star. Ayurveda encourages us to align ourselves with the planets, stars, and their motions. The idea behind aligning with the cycles of time is that what you do each day has the capacity to influence your entire life span.

Adjusting a yoga practice and sadhana according to time of day, season, and one's age is one of the unique aspects of how Ayurvedic wisdom can be integrated with yoga. Practicing yoga in alignment with the wisdom of nature empowers us and brings about deeper experience and eventually greater awareness. As people develop more awareness of the workings of yoga and Ayurveda, the yoga practices of modern times, which are so often mindless and robotic, can potentially become more aligned with common-sense wisdom and yield greater results.

The morning period from 6am to 10am is water (kapha) predominant. The mid-day period between 10am and 2pm is fire (pitta) predominant. The late afternoon period from 2pm to 6pm is vata predominant. These same time zones continue and repeat themselves at night from 6pm – 10pm (kapha), 10pm – 2am (pitta), and 2am – 6am (vata). These times are so sensitively aligned that, in clinical Ayurveda, procedures are applied during specific times to influence the doshas specifically. This tells us what is best to do during certain times to balance our health, and also what things to avoid so as not to aggravate our health.

For example, if you want to develop greater strength of discipline, overcome depression, lose weight, and improve circulation and digestive power, then make an effort during the morning kapha period. If you want to balance pitta, avoid over-activity, intense exercise, skipping lunch, and traffic jams during the mid-day period. If you are interested in improving concentration, calming the mind, reducing anxiety, and improving digestive regularity, then from 2pm to 6pm it is helpful to go for a walk, take a moment to breathe, chant mantras or meditate, eat dinner, and read a book. The evening is a time to rest and sleep, allowing the body a chance to restore. The kapha period between 6pm and 10pm prepares us for slowing down. It is ideal if we can go to sleep during this period. We can notice that our physical behavior and mental attitudes are usually very much characteristic of the current time period.

Dosha Life Cycles

As with the periods of the day, the doshas also find their place in the span of an entire lifetime. The kapha period is dominant from birth to sixteen years of age, reflecting the natural development of the tissues and the body as a whole. From sixteen to fifty years of age, the element of fire is predominant, reflecting the mind's pursuit of a goal. These years represent a proactive period of searching and yearning to fulfill desires. Work is important, the body is strong, and the mind is inspired. After age fifty, the air element becomes predominant and begins to wither the body away. The body becomes gradually dryer and more sensitive, and starts to shrink in size.

These time periods for the most part are measured against the function of the agni or digestive strength. The life cycle is simply an elongated day with the slowest metabolism in the morning period and the strongest metabolic strength during the middle of the day or life. As we move towards the end of the day or life, the metabolic strength begins gradually to reduce. Even though the mantra of Vedanta[147] states that we are not the body or the mind, it is interesting to see that the relationship between the mind and body does shift as the soul remains in the body for a greater length of time.

The Wisdom of Culture

On my first sojourn in India many years ago, I learned that yoga and Ayurveda have been maintained as an unbroken tradition for thousands of years, mainly through the practice of devotion. Before its recent renaissance, Ayurveda had become integrated into the culture through many spiritual festivals, rituals associated with birth, marriage, and death, and other periods of the year that match specific astrological positions. The entire country is so imbued with devotion for God in many forms that it has cultivated a natural appreciation for life and family, a love for nature, and camaraderie with mankind. These bonds are the essence of how, over thousands of years, yoga and Ayurveda have saturated the whole society, not just limited to the Vedic-Hindu people. How can natural law be segregated from any soul? The thin veil of ignorance cannot withstand the penetrating force of wisdom. These practices speak to the wise with Mother Nature's eternal song, and they guide those in pain with the consoling quality of conformity with natural law.

On a quiet and chilly December afternoon, I was enjoying a quiet walk along a dirt road in the small mountain village of Dwarahat in northern India. I passed a school with well-dressed kids playing outside during recess. I then walked past a humble family home with no glass windows, only wood shutters to keep out the cold. As I walked further, I enjoyed a clearing with open vistas of great mountain peaks. As I took a deep breath, I was consumed by the stupendous mountains, the Himalayas, immersing my entire being.

After a moment, I continued on and walked up to a group of schoolboys and young men, some in their teens and early twenties. After they asked me many questions, I got a chance to bring up some of the spiritual topics that drew me to India. I was very impressed by their deep knowledge of such eternal truths as karma, rebirth, gods, and gurus. As the conversation continued I became more and more intrigued about where their understanding of such sacred principles had come from. I was fascinated by hearing them speak eloquently of

---

147 "Mind, nor intellect, nor ego, feeling; Sky nor earth nor metals am I. I am He, I am He, Blessed Spirit, I am He! No birth, no death, no caste have I; Father, mother, have I none. I am He, I am He, Blessed Spirit, I am He! Beyond the flights of fancy, formless am I, Permeating the limbs of all life; Bondage I do not fear; I am free, ever free, I am He, I am He, Blessed Spirit, I am He!" Sanskrit chant of Adi Shankara, English translation by Paramahansa Yogananda in *Autobiography of a Yogi* (Self-Realization Fellowship, Los Angeles, Calif.)

epic scriptures such as the Bhagavad Gita and the Ramayana, which explained the core universal truths of the world's spiritual traditions. At the moment, I felt ignorant and not sure how they could possibly be so wise, as I was only a few years older than some of them. Finally, I asked, "How do you do it? How do you know all of this?" With a smile on their faces they responded, "It's our life. We don't know any other way. This is the way that we live." It was at that precise moment that I realized the importance of lifestyle and its relationship to being a spiritual person.

Daily Routine

Health begins with how we live each day, with how we start and end each day being the most important. The daily routine is the primary basis for balanced living and will ultimately determine the quality of one's life. It is in this twenty-four hour period that a person can develop habits and, potentially, the strength and discipline necessary for overcoming the challenges and health issues that life can often unexpectedly bring.

The Sanskrit term *dinacharya* (daily routine) combines two words: *dina* means day and *charya* means a practice or observance. The choices that a person makes on a daily basis will have a substantial influence on who they become. Yogananda's guru, Swami Sri Yukteswar, once said, "Everything in future will improve if you are making a spiritual effort now."[148] The daily routine is the single most important teaching of Ayurveda, both in health and spirituality. It is the only true way to reclaim the health and happiness lost in our culture from the influence of a scanty collective consciousness that fabricates poor habits, mental conditions like nervousness, depression, and laziness, and a fragmented mind-body relationship. We cannot force spirituality upon anyone, but we can teach people to embrace a way of living that aligns them with a more natural state of being that will eventually increase their quality of health and awareness.

When Yogananda came to the West, he emphasized the importance of teaching people "How to Live" as a way towards finding real contentment or santosha. Nothing but a living relationship with God can ever bring us lasting fulfillment and happiness. Trying to control or force a system of health upon people will never work and will only take people further away from knowing who they really are.

Living a life in accord with our true nature on a daily basis is one of the greatest

---

148 *Autobiography of a Yogi* by Paramahansa Yogananda (Self-Realization Fellowship, Los Angeles, Calif.)

blessings of Ayurveda. The fundamental principles of dinacharya are rooted in the cycles of the earth-moon and sun, which influence the vibratory qualities of the water, fire, and air elements. Each day begins by honoring the sun, as it is the life energy, the core of every human being's will to live and seek the highest quality of life. As it rises from the eastern sky, it is also rising within us as an energetic force. We must honor the sun as the eye of our spirit, and see its radiance spread throughout the kaleidoscope of colors in nature.

Ayurvedically speaking, there are two main shifts in the sun's position that affect both the daily and seasonal routine. One is called *adana* or the receiving period, when the Sun is taking its northern course in the sky. This is the time from the winter solstice, through the entire winter and spring, to the summer solstice, when the sun gets further north in the sky in the northern hemisphere. (The same occurs in the southern hemisphere, except in the opposite direction.) This is the warmer period of the year, when there is more rain and stronger sunlight. During this phase, the earth and its small replica, the human being, are more receptive to absorbing prana and cosmic intelligence or mahat, which are carried in varying proportions in the elements of air and fire.

The *visarga* or releasing position is when the sun takes the southern course in the sky. This is the time from the summer solstice, through the entire summer and fall, to the winter solstice, when the sun is receding to the south. Lunar energies become predominant, temperatures begin to decrease, and tropical and sub-subtropical areas receive a great deal of water. These climates are usually humid and experience large amounts of rainfall. During the visarga phase, the element of fire or agni decreases in the sunlight. This becomes a special period to embrace the moon's energies, which are cooling and restorative and now more readily available to replenish us.

These two main phases of agni (solar or receiving) and soma (lunar or releasing), along with the force of vayu (wind or shifting), are responsible for the cycles of time, the seasons, the fluctuations of the doshas, and the overall function and feeling of the body. In the ancient Vedic era, these energies were revered as aspects of God or Divinity. Ancient people were constantly aware of these changing patterns and their relationship to health, agriculture, and spiritual rituals. The truth is that we feel differently at various times of the year. Our interests and capacities change. We are more physical or agni in the summer, and more reflective, contemplative, or soma in the winter.

The ancient wisdom of Ayurveda and yoga provides us with many therapeutic practices necessary for balancing the mind-body relationship, and yogic disciplines for peace of mind. The list of techniques below has been set forth in an ideal order, and includes many suggestions for integrating the practices into your lifestyle. Each person must find their own ways of integrating these techniques in the most practical manner, given capacity and lifestyle.

1. **Awaking at Sunrise** – To align ourselves with the master force of the universe. For higher esoteric purposes, yogis rise at the sacred time of creation or *Brahma Muhurta* to perform rituals like *aarathi* (candle-lighting) as an offering to their chosen deity or image of God, invoking the Divine presence into their morning sadhana. This is an ideal time for yoga asana and pranayama, which discipline the mind-body relationship. End your practice with a period of meditation, according to your capacity. 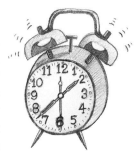 Visualize the sun rising from the base of your spine to the top, settling at the third eye. This can be done several times to relax the mind, enhance concentration, and increase the flow of prana in the nadis. Then end with moments of deep prayer, sharing your love, compassion for others, and gratitude for all that blessings in your life.

   Optional practice: Depending on how you feel, another option before beginning sadhana is to go for a short but brisk walk outside to circulate the blood and oxygen and warm up before doing asana. This also helps clear any congestion in the chest or nasal cavity.

2. **Cleansing Practices:** These are important parts of a regular Ayurvedic dinacharya. They are gentle and help cleanse some of the main senses whose organs are located in the head, such as sight, smell, and taste.

   A. **Tongue-Scraping** – The tongue should be gently scraped daily before brushing the teeth. This simple procedure removes dead bacteria, refreshes the breath, and stimulates the internal organs and digestion. The best scrapers are usually made of silver or copper. A small spoon can also be used.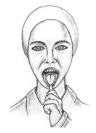

   B. **Tooth-Brushing** – Brushing with a soft-bristle brush massages the gums. A small amount of neem herb powder can be added if you can bear the bitter taste. Flossing is best done in evenings to give the gums a six- to eight-hour break from food between the teeth. To remove particles and bacteria that cause bad breath, use astringent pungent and bitter herbs such as neem, cardamom, and cinnamon in bark or powder form made into a paste. Toothpaste formulas with these types of ingredients are available from various Ayurveda companies.

C. **Medicated Eyewash** – To stimulate secretion and promote cleansing. The eyes are the windows to the soul and should be kept clean and clear, especially in urban environments where the air quality is poor. This can be done with a tea brewed with the herbal formula triphala: A half teaspoon should be boiled and the water than strained and cooled. This is recommended for all dosha types. In the evenings, a soothing gentle massage of the eyelids and surrounding areas with ghee (clarified butter) allows the eyes to restore themselves after excess sun or computer use. Ghee drops can also be added directly into the eyes, but should not be too warm. Rose water, made from rose petals, is very good for pitta types. Be careful not to use commercial brands that use chemicals to create the rose scent.

D. **Nasal Cleansing** – Finely powdered pure salt or sea salt is put in a special neti pot, dissolved in warm water and poured through one nostril at a time. Use of a neti pot to flush the nose with saline water is a great way to avoid allergies, congestion, and headaches. Neti pots can be purchased at some health food stores. The nose is considered one of the most important orifices in the body, as it supports the proper functioning of the four senses located in the head. This is an important therapy for kapha management. It is best done early in the morning, shortly after rising.

When not to use a neti pot:

- Do not use the pot if you have a sinus infection or severely blocked sinuses. It is best to wait for the nasal passages to be mostly clear before use.
- During a nose bleed, neti-pot rinses should be avoided, as the salt can further aggravate the problem.
- Do not use the pot if the nose is fractured.

3. **Self-Massage** – Abhyanga is the most popular practice of a balanced Ayurvedic lifestyle. It benefits everything from nervous to muscular, skeletal, digestive, and respiratory systems. Abhyanga nourishes all the dhatus and is an effective form of rasayana or restorative practice. It keeps the skin

from drying and improves joint mobility and muscular flexibility. As mentioned earlier, abhyanga's benefits are enhanced when performed before asana practice, as this allows oils to seep in deeper before asana heats the body, induces sweat, and purifies the tissues.

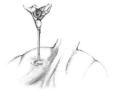

4. **Oil-Pulling** – This practice is called *gandusha* in Sanskrit and involves 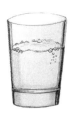 swishing oil in the mouth for a period of 10-20 minutes. This is an excellent practice for the gums and also strengthens the teeth and settles the nerves around the mouth and face. A prepared blend of sesame oil and neem oil is very good for this. Plain sesame oil is fine too.

5. **Nose Oil** – After rinsing the nostrils with the neti pot, it is best to add oil drops (*nasya*) that blend herbs and oils to promote proper sensory and mental acuity and function. Nasya also enhances the effects of meditation: as the oils drip back through the nasal cavity, they calm the sensitive nerves that influence brain function and the central nervous system. It is best to administer the oil using a small, one-ounce dropper bottle while lying down on a flat surface. Tilt the head back so the nostrils point upwards.

Add two to four drops in each nostril, and then perform short and quick inhalations until you feel the oil reaching the throat. It is also very helpful to massage and pinch the nose with the thumb and index finger several times, so the walls of the nose absorb the oil. I have developed a tri-doshic formula available on my website that enhances the practice of pranayama.

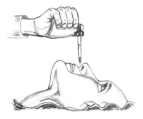

6. **Fluids** – It is best to drink room-temperature water throughout the day. Cold water should be avoided, especially while eating food, as this dampens the digestive fire. Warm water is also good, as it acclimates well to the gastro-intestinal tract. Copper cups, known as *tamara jal,* are recommended for drinking water. Leave the water in the cup for eight hours or overnight and drink it upon rising in the morning. The water thereby becomes infused with an important mineral that benefits digestion, has a peristaltic quality, cleanses the kidneys, and kills bacteria. Stimulants like caffeine should be avoided, especially first thing in the morning, as this creates dependency, taxes the adrenals, and can create hyperacidity. For general cleansing purposes, warm

water with a fresh wedge of ginger, one teaspoon of honey, and a squeeze of lemon is beneficial for the doshas and balances kapha.

7. **Abdominal Undulations** – Nauli is one of Hatha Yoga's purification rites. It is described in detail in the chapter on yoga asana. This exercise is ideal in the morning time to encourage the bowels to move and improve circulation.

8. **Exercise** – The key aspect of exercise is the effect it has on 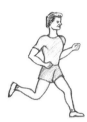 the cardiovascular system. While exercise is vital in promoting circulation and maintaining health, it is important to gauge exercise so that it does not damage the body or deplete ojas. Many people confuse adrenal with real life-force energy. Ayurveda recommends walking over running. Hiking is also good, as going uphill raises the heart rate and strengthens the inner organs and outer muscles.

9. **Sweat Therapy** – Sweat is an important bodily function that is largely overlooked. I typically recommend that a person attain at least one good sweat per week for general health maintenance.

10. **Yoga** – Asanas are good to do in the morning time. If you want to get more effective results, then it is best to begin them before 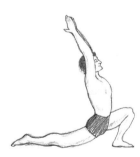 doing anything else, as the body is fully restored in the morning. Some variations, like combining abhyanga and some of the oil practices, can be done prior to asana. Pranayama is simple to do and can be practiced for a few minutes after abhyanga, or along with asana practice. Kapalbhati or the "punch breath" is best done in the morning, as it has a punching action on the lungs that pushes out stagnant kapha dosha. Bastrika or bellows breathing also has a rajasic or stimulating action that promotes circulation and increases digestive strength. If you are doing these just before meditation, it is important to introduce Nadi Shodhana or alternate-nostril breathing to calm the breath and balance the lunar and solar channels. These are all described in greater detail in the chapter on pranayama. Vata types benefit by warming up before yoga with either a hot shower or an oil massage. Pitta and kapha types usually warm up more easily, so this may not be as important for them.

11. **Meditation** – This is the ideal practice for connecting the body, mind, and spirit. Many people do not realize the amount of energy that meditation requires. This is why it is so effective in the morning. The mind is also calmer then and this makes it easier for many to sit in stillness. Meditation is greatly enhanced when asana is done beforehand, as was originally intended, although it is not always necessary to do asana before meditation. When the day begins with meditation, it leaves us with a residue of peace that lasts throughout the day.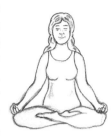

12. **Meals** (Breakfast, Lunch, and Dinner) – To maintain metabolic balance and digestive strength, establishing consistent meal times is necessary to support the mind-body relationship. Meal times are coordinated to the timing of the doshas and the way the metabolism shifts from morning to evening.

13. **Menses Pointers**
    A. Avoid any intense activity that is heating to the body, such as asana, inversions, running, sports, etc.
    B. Avoid alcohol.
    C. Avoid sex.
    D. Avoid detoxes like pancha karma, fasting, or stimulating therapies.
    E. Avoid strongly spiced foods.
    F. Avoid ceremonies that expose menstrual energies.
    G. Do read, write, and meditate.
    H. Walking is also good.
    I. Cooking and taking the Ayurvedic medicine tikta grihta (shatavari ghee) is good in supporting the menstruation process.

14. **Mini Daily Tune-Ups** – There are a number of ways to keep ourselves in balance and our consciousness spiritually attuned while going on with our daily activities. The key to living a balanced and healthy life is to find ways to integrate these practices into our daily routines. There is no perfect time to begin doing yoga. There is no ideal situation or job that will help us do these things. We must simply choose to do them. The time is already there: it's just a matter of what you decide to do inside it. Here are a few simple things that anyone can integrate into their lifestyle.

- **Mantra** – The Hindu-Yoga beaded necklace is called a mala and has 108 beads. It can be used to keep count of a mantra sadhana or practice japa mantra. At any time, one can sit quietly and silently repeat a chosen mantra to clear the mind. This also improves concentration. I like to do several rounds of this before meditation.

- **Alternate-Nostril Breathing** (Nadi Shodhana) – This is effective in balancing the mind, calming the heart, and releasing stress. This is a relaxing form of breathing that can be done quietly. It reminds us how wonderful it is to breathe deeply and slowly. We often forget this when in front of a computer or speaking on the phone.

- **Kapha Busters** (three spinal directions) – This is an easy-to-do series of repetitive spinal movements that promote circulation, warm up the body, and release stress. Whether you sit at a desk for many hours a day or work standing up, these exercises can release muscular kinks and decompress the mind.

- **After Dinner** - To promote digestion and ease pressure off the liver, lie in a left-lateral position with the head propped up with either the arm or a pillow. Positioning the left side down places the ascending colon, on the right side of the abdomen, over the descending colon on the left side. This activates the solar nadi to promote digestion. Hold this position from 10 to 20 minutes.

- **Pre-Sleep** – Massaging a small amount of warm coconut, sesame, or almond oil on the top of head or entire scalp before going to bed promotes sound sleep. The palms of the hands and soles of the feet can also be massaged to calm the nervous system. These five points, like the fingers of each hand and toes of each foot, represent the five elements.

- **To Fall Asleep** – As you lie in bed with eyes closed facing upwards, begin to observe the natural rhythm of your involuntary breath. As the breath flows in, mentally repeat the mantra *Hum,* and as the breath flows outwards mentally repeat *Sa*. Do this consistently until the mind becomes very slow or you simply fall asleep. The mantra *Aum Shanti* can also be used to promote peace of mind. For vata types or imbalances, it is best to sleep flat on the back or on the left side. For pitta types or related conditions, it is best to sleep on right side, which keeps the body and systems cooler. It is best if kaphas sleep on the left side.

- **Waking Up** – Let your first thought be of God. Take a few minutes to offer some prayers of gratitude to God as you embark on your day. Then think of positive aspects of your life and other inspiring thoughts of things you have to look forward to. This is a key time to set the right attitude for the entire day. Affirmations are also good to make at this time. Memorize some words that guide you and arouse the Divine qualities of your soul.

Seasonal Routine

In keeping to a daily routine of some sort, we can avoid being taken over by society's negative or tamasic qualities. Routines are great aids to increasing our resilience to the weather shifts that occur from one season to another. These seasonal shifts or *ritu sandi* are transitional periods that last about two weeks from the end of one season to the beginning of another. Viral infections such as influenza are common and particularly sneak into the system either during these transitional periods or when the body's immune defense system has been weakened from stress or low digestive fire.

Dependency on antibiotic medications also weakens our overall immunity. This has become another prevalent issue today, with pharmacies and the media advertising the purported necessity for these drugs with the message that they will protect you from disease. I don't completely disagree with use of such prescriptions, but I do disagree with dependency on such substances for fighting diseases, and the lack of responsible living that creates the health problems we are trying to avoid in the first place. Ayurveda teaches us that how we live matters and plays a major role in how we think, look, feel, and act. We must begin to take more responsibility for our lives, knowing that health comes from within and is maintained by making conscious, healthy lifestyle choices.

The traditional seasonal structure in India is based on six seasons of two months each and has some differences from American climate and weather. The two most important things are to understand the climate you live in, how it affects the doshas, and what your constitution or prakriti and imbalances or vikriti are. What I often tell my clients and students is not to become overwhelmed with trying to do so much. Begin with one or two things each season, and try to implement those changes consistently through the entire year. How we distribute our healthy lifestyle changes throughout the entire year is more important than trying to do a lot in one season and then dropping everything in next.

For example, if you know that it is beneficial for you as a kapha type to get up earlier in the winter, begin with this perhaps three times per week and see it through the entire winter and into the spring, rather than trying to get up early every day, when you know that may be a big challenge right at the beginning. Extremes don't work and don't last. Remember: if you trained yourself out of balance, you must retrain yourself back into balance. The body and mind are like a puppy dog that requires consistent training—or else the puppy does naughty things. So the mind-body, being like a restless and unconscious puppy, also requires gradual and persistent adjustments to re-groove new patterns into the brain.

Patterns of the Doshas and the Seasons

The doshas follow seasonal patterns:

- **Spring** – Kapha mostly accumulates in spring as, in some cases, does vata, depending on the geographical area. The coolness of spring can increase both these doshas. Phlegm and congestion build up for kaphas, while vatas start feeling sensitive to temperature and digestion begins to weaken.

- **Summer** – Pitta is mostly accumulated in summer and appears as acid indigestion and skin flare-ups.

- **Fall/Autumn** – Vata mainly accumulates in fall with the onset of cooler and dryer weather. Cracking joints, dry skin, and constipation are common symptoms.

- **Winter** – Kapha mostly accumulates with cold and wet weather.

With knowledge of what how the seasons affect the doshas, one can ward off imbalances. If daily routine (*dinacharya*) and seasonal routine (*ritucharya*) are not followed, imbalances for each dosha begin appearing in the following season. In many cases, symptoms of imbalance do not require an entire season to begin appearing. This is particularly the case with individuals who have not been following a healthy lifestyle. It could be a change in temperature or weather, an emotional episode, or a meal that causes the vikriti and its symptoms to appear suddenly. Seasonal adjustments must be made according to the area one lives in. Therefore, it is important to know your climate and its typical characteristics, so that proper Ayurvedic practices can be implemented. The details below reflect general seasonal qualities, which will vary from place to place.

Basic Seasonal Guidelines to Maintain Balance of the Doshas

Spring Season

General details:
This is the best season to cleanse or perform a comprehensive detoxification like pancha karma. As temperatures get warmer, the five pranic forces become more enlivened and udana (upward-moving prana) especially increases. Digestive strength increases a bit as well, so there is more support to flush out the bowels, stomach, and lungs from any residue of ama.

Yoga:
In yoga practice, one can emphasize inversions, sequences, standing poses, and back bends, all of which are heating, promote sweat, and assist in cleansing the body. Oil massage prior to practicing asana in a warm room is a great way to promote sweat that purges the tissues. Kapalbhati and Bastrika pranayama are excellent for reducing kapha in the spring.

Diet:
A kapha-balancing diet is good to follow, with some consideration of vata if that is part of one's constitution. Avoid heavy, sweet, and salty foods; avoid starches at dinner time; eat smaller meals rather than bulky ones; drink warm ginger, honey, and lemon tea several times a day; do a fast one day per week on fresh juices and hot herbal teas; use spices like cinnamon, ginger, mustard seeds, turmeric, black pepper, and cayenne. Mustard and sesame oils are also indicated.

Exercise:
All types of exercise that stimulate the cardiovascular system are good. Heart and lung exercises done a minimum of three to four times per week are appropriate.

Therapies:
Light oil massage with sesame, mustard, or kapha-blend oil is recommended, followed by vinyasa yoga and a sauna, steam, or hot shower. This is very important and ideally should be done two to three times per week. Peppermint and eucalyptus oils are stimulating, and camphor opens up the lungs.

Summer Season

General details:
This is the season to be cautious of pitta dosha. The key is to stay cool and

never allow the body to overheat. It is important to avoid direct, prolonged exposure to the sun. Wear a hat to keep the head cool, and sunglasses to avoid straining the eyes when the sun is bright. Practice moderation in every aspect of your life, including work, exercise, and socializing. Early to bed and early to rise are good to keep the body resting while the moon's energies are predominant. Full-moon bathing and even sleeping outside on the full moon are recommended. Walking barefoot in the grass is cooling and soothing. The Ayurvedic scriptures recommend a short nap in the afternoon to restore the ojas from the draining power of the sun. This recommendation is limited to the summer season.

Yoga:
Practice of yoga asana should be reduced to a minimum, especially heating balancing postures and inversions. Floor postures, forward bends, seated twists, and practices that stay near the earth or the floor and are more cooling are appropriate. Practice in early morning or early evening. Enjoy good Savasana periods and meditation, and whisper or silently repeat mantras. Alternate-nostril breathing, Sheetali, and Brahmari pranayama are recommended.

Diet:
Hot, pungent spices should be avoided. Never miss meals, especially lunch, and avoid overeating. Eat mainly bitter and sweet-tasting foods, and drink fluids such as coconut water, pomegranate or aloe vera juice, and water that has sat overnight in a copper vessel with a pearl or moonstone inside. Avoid excess fluids with meals. Salads are great, and spices such as saffron, turmeric, cumin, coriander, and fennel can be used lightly. Ghee is excellent and coconut and olive oils are also good.

Exercise:
Gentle exercise, such as walking, swimming, and bicycling is good, but in the early morning or evening only. Try to keep heart rate from going up too high, to 130 beats per minute or more, to avoid over-heating the body. Perspire slightly and gradually if possible. Movement arts like t'ai chi and qi gong are excellent, as is dancing. All exercise should be done with a light, spirited, and non-competitive attitude.

Therapies:
Massage with coconut or narayan oil made with shatavari is excellent for pitta types, as are shirodhara (warm oil streaming on the forehead), rose water misting, and a ghee massage of the eyes. Massaging coconut oil on the head and soles of the feet at bedtime is great for relaxing the nervous system. It

is wonderful to rest rose-water cotton pads or sliced cucumbers on the eyes in the evening. Aromatherapy with rose, vetiver, blue chamomile, lavender, geranium, and sandalwood is soothing and relaxing.

Fall Season

General details:
In most places, the early fall is still quite warm. In subtropical and tropical areas like India and the southern half of the United States, it can be very hot and often warmer than summer. After months of hot weather and plenty of perspiration, it is common that vata types become dried out. Because of this drying aspect, it is important to manage vata and pitta dosha in the early part of the season.

Fall, especially just before the onset of winter, is considered to be a crucial time for managing vata because both fall and winter have a strong capacity to increase vata and weaken the tissues. Pitta types may find themselves even more sensitive and a bit temperamental in the fall, after months of hot-weather exposure in the summer. This is typically the season when most doshic imbalances begin, as vata is the master dosha and commonly pushes pitta and kapha out of balance. Limiting exposure to the elements is important, particularly wind and excess sunlight. Adhering to a structured schedule in lifestyle, work, and dinacharya, the daily self-care routine, is vitally important during the fall season. It is probably a good idea to avoid taking on any new projects during this time and keep life as simple as possible. Avoid or reduce exposure to the media, late-night use of the computer, and gossip. No news is good news!

Yoga:
Sadhana is key during this time, especially early in the morning. Pranayama, mantra, and meditation keep a peaceful and sattvic mind throughout the entire day. Asana for both vata and pitta conditions is still useful, but keep it simple and more focused on stretching and releasing tension than on heating up and sweating. Vata in the body creates tightness, while pitta creates tension. So spinal poses like Paschimottanasana (seated forward bend), Halasana (plow), and Ardha Matsyendrasana (seated spinal twist) are good as part of dinacharya and preparation for meditation. Once the body has limbered up a bit, weaving in some pranayama will be effective in calming the mind.

Diet:
In autumn, the main diet to adhere to overall is vata, with sweet, sour, and salty types of foods. Warm spices like cumin, cinnamon, ginger, fennel, and

licorice are good for the digestion. Plenty of warm fluids in the form of herbal teas, fresh juices, and even nourishing-type smoothies are recommended. It is best not to fast during this season if vata is your main constitution. Focus mainly on warm and cooked foods that are moderately spiced, and include ghee and sesame and olive oils.

Exercise:
Walking is best and hiking is also good to keep the legs strong. I regularly recommend some weight-lifting, about once per week, to keep the muscles and tissues strong. Too much asana can make vata body types very thin and weak. Weight-bearing or cross-training type exercises are very helpful for such people.

Therapies:
Abyanga and nasya (nasal oil) are incredibly beneficial treatments that should be done either on a daily or, at the very least, weekly basis. If vata is already out of balance (vikriti) then enema therapy (*basti chikitsa*) is the best way to manage this sensitive dosha. When downward flow or apana becomes excessive, it can be unblocked through enemas.

Winter Season

General details:
As the coldest season of the year, winter is a big challenge for those with kapha in the constitution. There should also be some consideration for vata types, as cold temperatures increase that dosha. The key to success is to keep the mind inspired and positive and the circulation moving. This means getting outside as much as is possible, given unpredictable winter weather. This season becomes like a battle to fight off laziness, fatigue, and a slowing digestive system that is prone to accumulating ama, which often leads to congestion and coughs. Staying warm is very important.

Yoga:
Yoga asana sadhana is probably one of the most important factors, along with diet, in managing kapha, because both are done indoors. A heating practice that promotes plenty of sweating, such as vinyasa, inversions, and balancing postures is appropriate. This can be infused with detoxifying pranayama, such as Kapalbhati, Bastrika, and the double breath. Chair pose and its variations are excellent. Dancing Shiva pose, headstand, and handstand are some of many postures that can keep kapha in balance. It is helpful to heat up the room or practice in front of a fireplace to open up the skin pores and induce sweat. The practice needs to be consistent and persistent, with little let-up.

End with a short cool-down before transitioning into meditation. Savasana is counter-indicated. The best time to practice is early morning, even before sunrise. Practice should be done a minimum of three to four times per week, and some weeks on a daily basis.

Diet:

A kapha diet should consist mainly of spicy or pungent and bitter foods. To keep the metabolism strong and active, it is helpful to eat smaller meals three to four times per day. Another helpful practice is to drink warm spiced tea, with ginger or cumin, coriander, and fennel, several times per day to keep the gastro-intestinal tract flowing. Foods should be warm and cooked for easier digestion, and fluid consumption during meals should be reduced to one cup to avoid diluting digestive enzymes in the stomach. Dry foods are also good to keep kapha in balance, as they prevent moisture from increasing.

Exercise:

Exercise for kapha dosha can be increased in the winter and done in shorter bursts, with emphasis on sweating. Cardiovascular exercise is vital to keep circulation flowing during the months from December to March, when it can get very slow and weak. People commonly misinterpret household chores like walking the dog, cleaning the house, and doing laundry as effective forms of exercise. Exercise must raise the resting heart rate for at least 30 minutes five times per week. Another option is to do more vigorous exercise like hiking, bicycling, jumping rope, or a heated yoga practice with no rests.

Therapies:

The best overall therapy is sweating or svedhana. Fat is diminished most effectively through heat that produces sweat. Saunas, steam baths, and hot yoga are all good, but one must also be cautioned against excessive water loss if there is vata dosha in the prakriti. Sweating is even more beneficial when preceded by abhyanga, and should be done with strong and stimulating strokes and a small amount of mustard or sesame oil.

Doshas and Physiology

The yogic and Ayurvedic lifestyle includes a number of practices that can be integrated into either the daily or seasonal routine to maintain balance of the doshas and to address specific symptoms caused by imbalances or environmental changes. The use of oils in massage is one of the unique aspects of Ayurveda and works well with yoga postures and breathing techniques. The oils can also be applied prior to exercise of any type. The doshas have their own distinct influence on the various systems of the body, and some knowledge of this is helpful in establishing health routines. Although certain doshas tend to influence certain systems more than others, they each have their influence over all the systems, particularly vata, which controls all movement and circulation.

Respiratory System – As respiration influences circulation, in Ayurveda it is frequently called, or combined with, the circulatory system. Respiration is our link to life, and circulation improves the quality of organ function. Respiration is typically shallow and fast in vata types, strong in pitta types, and slow and deep in kapha types. Good circulation is essential to health, and heat and regular exercise help promote this. Everybody is different, and while some need to work continuously on maintaining good circulation, others do not. The skin is one of the best ways to measure this.

The quality of circulation of the blood reflects the nature of one's lifestyle, with blotchy skin or spotting the clearest indicator that a daily routine is not in place. Consistency in skin tone indicates good blood flow. Growths such as warts, cysts, moles, and skin tags can be correlated to excess kapha. Good respiration begins with good skin that can breathe, as the skin is the largest organ in the body. Kaphas are the best breathers and also have soft, porous, and moist skin tone. Pittas can have nice skin, but, when out of balance, it can appear redder in color. When aggravated and in more extreme conditions, rashes and adhesions appear. This can indicate forced respiration caused by extreme sports, anger, or fury in the mind. The mind is the ultimate influence on the respiratory system and this is where pranayama, mantra, and meditation can be used to keep the mind more consistently calm in all circumstances.

Vata – Pranayama, mantra, and meditation are critical and only effective when done with *consistency*. To improve respiration for vata types, I recommend first going to the mind. This can begin with the elimination of any type of multi-tasking. Emphasize attention focused on one task at a time. In pranayama, breathe deeply so that the lungs are completely expanded and contracted. Make inhalation and exhalation of equal length. For example, with alternate-nostril breathing (Nadi Shodhana), the inhalation through the left nostril should be identical in length to the exhalation through the right nostril.

In lifestyle, it is essential to integrate this quality of deep, mindful breathing into every activity, and most importantly when eating, speaking, having sexual intercourse, exercising, and just before bedtime and in the moments before falling asleep. The best mantra practice for vata uses the Hindu rosary or mala and includes one complete round of 108 repetitions two times per day, at sunrise and sunset. Meditation for improving respiration should be steady and consistent. Stillness should be emphasized above everything else. That means, if you are going to meditate for five minutes, do it without moving a muscle or even flinching once. This is more effective than meditating 20 minutes with a restless body. A calming and penetrating asana practice includes a plow (Halasana) and shoulder-stand (Sarvangasana) combination, followed by knee-to-chest pose (Pavanamuktasana) and then fish pose (Matsyasana). Lastly, do a seated forward-bending pose (Paschimottanasana). Hold each pose for about one minute. Corpse pose (Savasana) should be practiced for two to three minutes at the end of the series. The series should be repeated three to four times for effectiveness.

Pitta - One of the things I often notice with pittas during pranayama is they breathe with excessive force, sound, and jerking body movements. Since their circulation is the best of all types, the requirement is actually to do less and take the edge out of every breath. Alternate-nostril breathing has a neutralizing effect and is neither too heating nor cooling. Every breathing exercise should finish with one to two deep inhale-exhales and then a moment of relaxation.

I recommend devotional mantras done in kirtan style because of their less focused and more playful quality. This often leads to some dancing, which is a diffused type of respiratory exercise. Meditation is great as long as it does not get to the point where one becomes aggravated or frustrated. One common hindrance to good respiration is tension in the spine and back muscles. The seated spinal twist (Ardha Matsyendrasana) is ideal in this regard and should be done for one minute on each side, with a seated forward bend (Paschimottanasana) in between, followed by a minute of corpse pose (Savasana). The entire series can be repeated three to four times with good results.

Kapha – Pranayama like Kapalbhati (punch-breath), which has a punching or chopping quality, is best for removing stagnation in the lungs. Bastrika is also good when done quickly. Short sets of 24-36 repetitions should be followed with one to two deep inhale-exhales and then a moment of relaxation before beginning the next set. Kaphas do best chanting mantras out loud, while pittas do better repeating the words silently. The use of the breath to chant out loud improves circulation and vibrates the lungs, throat, and trachea, areas where kapha commonly builds up. Kaphas have the fewest issues with respiration, as they are generally deep breathers. However, because they breathe more slowly, like tortoises, their circulation can be a little slow, leading to poor flow, which can in turn lead to toxic build-up or ama. One simple asana combination is dancing Shiva pose (Nataraja) and chair pose with double breathing done five times. The entire series can be done three to four times, and abdominal undu-lations (Nauli) can also be added at the end. Rest can be done for about one minute by standing with the feet together and arms to the sides of the body.

Digestive System – Ayurveda views the digestive process as the key to health and wellness. Diet plays a vital role in this. Yoga exercises are also a direct means of managing the quality of our digestion. It is important to understand the general nature of this very sensitive system, how it functions according to your constitution, how it adapts to lifestyle changes, and how it reacts to foods and yoga. The mind is a major influence on the digestive function, particularly if it is tamasic or rajasic and constantly disturbed by propulsive emotions. Emotions of any sort have a disruptive effect on digestion and these vary depending on the doshas. Emotions arise as a symptom of an imbalance of the doshas or vikriti state. Eating food during any type of strong emotional mood is not recommended, as this can lead to toxic build-up from foods not properly assimilated. The ideal time to eat is after yoga and meditation, when the mind is serene. A focused mind that is not disturbed by the mental movies caused by emotions is sattvic. A sattvic mind gives strength or agni and vitality to the digestive process.

Vata – For vata types, deep and natural breathing is necessary to keep abdominal nerves relaxed. In yoga practice, this can be done through use of the diaphragm. Regardless of the pranayama technique, the breath needs to originate from a full lung capacity. To enhance this, a belly massage with a vata body oil should be done to relax the nerves and enhance the depth of the breath. Speech also plays a role in digestive function. If the mind is burdened by fear, the breath will shorten, as this contracts the throat and abdomen, creating a restricting effect on the speech and general expression. Any disturbance to the mind, whether it comes from an emotion or lack of focus, will have a contractive effect on the organs and their function. In many instances in my consultations, I have correlated digestive issues like constipation, which is the most common vata disturbance, with fear of speaking out or inability to express oneself.

Mantra can increase the power of concentration, dissolve fear, and promote good digestion. As vata has a wind-like quality that is moving and erratic, vata has the most sensitive digestive process. It can relay inconsistent nerve impulses that affect the mechanical operation of the colon, stomach, and intestines. In general, all types of yoga asana are good for vata digestion because they produce heat and promote circulation. Regular meal times are very important in keeping the digestive clock regular. Food should ideally be eaten in silence, with some exposure to the natural elements, in a quiet atmosphere and without television or even reading, which prevent the mind from actually enjoying food. Vatas need to learn to eat slowly and without disturbance from modern gadgets.

Pitta – Digestion for pitta types is usually strong and functions best in cooler climates. While a warm and comfortable environment is important for vata, a shady and breezy one is soothing and more conducive to pitta. The main concern with pranayama is doing it in shorter intervals and a softer manner, without tension in the chest, back, or face. Another thing to consider when practicing yoga exercises of any type is to avoid getting too heated. This reflects the overall theme of moderation and softening of attitude towards practice. Devotional mantras and singing uplifting carols send harmonious vibrations to the intestines. Meditation in general induces the moon's energy to rise, cooling the mind and relaxing the entire gastro-intestinal tract. Meditation is more specifically beneficial when done before eating lunch, counter-balancing the sun's strong effect on the digestive process. Coconut oil rubbed on the abdomen in the summer is a simple therapy for curbing pitta, which is often on the edge of spilling over during this season. A diffused approach to yoga sadhana and lifestyle is beneficial for balancing pitta digestion.

Kapha – A rajasic breathing technique like Kapalabhati helps activate secretion of digestive enzymes, igniting agni and heating the body. While pittas need to take a more passive approach to maintaining balanced digestion, kaphas need to be proactive. Inversions like headstand or handstand combined with Kapalabhati are beneficial. Nauli (abdominal undulations) can also be followed with Kapalabhati done on an empty stomach, ideally in the morning between 6 and 8am, after meditating, and just before breakfast. Stacking such techniques as pranayama, mantra, and meditation is good for kapha digestion. So are exercises that combine asana and pranayama with sports and other fitness approaches. Since circulation plays an important role for kapha dosha and health in general, any exercise or discipline done with continuity is beneficial. Warming kapha oil blends or plain sesame or mustard oil can be massaged onto the abdomen prior to doing any of the exercises I have just mentioned. An integral approach is key to maintaining a strong digestion.

Nervous System – The digestive system is responsive to asana, diet, and environment, and the nervous system informs us of what is happening in the body. It consistently guides us in maintaining a balanced mind-body relationship that promotes spiritual evolution. Spiritually, the nervous system, when balanced, provides us with the sensitivity to transmit streams of consciousness, expand our awareness, and develop our intuition. Physically, the nerves are responsible for influencing vata dosha. They are a complex and often unpredictable aspect of our anatomy and physiology.

As with the digestive system, the mind and our environment are enormous influences on the nerves and are strongly linked to the brain and the spine. Caring for the nervous system is of particular consideration in this era of technological advancement, which isolates both mind and body with mindless gadgets that further divorce us from nature's elements. In my consultations, I often ask my clients how often they are outside, in the sense that they are feeling sunlight on the skin or the feet or hands touching earth, experiencing the smell of rain, swimming in a lake, river, or ocean, and so forth. Many go months without such experiences and an array of health issues result.

The nervous system gives us the capacity to enjoy life and, alternately, can make us aware of discord in the body and brain. The management of the nervous system in yoga is done through the mystical surrendering process of pratyahara, which is one of the principal steps in Patanjali's ashtanga yoga model. It is prana that connects the soul and subtle or astral body. It also influences the mind at the level of deep sleep and subconscious and conscious states. All three levels of consciousness are greatly influenced by the central nervous system. Many of the neurological issues we see today, such as Parkinson's disease, Alzheimer's, and even muscular dystrophy, can be attributed to dysfunction of the nervous system caused by vata and pitta dosha excess.

Vata – Vata relates with the nervous system through the force of prana, its capacities and balanced functioning in the body. The regular practice of asana is essential to balancing the nerves, particularly the ganglia and nerves along the spine. Asana sequences like Surya Namaskar are good for increasing flow in the nerve bundles in the lumbar spine, hips, and legs. Many seated positions like Gomukhasana (cow-face pose) and Ardha Matsyendrasana (spinal twist) specifically target the lower spine and hip areas. Abhyanga or oil massage is one of the most beneficial therapies for maintaining healthy and balanced nerves.

Shriodhara, the classic Ayurvedic treatment that involves pouring a warm stream of oil over the forehead, is on-target for calming the nerves and brain. Nadi Shodhana (alternate-nostril) pranayama is another important tool for managing the prana-mind-nerves link and balancing the two aspects of the mind. For example, a mind in which solar energy flowing through the pingala nadi and brain synapses is predominant experiences a rajasic or agitated state in the nerves. A mind in which lunar energy, flowing through the ida nadi and even subtler brain synapses, experiences nervous hypersensitivity, can be seen in fluctuations in adjusting to temperature and sound.

Regular exposure through lifestyle to the five elements is the broadest thera-peutic practice that can be done by anyone in supporting the nervous system. Meditation or focused stillness serves as the vehicle that bridges the mind and nervous system into the mystical experience of pratyahara, which withdraws the life-current energy normally pulled outwards by the senses back into the restful sanctuary of the chakras or astral body, and further inwards towards contact with the soul. This topic is addressed more in depth in other passages on relaxation.

Pitta – The nervous system benefits greatly by the pitta heat known as the fire of the elements (*bhuta agnis*), the fire of digestion (jatharagni), and the fire of the body's tissue layers (*dhatu agnis*). These thirteen fires, in total, play a vital role in the function of the central nervous system and the body's capacity to rest and restore. If pitta is high, it has a wasting and depleting action on the body that dulls the nerves' ability to send proper signals linking the brain and spine, and the brain and organs. In a way, heat deforms the flow through the nerves by depleting the prana found in the blood's red corpuscles. Thus, pitta indirectly affects the nervous system through the blood, and both blood and nerves determine the health of the entire body. The modern era's health issues afflict the nervous system and bloodstream, and lifestyle has much to do with this. The former is weakened by an unfocused mind lacking real power of attention, while the latter is destroyed by excess work, stress, and lack of proper rest.

Kapha - A kapha constitution provides a shield that protects the nerves from the factors that typically disturb vata and pitta. Adipose fat is mainly a con-centrated layer of water under the skin and around certain organs. Its oily or greasy quality shields the nerves from environmental disturbances. However, in excess, this can create sensory dullness and mentally can put kaphas out of touch with others. It can also dampen the nerves' receptivity to stimulating therapies that keep kaphas' often-stagnant blood circulation flowing and di-gestive enzymes secreting.

This explains the issues surrounding kapha dosha and weight gain. The in-telligence network between the stomach nerves and the brain is diluted by excess water. Its cool quality in the stomach blocks the nerve networks that signal the brain when the stomach is actually full. This is why kaphas graze like a cow, eating small quantities of food at frequent and irregular intervals throughout the day. Kaphas are like vata in that they need to keep the body warm. However, kapha types also need to sweat and stimulate the body in order to remove excess water and fat. Inverted asanas, pranayama like Kapalabhati and Bastrika done quickly and strongly, and a proactive approach to lifestyle that includes multi-disciplinary activities are essential for balancing the kapha nervous system.

Muscular, Skeletal, and Lymphatic Systems – These systems play a very practical role in our daily lives. They inform our capacity for performing physical tasks of all types, including working, traveling, and the body's enjoyment of pleasure and satisfaction. The skeletal system is the framework of the body, enabling it to support the muscles. It also determines the body's shape, height, and size. The main issue we have in today's gadget, button-pushing culture is disuse of the body, unlike in ancient times when people built their own homes and walked to work, and families grew their food. Today, everything comes to us in a package, which has its distinct effects on the body related to the doshas. Structured and scheduled exercise routines have become necessary for many of us to maintain the health and wellness of our bones and muscles. There are number of interesting exercises and principles that can be integrated into our lifestyles to keep a healthy balance of these vital systems.

Vata – There are two approaches to consider when working with the muscles and bones: subtle or internal and gross or external. Subtle or internal therapies that can affect the skeletal system, the alignment of the spinal column, bone density, and mobility balance the pranas. Lymph is rarely an issue for vata, as lymph is literally water and excess vata is excess dryness, although vata can block and reduce circulation through the lymph nodes.

Once again, pranayama techniques provide an internal means for healing the entire skeletal system. Poor breathing patterns can reduce oxygenation and distribution of quality blood, which then reduces joint mobility, increases cracking of the joints, and dries the bones, creating common diseases such as osteoporosis and osteoarthritis. Shallow breathing reduces circulation and has a tightening effect on the body's muscles, further restricting joint function and flexion. On the subtle level of breathing, it is essential to expand natural breathing patterns, deepening the breath with conscious awareness to promote circulation, good-quality oxygen, and hemoglobin, which is responsible for transporting oxygen in the blood.

Another form of healing is to guide the prana internally by concentrating the mind on a specific area in the body and tensing the muscles. This is a signature feature of Yogananda's teachings[149] on healing through the power of

---

149   Energization techniques for recharging the body battery as part of an integral system of preparing the mind-body for meditation can be found in Paramahansa Yogananda's *Self-Realization Fellowship Lessons*.

the mind-body relationship. It is an esoteric and profound extension of the muscle-control practices and demonstrations that were developed in Bengal during the physical culture era of the late 1800s and early 1900s. It subtly energizes the 108 pranic power points known as marmas in Ayurvedic healing.

On the gross level, asanas held in a static or sequenced manner, followed by a period of rest, are helpful in building muscle strength. Chair pose (Utkatasana) helps build up skinny vata legs, while plank (Dandasana) and tiger pose (Bagghrasana) build the upper torso, arms, and shoulders. These should be practiced in short durations of 15 to 30 seconds each, in three to four repetitive sets. Externally, abhyanga and warm oil massage are a tremendous support for both the muscles and bones. A specific type of oil called mahanarayan is used for vata conditions that affect the muscle and bone tissues. In summary, for the long-term balance and strength of these tissues, a dual approach that considers both internal and external means complements Ayurvedic healing.

Pitta - Fire in the muscles has an overall positive effect, making them supple and flexible. In the bones, joints, and spine, balanced pitta creates good mobility and strength. Excess pitta creates inflammatory conditions like arthritis in the joints or inflammation in infected lymph nodes. Some of the main causes of this are spicy and acidic diets, excess stress, and extreme forms of bodily exercise. Balancing pitta always involves moderation and lifestyle simplification. In balancing the muscular system, yoga of a more soothing and relaxing type should be done, like moon salutations (Chandra Namaskar), floor postures like seated forward bend (Paschimottanasana), head-to-knee pose (Janushirasana), plow (Halasana), and seated spinal twist (Ardhamatsyendrasana).

High pitta creates tension in the muscles and makes athletes vulnerable to strains. The posture followed by rest approach is essential for pittas who are integrating yoga asana into a holistic lifestyle routine. Aloe vera gel can be rubbed onto the body to keep it cool, castor oil can be used for reducing inflammation, and brahmi oil in a coconut base is cooling and restorative. Meditation should be practiced with a focus on surrendering. This is the best long-term discipline for managing pitta in the muscles and joints. It is important to understand that Ayurveda as natural medicine works slowly and not just superficially, on the physical level, but aims at repairing patterns that disrupt the mind-body relationship by means of reflection and surrender. The elements are constantly fluctuating within us, and managing these forces naturally is only a matter of adjusting our routines and lifestyle accordingly.

Kapha – Water, with its soft and oily qualities, creates great muscular flexibility, producing high moisture and a damp skin. In yoga classes, I have witnessed that kapha becomes an obstacle in asana because extra fat and greater muscle density make it harder to perform twisting positions and inversions, and to hold standing postures, which takes a lot of muscular conditioning. The key to success with kapha is again heat, which produces sweat, reduces fat, and lightens the load, so to speak. As long as pitta is in balance, heat serves to promote lymphatic drainage and improve overall function of the circulatory system. Gentle pressure applied to the lymph nodes during massage is very helpful in promoting their function.

Endocrine System / Immune System – The endocrine is probably the most complex, delicate, and vulnerable of the body's systems, as it deals with the glands and secretion of hormones that affect everything from fertility to metabolism. The endocrine glands influence the autonomic nervous system and control respiration and the heartbeat, all of which influence the body's immunity.

The term "immune system" is commonly used to describe the body's ability to ward off viruses and bacteria. We often speak of immunity as if it were a battery that requires recharging after depletion through excess work, worry, stress, and poor dietary habits. The immune system is not a tangible organ, but represents a link to the life current known as ojas in Ayurvedic medicine. Both the endocrine system and immunity are threatened by the modern lifestyle more than ever before, largely owing to today's instant-gratification mentality. The speed of our lives and the amount of responsibility in modern life leads to a breakdown of these two systems. The hormones secreted in our bodies are like a natural internal pharmacy that regulates our overall well-being and the balance of mind and emotions. Yoga, Ayurvedic lifestyle, maintaining a positive attitude towards life, and having a clear purpose are required to keep these systems fully and properly functioning. In endocrine function, the pineal gland can be linked to the ajna chakra, the astral body's spiritual eye. The body's different glands (hypothalamus, parathyroid, pineal, pituitary, thyroid, thymus, ovaries, pancreas, suprarenal, testes, uterus) can be associated with the chakras of the astral body.

The endocrine-immune systems are interlinked and quite sensitive, as they are influenced by the central nervous system and chemical receptors in the blood., That being said, hormonal balance relies much on the state of the mind. Ayurvedic psychology (*manasa shastra)* takes its wisdom from Vedanta's core principles, which provide the framework for understanding the mind and how to manage it. Such principles include discipline (tapasya), introspection and reflection (svadhyaya), surrender to God (ishwara pranidhana), the qualities of the mind (gunas)—sattva, rajas and tamas—and the power of attaining a witnessing (*sakshi bhava*) attitude towards life.

Vata – One of the key factors in hormonal balance is dependent on vata dosha, due to its correlation with the nervous system. A structured daily routine is a great place to start, because if we lose balance in our day, the entire week changes, which can in turn affect the balance of our entire month. More extended periods of stress and excessive stimulation to the nervous system can lead to chronic fatigue syndrome. Counter-acting this begins with managing vata and is all about the mind. In India, they refer to stress of this type as the "hurry, worry, curry" syndrome. The global lesson is to slow down the pace of our lives and simplify how we live and the choices we make. In general, yoga asana can be very helpful in addressing the causes of patterned, subconscious behavior, as can meditation and introspection.

Pitta - The fire of excess is what fuels pitta, driving the mind and body in everything they encounter as a way of releasing energy. As a practitioner of Ayurveda, I have discovered the majority of thyroid conditions and cases of infertility and chronic fatigue are related to high pitta. In this regard, yoga asana must be moderated, particularly in the summer, when it becomes even more depleting. Pittas do well practicing yoga early in morning or later in the evening, when temperatures are cooler, and avoiding excessively long practice. It is better to break up any task into shorter sessions. Chronic fatigue issues are more common today than ever before, and many people do not realize they are exhausted or lack real energy. Energy is often related to adrenaline. Today's workout fads focus on short intense sessions, "fast-food" exercise crammed into a lifestyle. Such turn-and-burn activities rely on adrenal function over time. The adrenal cortex produces vital life hormones such as cortisol and aldosterone. The former is a response to stress and the latter controls blood pressure. Adrenaline, produced in the adrenal medulla at the center of the gland, is also an anti-stress hormone. Both the adrenal medulla and the adrenal cortex that surrounds it are directly related to pitta. Any sign of apathy may be an initial indicator that pitta is out of balance.

Kapha – As kapha dosha strongly influences the upper chest and neck, it creates overall strength and greater muscle, bone, and fat density, not seen in vata or pitta types. With kapha, adrenal fatigue can arise during or after acute or chronic infections, especially respiratory infections such as influenza, bronchitis, or pneumonia. Such issues weigh the mind down and slow the metabolism, gradually increasing body fat and slowing the circulation vital to endocrine functionality. Circulation is the key issue for kaphas with regards to all systemic functions, and is essential to their psychological wellbeing.

The levels of certain hormones, such as thyroid-stimulating hormone or TSH, which is released by the pituitary gland, and the triiodothyronine (T3) and thyroxine (T4) produced by the thyroid, influence depression as well as binge eating disorders. There are four essential components for working with kapha and maintaining hormonal balance. Strong asana that includes some vinyasa and inversions like plow, shoulder stand, and headstand, should be practiced. Pranayama like Kapalabhati and Bastrika are excellent for increasing circulation, producing new blood cells, and increasing hemoglobin. Application of Ayurvedic herbal oils such as narayan, made with shatavari and sesame, combined with sauna or used prior to asana practice, is an important part of an integral healing approach.

The beauty of these teachings is that there is really no limitation to the number of factors that can be considered in establishing balance of the doshas and promoting a healthy life. As I have discussed, the main tools for balancing the body begin with the body itself. Asana and breath-work promote physical balance. Oils, herbs, massage, diet, and sweating systems such as sauna, full-body steaming, and local steaming, complement treatment in crucial ways that make Ayurveda effective medicine because of its inclusive approach. It is important to keep in mind that every case or condition should be considered unique and related to all the factors in this inclusive system. This includes age, geography, health history, and the particular details unique to each person's condition. Natural medicine reminds us that healing takes time. Its course, like the surrounding circumstances, is different and unique to every person. Ayurveda and Western (allopathic) medicine can come together within a unified framework to promote lasting health with minimal side-effects. Each system can be considered according to its merits in promoting social responsibility in health and wellness while improving the quality of life. A better lifestyle affords all humanity the opportunity to create greater value and appreciation for human life, which can eventually extend to creating a life of purpose or dharma.

Food as Medicine

Diet is an enormous topic that needs to made simple, universal, and based on energetics. It should not be limited to a particular viewpoint, cultural bias, or individual. In Ayurveda and ancient traditions, food was always considered medicine and a gift from the gods. Ayurvedic wisdom confirms the assertion that food can heal us by saying, "The person who has the qualities of a physician should be appointed as Head of the kitchen."[150] The idea of food as mere sustenance developed during the dark ages. As cultures lost their connection

---

150   *Susruta Samhita*, Vol lll, Chap 1.

to the spirit, they also ceased to recognize that food is also part of the Divine order of things.

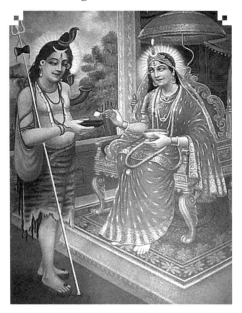

The topic of diet is probably the single most important factor in establishing health and wellness across the globe. Diet has become the most complicated feature of the urban lifestyle, with extensive options, variations, and poor food combinations that disturb the digestive process. There is no longer any debate that a whole plant-based diet is the most effective for balanced health and longevity. The increase in markets selling organic foods is not coincidental, as the importance of nutritional foods has become more widely recognized.

In an integral approach consistent with yoga, Ayurvedic diet subscribes to the concept that a balanced meal or diet is one that includes the six tastes. The six tastes correspond with the five elements and influence the related doshas. In Ayurveda, the tastes of various foods are associated with the elements and are managed according to an individual's constitution or imbalance. In this way, Ayurveda holds to the principle that there is no ideal diet for everyone to follow. How each person should eat depends on their own body type. Seasonal factors as well as age are also evaluated in deciding what foods are most important for each person.

A basic understanding of the tastes can help make diet more adaptable to your needs and serve to heal the body from diseases, injuries, and stress, as well as recover from daily exercise and work. In Ayurveda, all foods are categorized as either heating or cooling, aspects referred to collectively as *virya*. Ayurveda looks to natural food for building strength in the tissues or dhatus. It also considers food an important factor in purification of the body, unlike many modern approaches to detoxification, which starve the body with extreme juice fasts or other packaged- diet trends that include manufactured supplements. Ayurveda endorses cultivating a relationship with natural, unpackaged, locally sourced foods, as such practices will connect us to seasonal factors. It is also helpful to cultivate a geographical understanding of the climate's influence on the body. Diet should be simple, foods should be fresh, and we must eat with a calm state of mind and in a quiet and calm space.

Six Tastes (*Rasas*):

Sweet – These are starches and carbohydrates, such as bread, various grains, rice, and fruits, which are mostly composed of *earth* and *water* elements. Our bodies naturally crave sweets when we perspire from heat, as sweets increase water in the body and have a cooling quality (virya).

Salty – The seas are the main sources of salt, which is also derived from salt mines. Salt in its natural, crystalline mineral form is called rock salt. A specific type of rock salt commonly used in South Asia and India is *kala namak* or black salt, which has a pungent smell due to its high sulfur content. It is mostly composed of *water* and *fire* elements and helps the body retain water, especially during dry seasons like the fall. Salts have a heating effect (virya) on the body.

Sour – The process of fermentation, in which carbohydrates are converted to alcohol and carbon dioxide by combining yeast and bacteria, produces foods high in bacteria that are good for digestion. Such foods include pickled cucumbers, beets, radish, corn relish, Korean kimchi, sauerkraut, the popular kombucha teas, kefir, and Indian lassi, a yogurt drink often taken before dinner. Tempeh is also a great, fermented vegetarian food. These foods are pro-biotics and aid in producing healthy bacteria that provide a healthy and balanced digestion. Acidic fruits like oranges, cranberry, kiwi, lemon, limes, pineapple, strawberries, and grapefruit are some examples of sour-tasting foods. Sour foods are mainly composed of *earth* and *fire* and produce heat in the body. They should be avoided by pitta types who are out of balance.

Pungent – Black pepper, cayenne pepper, ginger, asafetida, cinnamon, cloves, and mustard seeds are some of spices that are pungent tasting. These produce heat and absorb water in the body. Pungents are composed mainly of *fire* and *air* and are best eaten by kapha types. In general, they should be moderated or reduced to a minimum during the summer. Pungents have a heating effect (virya) on the body.

Bitter – Generally, these types of foods are avoided because bitter tastes are not the most appealing to the palate. Bitter foods include coffee, which is also very acidic, unsweetened cocoa, South American yerba mate, olives, citrus peel, dandelion greens, arugula, bitter melon, bitter gourd, dill, Jerusalem artichokes, kale, saffron, fenugreek, calamus, sesame seeds, turmeric, chard, broccoli, brussel sprouts, and asparagus. Bitters are mostly composed of *air* and *ether* and are cooling (virya). They are therefore excellent for pitta types, with the exception of coffee, due to its acidic nature.

Astringent – Astringent foods are somewhat rare and have a drying effect on the body. Astringent tastes have an airy quality and effect, and therefore can increase vata rather quickly. Some astringent foods include the tannins in green or black tea, which have a diuretic effect on the body, and red wine. Most beans, which are known to be gassy and to increase vata, white potatoes, green bananas, pomegranate, most berries, including blueberries and cranberries, poppy seeds, and nutmeg are examples of astringent foods. These foods are mostly composed of *earth* and *air* and have a cooling effect (virya) on the body.

Vegetarianism

The dietary practice of vegetarianism is commonly associated with yoga, and has been part of this tradition since Vedic times. Vegetarianism found its place in the American counter-culture of the 1960s, and also has some connection to practitioners of mind-body medicine. Vegetarianism should not be restricted to yogis or other such groups, but should be established as a practice that embraces natural law. All living entities have an equal right to life. The expression "Holy Cow!" originates from the Vedic tradition, which honors the cow as sacred and symbolic of Divine Mother's love for her earthly children and the feeling capacity innate to women. It's no coincidence that in the United States more adult women are vegetarian than men.[151] Eating whole, plant-based type foods is a practice of living compassionately on this planet, particularly during these times when hunting for our food is rarely required.

In yoga, vegetarianism is born of the principle of ahimsa, which fosters respect and appreciation for all living things. Today, however, many people have chosen to become vegetarian based on scientific facts about its health benefits, rather than considering its practice from a moral and ethical perspective. In such cases, when the desire for meat-based foods is suppressed by logic, the habit eventually returns, due to subtle indwelling desires in the mind or vasanas. While samskaras reflect the habitual patterns set in place by the subconscious mind, vasanas fuel our actions from the unseen, subliminal portion of the mind. They give perpetual force to our behavior, until the mind's activity is arrested through pranayama, mantra, meditation, and proper lifestyle that adheres to the moral and ethical codes of conduct, the yamas and niyamas.

---

151   A study published by *Vegetarian Times* shows that 3.2 percent of U.S. adults, or 7.3 million people, follow a vegetarian-based diet. Vegetarian Research Group, Vegetarian Times, Harris Interactive Service Bureau. Research date: June 2013.

All of these can be defined as part of the core sadhana or disciplinary regimen. Outer sadhana is reflected in the yamas, niyamas, asana, and pranayama. It has great therapeutic value on the level of the body and emotions, and plays a vital factor in managing our patterns of eating and exerting discipline over the senses. In many cases, the decision to become vegetarian for health purposes can slowly bring about the understanding and compassion of ahimsa. Both sides, therapeutic and ethical, of the vegetarian diet can be equally valid reasons for making it a powerful, life-changing habit.

Many yogis make the foolish decision to eat meat as the result of thoughts born from actions connected to cravings and desires stemming from previous habit patterns. They do not exercise discernment, which empowers the mind with the capacity to discriminate (viveka) between what our biology actually needs and our conditioned psychology. Such statements as "Oh my body needs meat, it needs the protein" or "I cannot fast—going without food or missing any of my meals makes me dizzy and then I have no energy" are nonsense. They stem from excessive attachment to the body and misinterpretation of the body's actual nutritional needs due to mental conditioning or lack of discipline.

No living creature wants to be eaten. Most animals fear humans and vice-versa due to the fragmentation of our mind-body relationship and our separation from nature and the elements. An interesting contradiction exists between the basic human instinct of self-preservation and those who follow a non-vegetarian diet. While most people fear close encounters with animals and would not even consider the act of killing and butchering the animal, they often effortlessly savor the pleasure of eating meat to satisfy their gustatory desires. Everyone naturally cringes at the sight or smell of dead animal flesh, or when passing a butcher shop's trash bin. However, at the sight of a colorful fruit stand, our mouth salivates with delight. I think it's for this same reason that many groceries stock fruits and vegetables near the entrance of the store, while the meats are kept in the rear.

All violence stems from fear, and therefore fearlessness (*abhayam*)[152] is required to fully embrace the practice of ahimsa. In 1935, when Yogananda visited Mahatma Gandhi at his ashram, he asked him to give his definition of ahimsa. Gandhi said, "The avoidance of harm to any living creature in thought or deed." From both the yoga and Ayurveda perspectives, there are two main points to consider. The principle of ahimsa plays a pivotal role in the evolution of human consciousness, as respect for life does not exist apart from nature, but supports cultivating a relationship with the Divine through nature. Any

---

152   Bhagavad Gita, Chap, 16, verse 1.

practice of anger in thought, harsh language, or hurtful action towards any living creature comes from deep-seated internal fear. Many yogis have shown that a harmonious mind and loving heart change the entire vibration of the aura. Animals can sense this, and it removes their instinctual fight-or-flight behavior. Swami Rama Tirtha used to approach tigers and bears in the wild Himalayan foothills with complete fearlessness, and encountered no violence from these imposing creatures.

In Ayurveda, vegetarianism is generally endorsed for longevity and its sattvic quality, which promotes the evolution of life's mind-body-spirit triad. In some cases of chronic or debilitating diseases, use of various meats is considered effective in Ayurveda. However, this depends on the specific condition and other factors related to the doshas, the person's health history, and so on.

Vegetarianism, or a whole food, plant-based diet, is being endorsed by many doctors[153] of allopathic medicine for its effects in reversing heart disease, lowering cholesterol, and treating obesity, diabetes, and many other afflictions. Diet is one of the main things I emphasize in my Ayurvedic counseling, because everyone has to eat food. Much can be gained by teaching people a proper nutritional relationship with food, according to their dosha type and seasonal considerations. Diets don't work. However, awareness, discipline, and universal scientific principles do, and the Ayurvedic approach promotes accord with natural wisdom.

Why No! Onions and Garlic

Both yoga and Ayurveda endorse what is termed a sattvic or pure diet. The term "sattvic" with regards to diet means vegetarian, pure, natural, organic, and having a spiritually conscious relationship with food. This means that all foods are recognized as Divine and blessed by the compassionate goddess Annapurna. Ayurveda prioritizes balance of the doshas and living a relatively healthy life as prerequisites to the spiritual path.

As I previously mentioned, this may at times require eating "unsattvic" foods. Garlic (*rashona*), for example, is considered a very effective food as it contains all six tastes except sour. It is a strong detoxifier and improves respiration, blood, and lymphatic function, and can be helpful in fighting parasitic infections. However, it has a strong grounding affect and dulls the mind, which makes it tamasic rather than sattvic.

---

153 Dean Ornish, MD, author of *Reversing Heart Disease*. Caldwell B. Esselstyn, Jr., MD, of the Cleveland Clinic since 1968, was featured in the pro-vegetarian documentary *Forks Over Knives*.

Onions are also very strong in flavor, although less medicinal in effect. They also have a stimulating quality on both the physiology and the mind. In yoga, both garlic and onions are avoided because they disturb the mind and make it harder to attain its natural state of calm and peace. Therefore, for yogis practicing Raja Yoga, onions and garlic should be avoided as they make a sound meditation practice more difficult.

Keep in mind that avoiding such foods is not the key to success in experiencing mystical meditation. Nonetheless, it is one of many important factors that yoga looks towards for improving the meditative experience. What this means is that everything matters and nothing should be considered inconsequential on the path towards spiritual oneness. In the diets of many cultures, garlic and onions serve as a cheap flavoring, as these are among the least expensive foods on the market. If you have a habit of eating out, it will be very difficult to avoid these foods, as they are literally in everything. Avoiding them will inevitably turn the yogi towards cooking more at home, where the ideal sattvic meal can be more easily created.

Fasting

The practice of fasting is a valuable way to heal the body of many ailments, and serves as a type of austerity that promotes mind-body synergy. Fasting is also an effective way to increase the body's vital energy or ojas and strengthen immunity.

Eating solid foods requires much energy and digestive power. Along with over-eating and poor food combinations, both of which are very common today, this burdens the stomach and gastrointestinal tract, leaving behind traces of waste that become toxic. Liquid or fruit fasts are the most effective and common today. They include drinking hot teas and fresh fruit and vegetable juices. Triphala is a mild Ayurvedic formula that can be taken during a fast to promote cleansing of the bowels. It consists of three fruit powders, each of which brings balance to the doshas: haritaki (vata), amalaki (pitta), and bibitaki (kapha). It can be easily found at most health-food stores. There are some basic Ayurvedic guidelines that should be followed when fasting for the best results.

Three Main Considerations Before Starting a Fast:

- **Body type (prakriti) and any symptoms of imbalance (vikriti)** Knowledge of your constitution or any imbalances can be helpful in deciding which types of fruit and vegetable juices and herbal teas to fast on.

- **The season** – Fasting can be more effective with awareness of the season. For example, in summer time, vata and pitta types must be very careful not to dehydrate through excess sweating, and should also be cautious about excessive exercise or strenuous work, which can deplete them. Fasting for vata and pitta types during very hot or dry weather should be limited to one to two days maximum, or avoided altogether if there is an imbalance. Kapha types do best fasting in the winter or spring.

- **Duration** – Vata types can fast from one to two days, pitta types can go up to three days, and kapha types can fast for over three days. The duration of any fast will also depend on a secondary dosha in the constitution, especially with the dual types vata-kapha and pitta-kapha.

In choosing what types of juices and teas to fast on, the six tastes should be considered, just the same as with regular dietary practices. Kapha types will do well with pungent tastes added to morning teas. This includes the spices used in Indian chai: cinnamon, cardamom, cloves, ginger, and black peppercorns. Vata types do better with milder spices such as cumin, coriander, fennel, and licorice. Pitta teas can consists of coriander, hibiscus, peppermint leaf, rose flower, and licorice. An Ayurvedic herbal combination of ten roots, called dashmool, can be used as a powerful detoxifier. It reduces pain in the joints, promotes hydration, and builds strength in the tissues.

All fruit and vegetable fluids should be taken at room temperature, or slightly cooled if fasting during the summer. Tea or any fluid drunk in morning should be hot, as this relaxes and opens the bowels, loosens toxins in the stomach, and promotes circulation. When fasting in warmer climates, such as the sub-tropical, it is good to choose bitter fruits and vegetables.

When a new client comes to me for consultation, I often recommend fasting for one day per week or twice per month as a disciplinary exercise. This is a simple way to learn that "Man shall not live by bread alone, but by every word that proceedeth out of the mouth of God."[154] Fasting is a way to overcome the ego-mind's conditioning that food alone is what keeps us alive. Fasting is a practice of embracing Divine existence and promotes mental strength over the body. Fasting uplifts the mind, as it promotes sattva and increases inner radiance or tejas and the upward flow of prana. Fasting is a powerful ritual consistent with many of the world traditions, an observance of the highest type of purification.

---

154   Matthew 4:4.

In many of my cases, I have seen fasting reduce depression and increase sleep and concentration. Fasting is something that everyone can benefit from, although is not required for young children. Short fasts can be done by older teenagers as an austerity. However, it should not be done for more than one day, as their digestive fire is very strong. Fasting should be avoided during pregnancy, as nutrition for the developing fetus is critical. One of the most important points to consider when fasting is to double the fluid intake that would otherwise be consumed at meals. Room-temperature spring water is especially vital, so that the body maintains essential mineral nutrients while cleansing itself. The spring season has always been symbolic of renewal and purification, and fasting can be quite effective then for promoting greater health and wellness in your life.

Balancing Our Natural Urges

The body produces natural signs to inform us of the need to release the excess energy produced by our karma, mind, senses, and emotions. These urges are indicators that should not be ignored. If so, complications leading to imbalances of the doshas may occur. There are thirteen natural factors that keep the body functioning in balance. Any suppression of these will imbalance the mind-body synergy.

There are various symptoms that indicate some obstruction to these urges, and Ayurveda encourages us not only to avoid suppressing these, but more importantly to understand their relationship with the mind. The mind is responsible for how the body operates and any symptoms that arise are an opportunity for inner reflection and more intimate awareness of the higher Self. These urges greatly influence the balance of the doshas, and their proper functioning should not be disregarded. I have listed some simple remedies for issues resulting from suppression of these urges below. The term "suppression" means there has been either a voluntary or unconscious blockage of this function. Health issues related to these thirteen functions arise from mind-body fragmentation, which is a result of mental conditioning and poor lifestyle regimens.

Urine – Peacock (Mayurasana), bow (Dhanurasana) and cobra (Bhujangasana) stimulate the urinary bladder. Gentle steam, warm baths, massage, and enemas are also recommended.

Feces – Chair pose and spinal twist (Ardha Matsyendrasana) are good postures for massaging the colon. Warm baths are calming to the nerves, and clockwise abdominal massage with oil is helpful for moving the stool, as of course are enemas.

Semen – Rice, milk, stimulation, and massage or pressure on the *guda marma* or point between rectum and genitals, sexual intercourse, and dashmool enema are all recommended.

Flatulence – Lie down in a left-lateral position for few minutes, followed by the lithotomy position, commonly used during labor. Lying flat on the back with the legs pulled back to the sides of the torso relaxes the sphincter around the anus. The knees-to-chest yoga pose (Pavanamuktasana) is also effective in removing gas, because the pressure on the abdomen relaxes the intestinal wall. Running in place for 15 to 30 seconds and a balanced yoga practice are also usually effective.

Vomiting – This is a strong urge that, when suppressed, has strong adverse effects. Such interventions as fasting, smoking certain herbs,[155] blood-letting or leech therapy, yoga asana, and castor-oil purgation (virechana) are recommended.

Sneezing – Massaging the head and neck area, steam, Kapalabhati pranayama, nasal-oil drops, and a vata-pacifying diet are recommended.

Belching – This often indicates excess air in the stomach or indigestion. Yoga asana, walking, and combining forward and backward bends, as in the sun salutation, are appropriate.

Yawning – Vata treatments like shirodhara,[156] a vata-pacifying diet, and deep sleep are appropriate.

Hunger and Thirst – Eating of bulking foods like ghee, yogurt, milk, grains, and even meat would be required if the body has been exposed to harsh suppression of these urges. Oil-pulling and gargles are helpful in reducing the dryness in the throat produced by thirst. Sweet and salty tastes increase water retention and mineral absorption.

Tears – When the eyes tear, the fluid released through the ducts cleanses the eyes and has a calming effect on the nerve tissue, as tearing is a natural release of the nerves. Sleep is very important, as is calming herbal smoke and soothing chamomile tea.

---

155   In Ayurveda various herbs are used to inhale into the lungs to produce medicinal affects on the lungs, respiratory and nervous systems, and digestion. Note: This point does not refer to cannabis and its particular uses in recent times.

156   The word shirodhara comes from the Sanskrit words *shiro* (head) and *dhara* (flow), This is one of the most popular treatments in Ayurveda. It involves pouring a warm stream of oil over the forehead, which has a strong calming effect on the mind and nervous system.

Sleep – Only one thing can replace lack of sleep, and that is sleep itself. It has no substitute except enlightenment.

Breathing (after strong exercise and other exertion) – Lack of breathing sometimes occurs in those persons with poor cardiovascular conditioning, or those who exercise in places that lack fresh air or work in hazardous areas. Vata-balancing guidelines must be addressed in these cases.

Ayurvedic Parameters of Balanced Doshas and Signs of Spiritual Development

- Digestion – Strong digestive fire, passing at least one stool per day in the morning, and sometimes another in the afternoon.

- Abdomen - No feelings of discomfort or signs of distention, especially after eating.

- Sleep - Easy to fall sound asleep at night without interruption for five to eight hours. Napping only in summer time. At times, less sleep is required.

- Tongue – Clear, smooth, no white coating, natural pinkish color.

- Eyes - Clear, lustrous, no twitching, itchiness, or dryness.

- Skin - Nice luster, even-colored, no dryness or flaking around the joints.

- Mental Attitude - Good mental focus and concentration, able to listen and digest information before making a decision, cheerfulness, positive outlook in all circumstances. Fearless, equanimous, peaceful, and serene.

- Spine - Supple, straight, and erect, with good flexion and range of rotation.

- Body – Lightness and good strength, flexibility, and circulation. Luster in the eyes and no strong odor from the body.

- Character – Consistent in family, friendship, and work relationships and environments.

- Attitude – Adaptable to social, personal, and environmental changes. Avoids gossip and excessive socializing.

- Contentment – Able to do things alone, enjoy periods of silence and solitude, and maintain a simple lifestyle.

- Sex – A balanced sex life is important, as suppression of this urge can create health complications. Sexual intimacy is to be shared in marriage or in committed relationships only. Integral yoga practices are also helpful in transmuting sexual force into spiritual power through meditation.

- Spiritual – Yearning for enlightenment, a pull towards meditation, an attraction to nature and silence, enjoyment of solitude, absence of aversion towards anyone, a growing feeling that every form of life and the world are all Divine.

The Stages of Life

One of the fascinating things about life is observing the various stages that we go through from infancy onward. Our needs, interests, and perspectives on life change as we explore the mystery of living in this world. We often do not take account of the fact that we only have so long to live. We just presume our passing will come "later on" in life.

If we consider that the current world-wide life expectancy is about 66 years for both sexes, we might rethink how we live and the choices we make. I have always thought that the world would be a much different place if at birth we were also given the exact time of our death. If we knew the exact moment or even year of our physical death, would that change our attitudes, the choices we make, and how we treat others? It certainly would be a great experiment. I've noticed that people generally express greater humility and are more sincere and loving when their health is at risk. Vedic wisdom teaches us that life is a priceless gift, a Divine blessing, and an opportunity to learn and discover the hidden treasure within us.

The Ayurvedic texts or *samhitas* mention that life expectancy is 100 years or *varsha shata*. This claim of the ideal age is also found in the passage from the Yajur Veda, called the *"Jeevem Sharada Shatam"*: "Let us see the sun for 100 years, let us breathe for 100 years, let us live for 100 years."

Although the current life expectancy figure includes many third-world Asian, African, and South American countries, it does give us an indication that we do not have that much time on the planet. Regardless, people continue to live blindly, as if not knowing when we will die validates abusing the fundamental principles of health, ethics, and truth. Societal norms toss us into an endless cycle of desires, chasing ego-centered ideas until one is lost in boredom or no longer entertained by the show of life.

In modern times, we have fallen into the pattern of equating being successful with having money and acquiring things, only to learn the hard way that money cannot buy happiness. Luxuries can often keep us distracted from the real, if subtle, truths of life, which lie hidden behind the experiences we do not seem to understand. Life is tricky and, as we have all experienced, often unpredictable. We know of our true calling. We hear it in our inner voice. However, what is required to attain it is a real shift. This involves the great risk of going against the grain of our society's and often family's expectations, and overcoming our personal fears. In the end, the goal is the arrival of our truth, a greater understanding and awareness of who we really are. What seems initially to be a sacrifice is in reality not one at all, once we realize what has been gained. Sacrifices are blessings in disguise, because eventually the real value of a balanced life is discovered.

The wisdom of the Vedic traditions explains that if you balance your life between the spiritual, inner world of the yoga disciplines, and the natural outer world of the Ayurvedic disciplines and our daily responsibilities, in such a way that you are in accord with the stages of life, you will develop properly as a human being and spare yourself much wasted time. It is important to remember that as we end one life stage, we begin another. The ideal of service to humanity is a theme in all four stages. In every stage of life, we serve the Divine through our human interactions, while learning more about ourselves

These stages of human life were originally known as the ashramas, and provide the basis for living in the way that most efficiently heals the body, mind, and soul. The four stages of life are detailed below. Each has its own duties and responsibilities, which demonstrate our capacities and potentials for spiritual and human evolution. The first two phases are correlated to living in harmony with nature and our outer life with respect to personal development, social responsibility, and vocation. The second two stages deal with the spirit and our inner practices of learning to live "in the world but not of it." They include enjoying periods of solitude and the practice of silence, pranayama, mantra, and deep meditation. These are four periods of time all mankind must pass through in order to live a balanced life. Success lies in aligning oneself with the characteristics and responsibilities of each stage.

Student Stage

This student stage, known as *brahmacharya,* begins at approximately the age of seven, after a child has been raised and nurtured by loving parents and can begin to perform certain tasks on their own. This period lasts until the student has reached their mid-twenties or approximately twenty-five years of age. During this period, quality education should be attained, disciplinary skills developed, and a respect for elders established.

Vedic wisdom stipulates that parents are not the best teachers, because they either spoil the child or impose undesirable traits of their own. Children must be taught the qualities of character development at spiritual centers such as the ashram of an enlightened teacher-guru-preceptor. This may not be the most realistic and practical arrangement today, but, as spiritual ideals continue to expand in our society, a similar concept may develop.

In this setting, children are given initiation (*diksha*) and learn daily disciplinary practices, such as rising early, taking baths, chanting mantras such as the *gayatri japa* to the rising sun, and the study of scriptures and the sciences. In later years, the principles of business and self-defense are also taught, enabling the student to cope with all types of people and life circumstances.

Sending your child off to such a highly disciplined school may seem odd for many parents, but it eliminates a very common problem that children face today as they grow into adults, which is that they inherit their parents' habits and faults. A great deal of time is then spent undoing much of what the child has unfairly been exposed to. There is a somewhat sad expression that goes: "The first half of our lives is ruined by our parents. The second half is ruined by our children." Later in life, grown children return to their parents all that they were exposed to.

In the 1980s, two great educators and infant specialists named Magda Gerber and Tom Forrest, MD, a pediatric neurologist, began educating parents on the proper guidelines and principles of allowing infants creative exploration in a safe environment. Gerber says, "An infant always learns. The less we interfere with the natural process of learning, the more we can observe how much infants learn all the time." This type of education for parents can save children from often paralyzing narcissistic traits that can leave them clueless about who they really are or what great talents they may have buried within themselves.

Most importantly, students in this first, brahmacharya stage are given specific guidance on sexuality and how to use sexual energy morally, ethically, and for the purpose of procreation, as they begin the second stage of householder (*grihastha*). In modern times, sex has been confused with love. Seeking it in this way becomes a form of "mental masturbation" that is never satisfying and creates physical attachment, mental insecurity, and emotional instability. The term *brahm-acharya* literally means control or mastery over this creative energy.

Householder Stage

This stage is known as grihastha. Marriage vows are usually taken, as a stable home promotes creativity and influences all aspects of our life. Family life and partnership provide support for enduring the journey on the spiritual path. Rama and Sita of the epic Ramayama are the symbols of fidelity, unconditional love, and the balance of inner powers that enable us attain victory over maya, the world's illusions. What the previous stage teaches us is first to study and learn more about who we are as individuals. Then we will go into a relationship or marriage with a clearer understanding of what our needs really are. In this way, we are better able to choose a compatible partner. Those that think that they will find everlasting santosha or contentment through another person, and therefore postpone personal development to a later time, are mistaken. The first stage is primarily a preparation phase for a long-lasting marriage and success in the business world. This concept of social and personal development in the brahmacharya stage is consistent with the principles of the yamas and niyamas of the *Ashtanga Yoga Sutras,* in that lifestyle disciplines need to be in place to a certain degree in order for there to be sound spiritual progress in the techniques and practices of yoga.

Seclusion Stage

This third stage is called *vanaprastha* and serves as a preparation for the final stage, renunciation. The seclusion stage is a necessary step towards developing greater mastery over the senses. More time is spent away from family life and in seclusion, often studying scriptures, meditating, and practicing silence and solitude. Gradually, in this stage of life, more discipline over the creative sexual energy should be attained to transmute this energy and raise the kundalini upwards through the spinal charkas. In yoga, the natural urge to procreate is shifted into a process of controlling and redirecting the sexual energy. This can be done in conjunction with a comprehensive lifestyle that embraces spirituality. In this stage, a couple often returns for deeper study with a guru or spiritual teacher, in preparation for the highest renunciation.

Surrender Stage

The term *sannyas* is commonly used for those who take final vows of renunciation in an ashram or monastery. However, this is more than just joining an ashram and wearing a robe. It is the highest level of surrender to God. Practically speaking, sannyas means to give back to the world and completely surrender to the ideal of inner freedom and detachment from the worldly temperament. It is a great time to dedicate oneself to selfless service and guide others to a balanced, spiritual way of life.

Personal Relationships

One relationship that I have not discussed is that of an intimate, personal type. There are many types of relationships that we have in our lives, from family to friendships, work, intimate partnerships or marriage, and social acquaintances. Intimate relationships play the strongest role in our lives, because all souls are born into a new life with the innate desire to find the "one" love or partner we will share our life with. This instinctual desire produces a yearning in our hearts for living a balanced life.

Vedic wisdom propounds a four-fold balanced approach to life through the four aims, which are affection and intimacy (kama), work or vocation (artha), purposeful life (dharma), and spiritual liberation (moksha). Taken together, these four aims constitute a holistic lifestyle.

In the Yoga Tantra teachings, Shiva and Shakti, who represent the sun and moon, symbolize the supreme relationship in life. Esoterically speaking, such a relationship can be established by means of balancing the solar and lunar forces of prana that flow through the pingala and ida nadis or channels. The Shiva-Shakti union through yoga is established by virtue of practicing mantra, pranayama, and meditation, along with all the Hatha Yoga practices I have discussed earlier.

The culmination of yoga is union with God or the Divine. The big question for many is, who is the "one" and where do we find him or her. The basis for an intimate relationship or marriage is that we identify with the Divine in whomever we become attracted to. Through this way of noticing the Divine reflection in our partner, we save ourselves from "falling" in love, and rather experience the arising and growth of our spiritual life. When we recognize the Divine in our partner, we are focusing on the person's positive attributes and qualities. As we grow in spiritual consciousness, we learn to embrace the

Divine, which abides in all living things. Marriage or spiritual partnership is a commitment of accepting each other just as we are. Through mutual support, guidance, individual and shared sadhana, and natural lifestyle, such a personal relationship can greatly serve us in our spiritual development.

Chapter TEN

The Relationship of Spirit and Ecology

*The goal of life is to make your heartbeat match the beat of the
universe, to match your nature with Nature.*
Joseph Campbell (1904 – 1987).

Ecology as a Spiritual Primer

Ecology is a broad term for the relationships that living organisms have with
one another and the environment. Yoga and Ayurveda provide us the tools
and understanding to improve our spiritual ecosphere in such a way that our
surroundings, environment, and interactions with other living entities can
become doorways for spiritual growth and the healing of the mind and body.
Our world can be observed through scientific principles, which in turn can
give us an idea of how it operates and affects our lives. Although science has
only a limited grasp of our higher spiritual purpose or moksha dharma, it
can improve our lifestyle, health, and happiness through what we might call
spiritual ecology. The practical wisdom of the five elements is the backbone of
an Ayurvedic approach to creating a healthy mind-body relationship through
natural means. In what we might call Vedic ecology, the five elements are called
panchavati or "five forests." It is said that every village must keep a bundle of five
trees from the forest, with each tree representing one of the five great elements.

Ayurveda teaches us how to embrace Mother Nature, for she can transform and
enable us to enter the spiritual domain through the external world. While yoga
teaches us how to turn our attention inward to discover our true Self, Ayurveda
teaches us how we can heal ourselves by improving our relationship with the
external world by means of the spirit hidden within nature and the elements.

While environmentalism is often equated with ecology, it really only reflects a small aspect of our cultural sociology. I use the terms *spiritual ecology* and *spirit-ecos* to refer to the way in which our lifestyle, understanding of nature's basic laws, and life purpose are all interrelated. Culturally speaking, we could say that people are becoming more "spiritual," rather than "religious," through a renewed communal ecology. Improving our personal relationship with our ecology naturally promotes the principles and values that uphold any true religion.

Spirit-ecos brings the world together to learn a common language and establish an eternal relationship with Divine Mother, which can guide us into a unified dimension of consciousness. Spirit-ecos helps us comprehend that our personal choices and actions impact global ecology. Spirit-ecos is about acquiring greater personal accountability. Ecologists and some in spiritual circles speak about healing the planet, this being an indirect way of saying we need to heal humanity. Ecological responsibility begins with education and simple living. This can both increase spirituality on the planet and affect how we produce.

I believe the work of Vandana Shiva,[157] for example, is part of a global movement that has become aware of the important relationship between humanity and nature. It can be said that ecology begins with how we grow our food, as this is the most direct relationship we have with nature, and in turn influences our health and the global environment we all share. Some are fortunate enough to reflect and discover that spirit is who they actually are. Others find spirit hidden in the collective consciousness of oneness revealed by Mother Earth's relationship with her father, the sun, and her mother, the moon. This relationship is both one-in-three and three-in-one.

Integral Ecology

The partnership of the sun and moon has always played an integral role in Vedic culture. In yoga, the Shiva and Shakti paradigm is symbolized by Mount Kailash and Lake Manasarova,[158] which are found next to one another in western Tibet. Ayurveda propounds the stabilizing effects nature and the five elements

---

157   An Indian environmental activist and anti-globalization author.
158   The name "Manasarovara" is a combination of two Sanskrit words, "manas" meaning mind and "sarovara" meaning lake. It was created in the mind of Lord Brahma and symbolizes the womb of life, as it is the source of the four great rivers of India, the Brahmaputra, Ghaghara, Indus, and Sutlej. Mount Kailash is symbolic of the heights of consciousness hidden within the human body, and also represents liberation. Both Mount Kailash and Lake Manasarovara are pilgrimage sites, attracting many Hindu yogic devotees from all over the world. It also has strong connections to the Buddhist religion, as the Buddha was said to have meditated there and visited nearby areas.

have on the mind-body relationship. Vedic ecology elucidates the idea of the three aspects of the forest, the organic, abundant, and spiritual, as a metaphor for the earth. The wisdom of Vedic ecology is based on a four-fold integrative system that includes trees, animals, water, and humans. The fundamental principle of Vedic ecology is that these four tenets are integrated equally and not segregated one from another.

Four Tenets of Vedic Ecology

Trees – Trees naturally symbolize the forest and also represent each of the five elements. Vedic culture has always been connected to trees through the guru-disciple relationship, which includes initiation and the sharing of the wisdom of universal law. The tree can be considered the guru or elder of the forest. In yogic thought, the tree is seen as upturned, with its roots representing the entry of consciousness into the head or medulla oblongata. Trees help us learn, providing direct connection to the inner vibrations of the earth. They also furnish humans with shade in the summer, and serve as an umbrella in the rain. Trees cast an aura of strength and have a majestic quality that often leaves us in awe. Trees are to be acknowledged in the construction of villages, and their placement, direction, and quality must be considered.

Vedic architecture or *vastu* is an important branch of the ancient Indian learning that applies the principles of the five elements to structures and their relationship with nature. It is similar to Chinese feng shui, although older, and contains concepts also found in Ayurveda and yoga. Vastu embraces the relationship between physical structures and the earth, and also deals with the influence of the sun and moon on their placement.

Animals – The Laws of Manu or *Manusmṛti* recognize that all living things are part of one eternal family. This includes the relationship between man and animals. As George Bernard Shaw said, "Animals are my friends...and I don't eat my friends."

All animals inhabit a wild forest or *mahavan* that maintains its original, organic state, untouched by humans. In the villages, the cow, with its gentle nature, is in the closest proximity with humans. The cow is symbolic of Mother Prakriti or Mother Nature, and signifies the maternal quality of nurturing home and family. Homes always had a special room for the cow. While some of this still exists in India today, it is not as common. Even after World War II, cows still roamed the streets of major cities like Delhi and Kolkata, although the government has recently enacted laws segregating them into special areas to reduce accidents and improve hygiene and water purity. Oxen and bulls are still used instead of machinery in small rural farms for various agricultural purposes. However, elsewhere in today's world, animals are incarcerated in places we call zoos, and placed behind bars, walls, and fences to be stared at and ridiculed, deepening the great divide that now exists between humans and animals.

Water – Water in the form of rivers, streams, and lakes brings life to trees and provides a rich source of minerals for crops and herbs. Water brings prosperity, fertility, and cleanliness, and improves hygiene. Water is the element connected to the god Vishnu, being the force of preservation that provides a sense of support, nurturing families and villagers. Harvesting rainwater is an ecological practice. Rainwater is precious and contains the energy of the heavens.

Humans – A balanced lifestyle depends on an amalgamation of humans, trees, animals, and water. The human being is spirit incarnate. Through the laws of karma, mankind can find a life in harmony with nature. This integrative approach from long ago still appears today throughout Asian households, with many people in the same family sharing a home. In India and other parts of South Asia, it is very common to see young couples or adults living with their parents or grandparents.

In the Western world, this idea seems ludicrous and tortuous to some. Cities are filled with high-rise apartment buildings, boxes in the sky, where single people live separate from each other, their families, animals, and nature. With the advent of concrete in the last 150 years, humans in cities have become even more literally out of touch with the earth. A question I pose during lectures I give in major cities is, "How often do you touch the grass or the earth?" It is always remarkable to learn that many have had no contact with the earth in weeks, sometimes months. Major cities throughout the world pose a threat to sustainable living as long as humanity is separated from nature.

The Trinity of Nature, Spirit, and Forests

The reawakening of spirituality in the modern age must include a relationship with nature if it is to endure. The spiritual wisdom of the East is finding its place in the Western world after millennia of being confined to Asia. The material and technological advancements of the West are in great need of the unhurried values of the tradition-based societies of the East. A unified framework for balanced living has only recently arrived on Western shores, just as Asian cultures are beginning to follow in the footsteps of America.

Our entry into the bronze age or Dwapara Yuga is evident from the global recognition of yoga and, more specifically, with the sweeping interest in the alluring wisdom and colorful lifestyle of Indian culture. Presently, India has the second largest population in the world, only slightly behind China's. Even with the extreme diversity of its people, it remains a land devoted to the Divine. The seeds of this spiritual quality were planted in the forests long ago, during the early Vedic era. Ever since, spirit and nature have been inseparable in the culture.

The Hindu teachings mention three kinds of forest that are nature's ambassadors to the human spirit. The first is the natural, untamed forest or *mahavan,* where nature and all the elements remain intact. The mahavan provides support for life and abides in accord with the energy of preservation. This reflects the importance of conservation in a balanced and sustainable ecosystem. On the spiritual side, this corresponds to the god Vishnu, also known as Narayana, who is the preserver of the cosmos and all things.

The second type of forest is that of abundance, the *shrivan*, which is utilized for growing orchards and is farmed to provide fruits, vegetables, timber, and other commodities that produce wealth. This forest, where things of all sorts are created and re-created, is associated with the god Brahman, the force of creation and representative of the Supreme Reality. The word Brahman originates from the Sanskrit root *bṛh-*: "to swell, expand and grow."

The third type of forest is for sadhana. It provides a hermitage for stillness and austerities. The *tapovan* or forest of Shiva, the lord of yogis, is a place for seclusion, where the seeds of bad and selfish habits can be destroyed. The vibrations of nature and the elements are an enormous boon for meditation and introspection. In the tapovan, a sadhaka or aspirant can work with the maha prana in a unified manner, without the disturbing currents of gossip, commerce, and family life. As we grow in our understanding of nature and the spiritual significance it has in the evolution of mankind, we also embrace the original relationship of the sun, moon, and earth.

Dharma and Ecology

The word *dharma* is a very powerful term in Vedic wisdom used to describe various principles. Dharma is one of those words that encompass a broad spectrum of spiritual categories used in many contexts. The Sanskrit word dharma is derived from the root *dhar*, which means to support or uphold, and is mostly used in an ethical sense, as a principle of truth. There are many types of spiritual dharmas in yoga and related traditions such as Buddhism. For example Buddhism has its Three Jewels: the Buddha, meaning the mind's perfection in enlightenment; the Dharma, meaning the teachings and main principles of the Buddhist system; and the Sangha, meaning the support and guidance given through community.

Patanjali's eight limbs of yoga can be considered major "dharmas" of the yoga tradition. When we live our lives in accordance with these spiritual truths, we are following our highest dharma, and synchronizing our individual consciousness with cosmic, universal intelligence. As we grow into spirit-ecos, our dharma is naturally revealed. The highest dharma of life is the evolution of the soul, and as long as we disregard our ecology, we are also ignoring the very fabric of our existence. Dharma and ecology play vital roles in creating peaceful societies.

Living in accord with universal principles provides us with guidance leading to our finding a sacred place within ourselves. This sacred alignment is about following our inner heart or conscience to bring about a balanced outer life. This balanced place in life lies between activity and passivity. In our active world, we fulfill our responsibilities in relationships, work, hobbies, and so on. In our more passive or interior world, we create time for introspection, inner study, and devotion for the Divine. The sacred space between these two aspects is the mythology of our lives, which can become a doorway into greater knowledge, health, and happiness.

Dharma explains that everything is interconnected and nothing is unaccounted for. Attuning to our life purpose can help us live in our truth. Any denial of truth keeps us bound to the cycles of birth and death or samsara. It is like thinking you are walking forward, when in fact whenever you take a step forward you take one step back. Not ever realizing it, you end up in the same place you have been for some time: nowhere.

People coming to Ayurveda for the first time are taking a huge step forward in improving the quality of their lives. They are beginning to realize that their inner life must be intrinsically connected to their outer life. The practice of Ayurveda is about aligning ourselves with the highest dharma, with the intention of balancing the body-mind relationship and reaching the highest place. When the body and mind do not honor their dharma, you can do all the yoga, meditation, and studying in the world, and it will still get you nowhere.

The moment there is a spark of interest in following your dharma, the opportunity must be seized, or it may not appear again for a long time. One of the challenges that our modern urban societies face is the obstacle of instant gratification, in which expectations of rapid returns leave us feeling empty-handed if we don't immediately reap the fruit of our actions. Ayurveda and yoga, as healing systems for the body, mind, and soul, are concerned with spiritual evolution. This takes time and is in fact calculated over many lifetimes. So if we create expectations measured by a worldly time scale, we are in trouble. True soul evolution will never satisfy the current state of mind that seeks instantaneous results for our efforts. The practice of yoga and Ayurvedic principles requires a sacrifice of time and the willingness to surrender all attachment to what you may believe to be the purpose of your existence. This is not to say that practice of these principles will not produce visible results in one life. It simply means that many of these changes happen on such a subtle level that, though things may be very different, such differences do not always manifest externally. As we evolve through a life of dharma we learn both to embrace and surrender to the Divine order of things.

Discovering Your Dharma

There is this place within ourselves that we can all discover. It is our very own abode of truth. This place feels true to our being and reveals itself in language that aligns with our deepest wishes. Few understand this and sometimes even those who understand question it. In spite of this, we still know what we must do to bring us what we need to fulfill our heart's deepest cravings.

I remember the empty feeling I had inside for many years in my mid-twenties when I worked on different jobs and business ventures that barely fulfilled even my material desires. No matter how hard I tried to work at these tasks, it felt like an invisible hand was pushing me further and further away from them. With great determination, I persisted and even created a list of goals and timelines for the next 15 to 20 years. In retrospect, not one of those goals came to fruition.

Although my life has led me to my dharma, in a way this did not come by choice. It was discovered through a constant craving for something more, the power of surrendering to the Divine hand. Behind each of life's experiences lies a new doorway for growth in our spiritual purpose. This is the most liberating feeling, a state of freedom that exists just beyond the flutter of our thoughts, emotions, and reactions. Through surrender, one gains the power of insight into one's true dharma, which, with sufficient detachment, is easily distinguished from the externalities of life.

Dharma represents a surrendering of our consciousness to the intangible and unknown. It involves the gradual annihilation of fear. Fearlessness is a vital trait for practicing meditation. Even if we do not have any training or experience, we can begin with sitting in stillness for a few minutes each day. Stillness is the doorway into the expansive domain of consciousness where knowledge, greater understanding, and compassion can be attained. Stillness lies beyond the mechanical gestures of the body and mind, and can lead to the experience of being in oneness.

The terms "stillness" or "doorway" are also metaphors for the experience when the meditator and the meditated become one. This can happen to the jnana yogi during the study of great scriptures, to the karma yogi who selflessly engages in any task in service to others, and to the bhakti yogi who dissolves the "I" into devotion for God. Swami Sivananada says that such tasks reveal the "silent witness, when emotions, moods, sentiments, arise in the mind, separate them, study their nature, dissect and analyze them. Don't identify yourself with them. The real 'I' is entirely distinct from them. It is the silent witness or *sakshi*." Such a feeling can connect us to the entirety of life, abundance, peace, and love.

Ecology of Relationships

Our sadhana supports our dharma and guides us through the barrage of fleeting moments we experience in the realm of time and space. In every moment of our day, by keeping awareness of our thoughts, the breath, and our intentions, we can find many opportunities to enter into the sacred space that is our highest truth. Marriage can also be a powerful sadhana bringing us into our dharma, if both people go beyond judgment and accept each other. In relationships, the challenge comes in not reacting when our partner acts unconsciously, but simply observing their behavior as part of their "ego ecology," a conditioned pattern developed over time in previous experiences. Each of us has planted our own landscape, and if couples can work from this place of understanding each other's ego ecologies, then the relationship can nurture both people in living and evolving towards enlightenment. When couples can live with each other in this manner, they can find freedom from the clutches of the ego, allowing the relationship to merge into the eternity of oneness. We can learn to see our sacred partnership as two unique and distinct landscapes that are part of one eco-system longing for sustainability and harmony.

In my view, one of the factors contributing to why many intimate relationships or marriages in the modern era do not endure is that people spend more time reacting than responding to each other. Communication is then based on emotional swings rather than truly listening and learning to observe. The love we feel for one person may be more intense than that we feel for another, but it is the same love that unites us all. Your partner's ecology and the loyalty you give to that partnership provide you the landscape for realizing this. The idea of finding the "right person" can be an escape and a vicious ego trap. What is important is to find a compatible ecology, where your spirit synchronizes with another's lifestyle. This is where your life's purpose or dharma and spiritual lifestyle or sadhana can abide in symmetry with one another.

I regularly meet people in my Ayurvedic consultations seeking to answer the question, "What is my dharma?" Other things that come up include: "I don't know why I have this job or why am I with this person." This is a sort of wandering through life with no real sense of responsibility, direction, or meaning. Many have a curiosity to know why certain things are happening with their health or why they don't sleep well. Some are afraid to explore the reasons. In these times, fear drives people to work for money, and many have relationships for the same reason, to meet their own expectations of life needing to appear a certain way. Consumerism creates a type of escapism that falsely veils us from emotional wounds. Over time, these buried emotions punish the body, its systems, and organs, and doshic imbalances or chronic diseases begin to appear.

One of the best things people can do to explore and potentially discover their higher purpose is to spend time alone, or go on a retreat that allows for introspective analysis. Introspection can be done anywhere, but is best done through reading, writing, or meditating, as these help withdraw the senses and internalize our awareness. "I am not solitary whilst I read and write, though nobody is with me."[159]

Our dharma can bring us financial support and also fulfill our higher nature as a soul seeking union with God. Rightly living with this intention is about taking responsibility for who we are and who we want to become. As we improve ourselves by searching for this sacred place, we also serve the world. As we discover more about ourselves, we give back to our ecology. It's a give-and-take relationship that must stay intact if there is to be a balanced evolution of human life on earth. In other words, we have both an inner and outer duty. It seems that when humans lack harmony within themselves because of *adharma* (lack of purpose), this manifests ecologically, as is evident on planet earth today. Without dharma, humans are prone to create lifestyles and choose relationships that are filled with complexities that burden nature and hinder evolution.

---

159   From the essay "Nature" in *The Essential Writings of Ralph Waldo Emerson.*

Spiritual Colonies

The yoga tradition has always endorsed the power of community or sangha. It is said that environment is our greatest influence, and, in surrounding ourselves with like-minded spiritual people, we support our evolution. This idea is somewhat based on the relationship humanity has had with temples or physical places of worship, devotion, and study. In visiting such energetically-charged structures, one develops an inner temple within our own spiritual hearts. The most important factors in creating a Vedic lifestyle are choosing the right activities, a simple and peaceful environment, and the people we surround ourselves with. We become what we do the most, and therefore the Vedic life endorses three pillars of spiritual evolution, which include cultivating knowledge (head), taking action (hands), and following our heart.

In today's urban societies, marked by capitalism and consumerism, the fractured mind-heart relationship is the deepest wound we have to heal. The mind-heart relationship, a deeper and more subtle extension of what I have discussed throughout this book as the mind-body synergy, is vital to living your dharma. The bedrock of a mind-heart relationship is a sound mind-body relationship that provides the initial stability necessary for entering into the quiet heart. The expression "follow your heart" has been buried out of existence and now exists more as a "follow your head" that perpetuates the divide between our spirit and ecology. More often than ever before, our urban societies have become emotionally bankrupt, so that many live on the basis of intellectual choices that conform to the standards of society.

One of the ideas of Paramahansa Yogananda's teachings on the evolution of mankind is the development of spiritual colonies where men, women, and children can live according to the universal principles that sustain spirit-ecos societies. In such colonies, wisdom, activity, and devotion are given equal importance for the development of mankind and maintaining a sustainable and harmonious relationship with nature. Prabhupada, founder of the famous Hare Krishna movement in America, started twelve such communities in Europe, North America, and India. Other organizations have endorsed the same concept. Living in such colonies could possibly eradicate the need for centralized government and allow people to live according to the universal laws of nature and karma.

Yoga and Ayurveda festivals and conferences have now emerged throughout the world as places where like-minded people can come together and enjoy the sacred language of spirituality. These types of events have existed in India for hundreds, if not thousands, of years. An example is the immense Kumbha Mela, where millions converge and plunge into holy rivers, hear discourses, and connect with fellow yogis. Much of what we see today in the yoga culture is spread out in bits and pieces, from vegetarian eateries and organic farms to yoga asana centers, kirtans, and retreat centers. Taken together, these are all integral parts of what makes up a spiritual colony.

Sun, Moon, and Earth

According to the Vedas, the system of yoga is born of the sun god and linked to a figure named Hiranyagarbha, the "golden egg" or light of consciousness. From that point, the great Yoga Darshana, one of the six schools of Indian philosophy, was disseminated through notable personages, such as the sage Vasishta, Bhagavan Krishna, Patanjali of the Yoga Sutras, and many others. One of the central themes of yoga is reverence for the sun by means of integral yogic techniques that awaken our lives from conditioned, fear-based thinking into awareness and love. The most obvious outer expression of sun worship in yoga is the sun salutation, which connects us to the sun's inspiring and luminous qualities.

However, yoga's elevated ideal is to direct all outer proficiency inward to become a seer of the inner sun or light that abides as the essence of the soul. In the yuga teachings of the cycles of human consciousness that I described early in this book, it is the proximity of the sun to its currently invisible partner star that determines the level or stage of consciousness that exists on earth. An infinite relationship exists between humanity and the light of the sun. Each day, when it shines on the earth, the sun is a bold reminder to countless numbers of people, cultures, and civilizations of the search for God or Ishvara referred to by Patanjali. The potential of our human existence lies in the power of our relationship to the sun-moon-earth, which is emblematic of the relationship we must embrace between the mind, body, and soul. The great saints and gurus have encouraged us to give more urgency to our life purpose and search for the Divine. The sun-moon-earth partnership signifies the power of evolution, change, surrender, and the harmonious existence inherent between humanity and nature.

As the growth of the global yoga community continues thriving with greater diversity and awareness, many throughout the world are expanding their horizons through conscious living. The eco-conscious community is now embracing the sun as the most valuable source of energy on the planet. There will come a time when the prime forces of nature, wind, light, and water, will produce all the energy required to support life on earth. The sun as the father of the solar system provides guidance, direction, attraction, and momentum for the moon, which the earth follows.

As spiritualists seek the light of their own truth, they must discover it by entering the heart of the moon. The spiritual heart is our link to the moon's feminine energies of feeling, intuition, and unconditional and eternal love. As the moon enjoys its tantalizing play while encircling the sun, it nourishes its child, the earth, along the way. I feel that the evolution of humanity rests upon embracing the qualities of the moon through reverence to the mother, women, and the qualities of nature. Such lunar qualities will be an enormous aid in eradicating war, famine, and the social inequalities that exist in both capitalist and Third World countries. As the child of sun and moon, the earth learns, evolves, and surrenders to them with grace. Yoga practices not only restore peace and harmony within us, but also encourage us to promote these ideals to all beings. This is reflected in the mantra "loka samasta sukhino bhavantu," which is basically a prayer that all beings in all realms have a happy and joyful life. This includes animals and all of creation.

In many ways, what I have tried to share in this book is that we can learn from the past. The ancient Vedas of the golden era provide us the most advanced principles for living harmoniously on earth, while fulfilling our greatest desire of experiencing Divine love. Love is the highest attribute of the soul. It is the force that moves the sun, moon, and earth, and keeps us seeking perfection, in relationship to ourselves and our achievements, and in our relationships with each other. Most important of all is our love for the One....as father, mother, friend, and beloved God. May the relationship of the sun, moon, and earth awaken your highest aspiration of life and bring you great health and happiness.

A

abhayam – fearlessness, regaining of non-dual consciousness.

abhimana – pride.

abhinivesha – desire to stay in the physical body which stems from spiritual ignorance; one of the five kleshas (afflictions).

abhyanga – self-massage, a staple practice of Ayurvedic lifestyle for preventing disorders of the doshas.

abhyasa – repeated practice, continuous effort in sadhana.

adana – receiving period.

advaita – non-dual branch of Vedanta.

agni – sacred fire, Vedic God, thirteen fires of health in Ayurveda.

ahamkara – ego or "I" consciousness.

ahara – taking in, absorption, food, intake of any sensory impression.

ahimsa – nonviolence, compassion.

akasha – ether, space.

ama – bodily toxins, undigested food waste.

ananda tandava – Shiva's dance of bliss.

apana – downward-flowing prana (energy), also called vayu, controls excretions.

ardha – half.

artha – vocation, job.

asana – posture, literally: "seat."

ashrama – life stage, period.

ashtanga – eight-limbed, eight.

ashti dhatu - bone and cartilage tissue.

asmita – egoism.

avatara – divine incarnation, liberated soul re-embodied to enlighten humanity.

avidya – ignorance.

Ayurveda – science of health, sister science of yoga.

B

bandha – body lock.

basti – medicated enema, treatment of pooling oil in any particular area of the body.

bastrika – bellows breathing, use of the diaphragm.

bhajan – India devotional song, chant.

bhakti – devotion to God.

Bhakti Yoga – devotional yoga.

bhava – feeling, mood, attitude, emotion.

bija – seed syllable or sound, vibration.

brahmacharya – celibacy or sexual moderation; also the "student" stage of life.

buddhi – higher mind, intuition; product of mahat.

C

chakra – subtle energy centers in the astral body.

chandra – moon.

chikitsa – treatment, therapy.

chitta – mind, consciousness.

D

devi – goddess.

dharana – power of attention or concentration.

dharma – life purpose.

dhatu – tissue.

dhyana – meditation.

diksha – initiation.

dinacharya – daily self-care routine.

dosha – constitutional type; also, mistake or fault.

dvesha – aversion.

G

granthi – energy knot or block related to the chakras.

grihastha – householder stage of life.

guna – quality or measure, related to level of consciousness or awareness.

H

hridaya – spiritual heart.

I

ida nadi – moon channel.

ishta devata – favored (personal) deity, personal image of the Divine.

ishvara pranidhana – commitment to the Divine, power of surrender, trust.

J

janma – conception, birth.

japa yoga mantra – repeating mantra during acts of service (seva).

jatharagni – digestive strength.

jiva – soul.

Jnana Yoga – yoga of knowledge, study of scriptures.

jyotish – Vedic astrology.

K

kaivalya – final liberation.

Kali Yuga – dark age.

kama – sensual affection, lust, emotional balance.

Kapalabhati – nasal-exhalation pranayama.

kapha – water and earth dosha.

karma – action and the result of action.

Karma Yoga – yoga of action and service.

kaya chikitsa – internal medicine.

kirtan – devotional music, chanting.

klesha – mental affliction.

kriya – purifying action.

Kriya Yoga – specialized and specific technique of pranayama revived by Mahavatar Babaji and disseminated in the West by Paramahansa Yogananda; includes an integral lifestyle approach that balances material and spiritual responsibilities.

kumbhaka – suspending, suspension of breath.

kundalini – sacred fire, awakened prana, serpent energy, awakened.

kutashta – spiritual eye.

M

mahat – cosmic intelligence.

majja dhatu - nerve tissue.

mala – Hindu rosary of 108 beads, used in mantra and pranayama practice.

malas – excretions.

mamsa dhatu – muscle tissue.

manas – sensory mind, outer/lower mind; the aspect of the mind that operates through the five senses and develops the conditioned and programmed habits associated with the ego.

manasa shastra – Ayurvedic psychology; section of teaching in classical Ayurveda dealing with the mind.

manda – slow, low; term used to describe digestive strength or capacity.

mantra – word, phrase, or sound repeated as a form of meditation.

marma – energy points throughout the body originally used in martial arts, yoga and in Ayurvedic medicine to promote pranic healing.

maya – force of illusion; ever-changing realm of life.

medas dhatu – fat tissue.

mitihara – moderation.

moksha – liberation.

mudra – gesture of body, hands, or eyes.

mukta –free, liberated.

murti – statue of a god.

N

nadi – pranic pathway, channel.

nadi shodhana – alternate-nostril breathing.

nasya – nasal oil.

nidana – causes of disease.

nirodha – ending, cessation, neutralizing.

niyama – personal code of conduct.

O

ojakshaya – diminished ojas (life sap).

ojas – life sap, vital energy, immunity.

P

pada – physical foot; section of a treatise.

parampara – succession, lineage.

pavana – gas.

pingala nadi – sun channel.

pitta – fire dosha.

prakriti – material nature; dosha constitutional type.

prana – life-force energy.

pancha karma – "five actions" detoxification therapy.

pranayama – breathing techniques.

pranvaha srota – respiratory channels that influence flow of prana.

pratyahara – sense withdrawal; relaxation techniques.

prema – love.

pronam – bow, prostration.

pruvakarma – preliminary practices.

puja – ceremony.

puraka – inhalation.

purnima – full moon.

purusha – essence of spirit, Self, and the universal principle; witness.

R

raga – attraction.

Raja Yoga – mind-training, meditative yoga, integral path of yoga.

rajasic – active, outward-bound energy.

rakta – blood tissue.

rasa – nutrition, "taste."

rasanyana – restorative, rejuvenating.

rashona – garlic.

rechaka – exhalation.

rishi – sage, seer.

ritucharya – seasonal self-care routine.

rupa – signs and symptoms of disease.

S

sadachara – good conduct.

sadhaka – spiritual aspirant or yogi.

sadhana – yogic discipline; spiritual practice or routine.

sakshi – state of witnessing.

sama – functional, balanced prana.

samadhi – contemplative trance, liberation, absorbtion, oneness.

samana prana – prana (vayu or wind) of balanced digestion; energy centered in the navel and abdominal region.

samhita – text; compilation of teaching or wisdom.

Samkhya – yoga and Ayurveda philosophy, includes the 24 cosmic principles (tattvas).

sampradaya – lineage; succession of teachings based on those of Self-Realized masters.

samsara – cycle of birth and death.

samskara – patterned or conditioned behavior.

samyama – union of concentration, meditation, and samadhi.

samyoga – union of mind and spirit.

sanatana dharma – eternal dharma; original term used to refer to Hinduism.

sangha – associations, community.

sannyas – renunciation, renunciate stage of life.

santosh – inner contentment.

sarira – body: term used to describe the three bodies: physical, astral, and causal.

sat – truth.

sat-chit-ananda – three-fold aspect of God as Existence, Consciousness and Bliss, the sustainer of life, the Absolute Self.

satguru – enlightened being committed to bringing emancipation to the disciple.

satmya – habituation; body's ability to adapt.

satsanga – spiritual discourse; group gathered in harmony of truth.

sattva guna – state of calmness; present and clear mind.

sattvic – calm, centered.

satya – truthfulness.

savasana – corpse pose, posture for experiencing pratyahara (sensory withdrawal), precursor to meditation.

seva – selfless service; primary aspect of the Karma and Bhakti Yoga paths.

shakti – power of kundalini, feminine energy, awakened prana.

shamana – palliation, practices to reduce disease.

shastra – book, treatise.

shat karmas – six cleansing rites of Hatha Yoga.

shirodhara – treatment consisting of pouring a warm stream of oil over the forehead.

shishya – disciple, student.

shodana – strong purification protocol.

shukra dhatu – reproductive fluid, sexual excretions of the genitals.

shunya – blankness or empty space.

siddhas – adepts.

siddhis – magical or spiritual powers; eight powers mentioned by sage Patanjali in the Yoga Sutras.

snehana – oleation, core component in Ayurvedic wellness and pancha karma; always combined with svedhana (sweating).

soma – moon, Vedic God, nectar energy often associated with amrita (ambrosia).

surya – sun.

sushumna – central pranic energy channel that carries the kundalini.

sva – individual, life.

svadhyaya – self-analysis, study, reflection.

svastha vritta – lifestyle treatment, preventative medicine.

svedhana – full-body steam bath; sweating; counterpart to abhyanga.

T

tamasic – slow, inert, dark, ignorant.

tanmatra chikitsa – therapies the work through the subtle energies.

Tantra – esoteric branch of yoga that includes Hatha Yoga practices based on the workings of Shiva and Shakti energies; book; tension.

tapasya – austerities, practice, discipline.

tattvas – cosmic principles associated with Samkhya yogic philosophy.

tejas – inner radiance; positive healing light.

titiksha – rising above the body and its sense enticements.

tri-dosha – balancing or applicable to all three doshas.

tyaga – attachment to outcome.

U

udana – upward-moving prana.

uttana – lifting.

V

vairgya – dispassion, detachment, state of mind prerequisite for experiencing samadhi.

vak – speech: power of language (Sanskrit) or Divine names.

vanaprastha – seclusion stage of life where, at approximately fifty years of age, one returns to deeper study and sadhana.

vasanas – subliminal desires.

vastu – Vedic architecture.

vata – air and ether dosha.

vayu – wind, force, Vedic God, another term for vata.

Vedas – ancient spiritual texts; wisdom of India's golden age.

Vedanta – Vedic philosophy, end of the vedas, unity perspective of yoga.

vidya – wisdom tradition.

vihara – releasing.

vikriti – imbalance.

vinyasa – fluid yoga sequences that connect movements with breathing.

vira – warrior, hero.

virechana – purgation, used mainly for pitta disorders.

virya – the heating or cooling quality of foods.

visarga – releasing period.

vishnunabhi – galactic sun.

viveka – discrimination.

vritti – mental fluctuations.

vihara chikitsa – healthy living, detached living.

vyana vayu - heart and lung prana that circulates throughout the body.

Y

yajna – sacrifice; fire ritual for removing karmas.

yama – control or mastery; code of social conduct.

yantra – geometric figure for meditation.

yoga – union, sacred science of uniting individual consciousness with cosmic consciousness.

yuga – epoch, cycle of world consciousness.

yukti vyapashraya – individualized Ayurvedic treatment protocol.

A

B

W

Y

Abhedananda, Brother. "Yoga Postures for Health." *Self-Realization Magazine,* Spring 2015.

Benson, Herbert. *The Relaxation Response.* New York: HarperTorch, 2000.

Bittman, Mark. "Rethinking the Meat Guzzler." New York *Times,* January 27, 2008.

Cruttenden, Walter. *Lost Star of Myth and Time.* Pittsburgh: St. Lynn's Press, 2005.

Das, P.S. *Yoga Panacea.* Kolkata: Dr. P.S. Das Yoga Research and Rehabilitation Centre, n.d.

Feuerstein, Georg. *The Shambhala Encyclopedia of Yoga.* Boulder, CO: Shambhala, 2000.

Frawley, David. *Gods, Sages and Kings.* Twin Lakes, WI: Lotus Press, 1991.

Frawley, David. *Mantra Yoga and Primal Sound.* Twin Lakes, WI: Lotus Press, 2010.

Frawley, David. *Yoga and Ayurveda.* Twin Lakes, WI; Lotus Press, 1999.

Frawley, David and Vasant Lad. *Yoga of Herbs.* Twin Lakes, WI; Lotus Press, 1986.

Gore, M.M. *Anatomy and Physiology of Yogic Practices.* New Delhi: New Age Publishers, 2014.

Johari, Harish. *Chakras.* Merrimac, MA: Destiny Publishers, 2000.

Joshi, Sunhil. *Ayurveda and Panchakarma.* Twin Lakes, WI: Lotus Press, 1997.

Jyotirmayanda, Swami. *International Yoga Guide.* Miami: Yoga Research Foundation, n.d.

Lad, Vasant. *The Complete Book of Ayurvedic Home Remedies.* New York: Harmony Books, 1999.

Lahiri Mahasaya. *The Scriptural Commentaries of Yogiraj Sri Sri Shyama Charan Lahiri Mahasaya.* Bloomington, IN: iUniverse, 2005.

Mata, Sri Daya. "Free Yourself from Tension." *Self-Realization Magazine,* n.d.

Miller, Alice. *The Drama of the Gifted Child.* New York: Basic Books, 2008.

Muktibodhanana, Swami. *Hatha Yoga Pradipika.* Munger: Bihar School of Yoga Books, 2013.

Prasada, Rama. *Patanjali's Yoga Sutras.* Philadelphia: Coronet Books, 2002.

Prime, Ranchor. *Vedic Ecology.* San Rafael, CA: Mandala Publishing, 2002.

Radha, Swami Sivananda. *Mantras: Words of Power.* Kootenay, BC: Timeless Books, 2011.

Ramakrishna, Sri. *The Gospel of Sri Ramakrishna*. New York: Ramakrishna-Vivekenanda Center, 1984.

Self-Realization Fellowship. *Rajarshi Janakananda*. Los Angeles: Self-Realization Fellowship Publishers, 1994.

Sharma, P.V. *Charaka Samhita*. Varanasi: Chaukhambha Orientalia, 2005.

Sharma, P.V. *Susruta Samhita*. Varanasi: Chaukhambha Orientalia, 2006.

Siegel, Daniel J. *Pocket Guide to Interpersonal Neurobiology*. New York: W.W. Norton, 2012.

Sivananda, Swami. *All About Hinduism*. Madhya Pradesh: Divine Life Society, 2003.

Sivananda, Swami. *Dhyana Yoga*. Madhya Pradesh: Divine Life Society, 2005.

Sivananda, Swami. *Japa Yoga*. Madhya Pradesh: Divine Life Society, 2005.

Sivananda, Swami. *The Science of Pranayama*. Madhya Pradesh: Divine Life Society, 2006.

Subramaniyaswami, Satguru Sivaya. *Dancing with Siva*. Kauai: Himalayan Academy Publications, 1997.

Tirtha, Swami Rama. *The Ayurveda Encyclopedia*. Bayville, NY: Sat Yuga Press, 2007.

Tirtha, Swami Rama. *In the Woods of God Realization*. Lucknow: Rama Tirtha Pratisthan, 1999.

Vasu, Srisa Chandra. *Gheranda Samhita*. Delhi: Dev Publishers, 2012.

Vasu, Srisa Chandra. *Siva Samhita*. Delhi: Dev Publishers, 2012.

Yoga Kosa. Pune: Kaivalyadhama Yoga Mandir, 2009.

Yogananda, Paramahansa. *The Divine Romance*. Los Angeles: Self-Realization Fellowship, 1986.

Yogananda, Paramahansa. *God Talks with Arjuna: The Bhagavad Gita*. Los Angeles: Self-Realization Fellowship, 2001.

Yoganada, Paramahansa. *The Great Light of God*. Los Angeles: Self-Realization Fellowship, 2006.

Yogananda, Paramahansa. *Man's Eternal Quest*. Los Angeles: Self-Realization Fellowship, 1982.

Yukteswar, Sri. *The Holy Science*. Los Angeles: Self-Realization Fellowship, 1990.

Waller, David. *The Perfect Man*. Brighton: Victorian Secrets, 2011.

World Watch Institute. www.worldwatch.org.

ABOUT THE AUTHOR

Yogi, mystic, and practitioner of Ayurveda, Mas has become one of the most influential yoga and Ayurveda teachers in the world and offers unique certification training programs throughout the USA, Asia, and India. Mas enjoys teaching integral yoga classes, offering health and wellness lectures and giving workshops that embrace core Ayurvedic principles. His work is primarily influenced by the lineage-based traditions of India, with prominence to the teachings of Yogananda and Sivananda. In 2014 he appeared in the triumphant film "Awake, The Life Of Yogananda" and as an Ayurvedic practitioner, he maintains an active international counseling practice that includes yoga and Vedic astrology. He is the founder/director of Dancing Shiva Yoga Ayurveda, an international non-profit educational organization and center based in Southern California.

About the Dancing Shiva School of Yoga & Ayurveda
www.dancingshiva.com

The original Dancing Shiva Yoga center opened in Los Angeles, California in 2001 and now operates mainly through affiliate centers and locations in the USA and internationally. Dancing Shiva has become recognized internationally through Mas Vidal's teachings and offers health and wellness Vedic counseling services as well as a variety of learning platforms, from online programs to retreat trainings, internships, and India pilgrimages. Dancing Shiva also offers clinical services (pancha karma) at various locations and events.

200 Hour Online Yoga & Ayurveda

Mas Vidal's Dancing Shiva provides the most comprehensive online yoga and Ayurveda studies program offered in the field today. A complete online and correspondence format allows students the opportunity to study individually, at their own pace and from their own computer. The course includes 108 hours of beautiful high definition (HD) video lectures, yoga classes, close up asana instruction, online testing, homework assignments and over 600 pages of written reading-study material. Certification is for 200 hours as a Yoga and Ayurveda Counselor. As long as you're online, you can be connected anytime.

250-Hour Yoga & Ayurveda Teacher Training Program

This is the original Yoga and Ayurveda program that unites both sciences into an authentic teaching approach and lifestyle-training course. It is mainly focused on application of proper asana and pranayama practice and integration of an Ayurvedic lifestyle. This 250-hour program is registered with the Yoga Alliance and certification is offered several times per year in California and at our affiliate locations internationally.

The program provides the foundation for becoming a yoga asana teacher or for those interested in deeper Ayurvedic studies. This course has been the cornerstone of the teachings at the Dancing Shiva center, and is influenced by the teachings of Paramahansa Yogananda and the Bengali yoga tradition, and other lineage-based organizations from India. The program also provides practical instruction on how yogic methodology and Ayurvedic lifestyle can be applied towards creating an effective meditation practice.

300 Hour Advanced Yoga & Ayurveda Programs

The advanced program modules provide a more comprehensive understanding of yoga and Ayurveda. Each advanced training, offers certification in 100-hour modules, and provides three levels of study with Mas Vidal and the Dancing Shiva faculty. This program is the most comprehensive approach of how yoga can be applied as a therapeutic system for healing the mind-body relationship. Each module provides a deeper exploration into the yoga and Ayurveda paradigm for those who have already completed or are currently enrolled in the 250-hour Dancing Shiva program. Participants with certifications from other schools or teachers are also invited to attend. Each module strongly adheres to a balanced relationship between therapeutics and spirituality. After completion of module levels 1 – 3, participants can combine their hours for registration with Yoga Alliance 500 RYT.

Ayurveda Health Counselor Certification

This special program provides students with the foundation principles for becoming a health counselor and is also an excellent course for those interested in medical–clinical study and practice of Ayurveda. The program is taught in the traditional gurukul (teacher-student) learning format of 1-3 students. It provides the core material taught in the first year curriculums at universities in India, accounting for a total of 250 hours of study.

India Programs and Pilgrimages

The Dancing Shiva school offers yearly yoga and Ayurveda programs and pilgrimages led by Mas Vidal. These programs take place at eco-villages, ashrams and sacred locations through out India. Dancing Shiva also offers Ayurveda programs in India at various schools and universities.

Traditional Study (Gurukul)

Each year, five individuals are accepted for private study-internship structure with Mas Vidal in the traditional manner of the Vedic tradition. Students are accepted on specific circumstances that will best benefit the student's ability to learn the material and experience personal healing. The criteria for acceptance into gurukul ranges from previous yogic experience, schedule and timing, and karmic factors as reflected in the astrological birth chart. The one-year training period is divided into four modules and is a combination of private tutorials (live or Skype), reading, yoga and Ayurveda exercises, attendance at special programs, conferences, or retreats, and assisting Mas on certain projects as an opportunity to learn. The schedule is adjusted according to each person, and the person can usually complete the certification within a one-year period or less.

Consultations and Vedic Counseling Services

Mas Vidal offers practical Vedic lifestyle counseling services to all types of clients. His capacity for promoting health and spiritual wellness originates from over twenty years of private practice and clinical experience, and is recognized internationally for his insightful wisdom that integrates yoga, Ayurveda and Jyotish (Vedic astrology). Initial sessions include review of the astrology birth chart, determination of the dosha
constitution and imbalances, lifestyle recommendations, specific prescriptions of diet, herbs, and yoga for creating balance of the physical, mental, and emotional bodies. The initial session provides the client with a comprehensive overview of health factors visible in the body, and unseen, as reflected in the birth chart, and also gives recommendations for beginning the Mas Vidal method of detoxification according to the wisdom of Ayurveda and modern scientific research. All sessions include a take-home booklet and a copy of the birth chart.

Mas Vidal's Optimum DVD Series

Experience ultimate yoga practices with Mas Vidal, which combine an integral approach to yoga with Ayurvedic principles. Each DVD emphasizes the importance of balancing your energies as per the science of tri-dosha. DVDs are available individually according to the elements of air, fire, and water, or the complete set can also be purchased on the dancingshiva.com website. In each

60-minute session on DVD, Mas Vidal teaches you how to practice yoga asana to work the physical body, use pranayama to heal the mind, and awaken the soul's inherent spiritual qualities in deep meditation.

The Strength & Balance "Air" DVD series is focused on strengthening the whole body, while also improving balance through the practice of a very sacred Salutation to the Moon, an ancient sequence of postures that align our inner energies. Included are various techniques and breathing exercises for calming and focusing the mind. This "air" series ends in a transformational meditation that brings the perfect balance between the body, mind, and soul. This is an important yoga practice for those wanting greater physical strength, a creative mind, and ultimate health. In Ayurveda, the intention of this yoga practice is to bring balance to vata dosha.

The Stretch & Relax "Fire" DVD series is focused on stretching the entire body to release tension and stress through the practice of a very sacred Salutation to the Sun, a complete sequence of postures that benefits the whole spine and heals the organs and major systems of the body. In this series, the body's inner fire is balanced through a combination of powerful postures and breathing techniques that bring you into real relaxation to truly transform your whole being and life. This "fire" series ends in a transformational meditation that brings the perfect balance between the body, mind, and soul. This is the ultimate yoga practice for those seeking a lean body and a peaceful mind. In Ayurveda, the intention of this yoga practice is to bring balance to pitta dosha.

The Tone & Shape "Water" DVD series is focused on toning and shaping the whole body through a combination of stimulating balancing postures and dynamic sequences that will make your body work out and sweat. Postures are combined with a very powerful breathing technique that stimulates digestion and improves the function of the cardiovascular system. This series ends in a transformational meditation that restores the mind-body relationship, building confidence and improving mental focus. This is a great practice for those looking to wake up and be challenged. In Ayurveda, the intention of this yoga practice is to bring balance to kapha dosha.

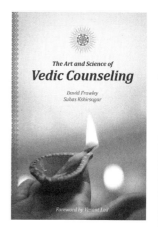